Connecticut Children's

Creating the Future 25th ANNIVERSARY

Honored to be your partners in care!

Pediatric Neurosurgery in Primary Care

Editors

JONATHAN MARTIN
GREG OLAVARRIA

PEDIATRIC CLINICS OF NORTH AMERICA

www.pediatric.theclinics.com

Consulting Editor
BONITA F. STANTON

August 2021 • Volume 68 • Number 4

ELSEVIER

1600 John F. Kennedy Boulevard • Suite 1800 • Philadelphia, Pennsylvania, 19103-2899

http://www.theclinics.com

THE PEDIATRIC CLINICS OF NORTH AMERICA Volume 68, Number 4
August 2021 ISSN 0031-3955, ISBN-13: 978-0-323-79635-4

Editor: Kerry Holland
Developmental Editor: Axell Ivan Jade M. Purificacion

The Pediatric Clinics of North America (ISSN 0031-3955) is published bimonthly by Elsevier Inc., 360 Park Avenue South, New York, NY 10010-1710. Months of issue are February, April, June, August, October, and December. Periodicals postage paid at New York, NY and additional mailing offices. Subscription prices are $250.00 per year (US individuals), $984.00 per year (US institutions), $315.00 per year (Canadian individuals), $1048.00 per year (Canadian institutions), $376.00 per year (international individuals), $1048.00 per year (international institutions), $100.00 per year (US students and residents), $100.00 per year (Canadian students and residents), and $165.00 per year (international residents and students). To receive students/resident rare, orders must be accompanied by name of affiliated institution, date of term, and the signature of program/residency coordinator on institution letterhead. Orders will be billed at individual rate until proof of status is received. Foreign air speed delivery is included in all *Clinics* subscription prices. All prices are subject to change without notice. **POSTMASTER:** Send address changes to *The Pediatric Clinics of North America*, Elsevier Health Sciences Division, Subscription Customer Service, 3251 Riverport Lane, Maryland Heights, MO 63043. **Customer Service: 1-800-654-2452 (US and Canada). From outside of the US and Canada: 1-314-447-8871. Fax: 1-314-447-8029. For print support, E-mail: JournalsCustomerService-usa@elsevier.com. For online support, E-mail: JournalsOnlineSupport-usa@elsevier.com.**

Reprints. For copies of 100 or more, of articles in this publication, please contact the Commercial Reprints Department, Elsevier Inc., 360 Park Avenue South, New York, NY 10010-1710. Tel.: 212-633-3874; Fax: 212-633-3820; E-mail: reprints@elsevier.com.

The Pediatric Clinics of North America is also published in Spanish by McGraw-Hill Inter-americana Editores S.A., Mexico City, Mexico; in Portuguese by Riechmann and Affonso Editores, Rua Comandante Coelho 1085, CEP 21250, Rio de Janeiro, Brazil; and in Greek by Althayia SA, Athens, Greece.

The Pediatric Clinics of North America is covered in *MEDLINE/PubMed (Index Medicus), Excerpta Medica, Current Contents, Current Contents/Clinical Medicine, Science Citation Index, ASCA, ISI/BIOMED*, and *BIOSIS*.

Printed in the United States of America.

PROGRAM OBJECTIVE

The goal of the *Pediatric Clinics of North America* is to keep practicing physicians and residents up to date with current clinical practice in pediatrics by providing timely articles reviewing the state-of-the-art in patient care.

TARGET AUDIENCE

All practicing pediatricians, physicians and healthcare professionals who provide patient care to pediatric patients.

LEARNING OBJECTIVES

Upon completion of this activity, participants will be able to:

1. Review pediatric neurological examination and diagnostic imaging studies pertinent to the nervous system.
2. Discuss common pediatric symptoms and imaging findings in order help to determine when to refer to a specialist.
3. Recognize the importance of collaborating with non-surgical and surgical specialists in managing complex pediatric diagnoses.

ACCREDITATIONS

Physician Credit

The Elsevier Office of Continuing Medical Education (EOCME) is accredited by the Accreditation Council for Continuing Medical Education (ACCME) to provide continuing medical education for physicians.

The EOCME designates this journal-based activity for a maximum of 16 *AMA PRA Category 1 Credit*(s)™. Physicians should claim only the credit commensurate with the extent of their participation in the activity.

All other healthcare professionals requesting continuing education credit for this this journal-based activity will be issued a certificate of participation.

ABP Maintenance of Certification Credit

Successful completion of this CME activity, which includes participation in the activity and individual assessment of and feedback to the learner, enables the learner to earn up to 16 MOC points in the American Board of Pediatrics' (ABP)

Maintenance of Certification (MOC) program. It is the CME activity provider's responsibility to submit learner completion information to ACCME for the purpose of granting ABP MOC credit.

DISCLOSURE OF CONFLICTS OF INTEREST

The EOCME assesses conflict of interest with its instructors, faculty, planners, and other individuals who are in a position to control the content of CME activities. All relevant conflicts of interest that are identified are thoroughly vetted by EOCME for fair balance, scientific objectivity, and patient care recommendations. EOCME is committed to providing its learners with CME activities that promote improvements or quality in healthcare and not a specific proprietary business or a commercial interest.

The planning committee, staff, authors and editors listed below have identified no financial relationships or relationships to products or devices they or their spouse/life partner have with commercial interest related to the content of this CME activity:

Gregory W. Albert, MD, MPH; Ashley T. Ashby, PA-C, MPAS; Randaline R. Barnett, MD; David F. Bauer, MD, MPH; Mandana Behbahani, MD; Alexandra D. Beier, DO; Ahmed Belal, MD; Luis E. Bello-Espinosa, MD; Jeffrey P. Blount, MD; Christopher M. Bonfield, MD; Markus J. Bookland, MD; Robin Bowman, MD; Jean-Paul Bryant, MSc; Regina Chavous-Gibson, MSN, RN; Scott W. Elton, MD; David S. Hersh, MD; Kerry Holland; Betsy D. Hopson, MHSA; Christopher D. Hughes, MD, MPH; Eric M. Jackson, MD; Andrew Jea, MD; Sarah C. Jernigan, MD, MPH; Sandi K. Lam, MD, MBA; Cormac O. Maher, MD; Francesco T. Mangano, DO; Jonathan E. Martin, MD; Rajkumar Mayakrishnann; Samuel G. McClugage, III, MD; Alaa Montaser, MD, PhD; Whitney E. Muhlestein, MD; Toba N. Niazi, MD; Greg Olavarria, MD; Smruti K. Patel, MD; Robert C. Pedersen, MD; Martin G. Piazza, MD; Rebecca A. Reynolds, MD; Brandon G. Rocque, MD, MS; Veronica J. Rooks, MD; Edward Smith, MD; Jignesh Tailor, MD, PhD; Rabia Tari, MD; Jonathan R. Wood, MD; Aaron M. Yengo-Kahn, MD; Mohamed A. Zaazoue, MD.

UNAPPROVED/OFF-LABEL USE DISCLOSURE

The EOCME requires CME faculty to disclose to the participants:

1. When products or procedures being discussed are off-label, unlabelled, experimental, and/or investigational (not US Food and Drug Administration [FDA] approved); and
2. Any limitations on the information presented, such as data that are preliminary or that represent ongoing research, interim analyses, and/or unsupported opinions. Faculty may discuss information about pharmaceutical agents that is outside of FDA-approved labelling. This information is intended solely for CME and is not intended to promote off-label use of these medications. If you have any questions, contact the medical affairs department of the manufacturer for the most recent prescribing information.

TO ENROLL

To enroll in the *Pediatric Clinics of North America* Continuing Medical Education program, call customer service at 1-800-654-2452 or sign up online at http://www.theclinics.com/home/cme. The CME program is available to subscribers for an additional annual fee of USD 324.00.

METHOD OF PARTICIPATION

In order to claim credit, participants must complete the following:

1. Complete enrolment as indicated above.
2. Read the activity.
3. Complete the CME Test and Evaluation. Participants must achieve a score of 70% on the test. All CME Tests and Evaluations must be completed online.

In order to claim MOC points, participants must complete the following:

1. Complete steps listed above for claiming CME credit
2. Provide your specialty board ID#, birth date (MM/DD), and attestation.
3. Online MOC submission is only available for the American Board of pediatrics' (ABP) Maintenance of Certification (MOC) program

CME INQUIRIES/SPECIAL NEEDS

For all CME inquiries or special needs, please contact elsevierCME@elsevier.com.

Contributors

CONSULTING EDITOR

BONITA F. STANTON, MD
Professor of Pediatrics and Founding Dean, Robert C. and Laura C. Garrett Endowed Chair, Hackensack Meridian School of Medicine, President, Academic Enterprise, Hackensack Meridian Health, Nutley, New Jersey

EDITORS

JONATHAN MARTIN, MD, FAAP, FACS, FANS
Paul M. Kanev Chair of Pediatric Neurosurgery, Division of Neurosurgery, Connecticut Children's, Associate Professor, Department of Surgery, University of Connecticut School of Medicine, Hartford, Connecticut

GREG OLAVARRIA, MD, FAANS, FAAP
Assistant Professor, UCF College of Medicine, Pediatric Neurosurgery, Arnold Palmer Hospital for Children, Orlando, Florida

AUTHORS

GREGORY W. ALBERT, MD, MPH, FAANS, FACS, FAAP
Lee and Bob Cress Endowed Chair in Pediatric Neurosurgery, Chief of Pediatric Neurosurgery, Arkansas Children's Hospital, Associate Professor of Neurosurgery, University of Arkansas for Medical Sciences, Little Rock, Arkansas

ASHLEY T. ASHBY, PA-C, MPAS
UF Pediatric Neurosurgery, Physician Assistant, Lucy Gooding Pediatric Neurosurgery Center, Wolfson Children's Hospital, Jacksonville, Florida

RANDALINE R. BARNETT, MD
Department of Neurological Surgery, The University of North Carolina at Chapel Hill, Chapel Hill, North Carolina

DAVID F. BAUER, MD MPH
Department of Neurosurgery, Baylor College of Medicine, Department of Surgery, Division of Pediatric Neurosurgery, Texas Children's Hospital, Houston, Texas

MANDANA BEHBAHANI, MD
Fellow, Division of Pediatric Neurosurgery, Lurie Children's Hospital and Northwestern University Feinberg School of Medicine, Chicago, Illinois

ALEXANDRA D. BEIER, DO, FACOS, FAAP
Surgical Director, Pediatric Epilepsy Program, Associate Professor of Neurosurgery and Pediatrics, Division of Pediatric Neurosurgery, University of Florida Health Jacksonville, Lucy Gooding Pediatric Neurosurgery Center, Wolfson Children's Hospital, Jacksonville, Florida

AHMED BELAL, MD
Department of Neurological Surgery, Indiana University School of Medicine, Indianapolis, Indiana

LUIS E. BELLO-ESPINOSA, MD
Division Head, Pediatric Neurology, Arnold Palmer Hospital for Children, Leon Neuroscience Center of Excellence, Orlando, Florida

JEFFREY P. BLOUNT, MD
Professor, Division of Pediatric Neurosurgery, Department of Neurosurgery, Children's of Alabama, The University of Alabama at Birmingham, Birmingham, Alabama

CHRISTOPHER M. BONFIELD, MD
Department of Neurosurgery, Vanderbilt University Medical Center, Medical Center North, Nashville, Tennessee

MARKUS J. BOOKLAND, MD
Assistant Professor of Pediatrics and Surgery, Division of Neurosurgery, Connecticut Children's, UConn School of Medicine, Hartford, Connecticut

ROBIN BOWMAN, MD
Associate Professor of Neurological Surgery, Director of Multidisciplinary Spina Bifida Center, Co-Director of Fetal Neurosurgery, Lurie Children's Hospital and Northwestern University Feinberg School of Medicine, Chicago, Illinois

JEAN-PAUL BRYANT, MSc
Miller School of Medicine, University of Miami, Miami, Florida

SCOTT W. ELTON, MD
Department of Neurological Surgery, The University of North Carolina at Chapel Hill, Chapel Hill, North Carolina

NICOLE E. HERNANDEZ, MS
Division of Pediatric Neurosurgery, Brain Institute, Nicklaus Children's Hospital, Miami, Florida, USA

DAVID S. HERSH, MD
Assistant Professor of Pediatrics and Surgery, Division of Neurosurgery, Connecticut Children's, UConn School of Medicine, Hartford, Connecticut

BETSY D. HOPSON, MHSA
Spina Bifida Program Director, Director of STEP Transition Program, Children's of Alabama, Birmingham, Alabama

CHRISTOPHER D. HUGHES, MD, MPH
Assistant Professor of Surgery, Divisions of Plastic Surgery and Craniofacial Surgery, Connecticut Children's, UConn School of Medicine, Hartford, Connecticut

ERIC M. JACKSON, MD
Associate Professor, Division of Pediatric Neurosurgery, Department of Neurosurgery, Johns Hopkins School of Medicine, Baltimore, Maryland

ANDREW JEA, MD
Department of Neurosurgery, University of Oklahoma College of Medicine, Oklahoma City, Oklahoma

SANDI K. LAM, MD, MBA
Professor of Neurological Surgery, Division Head, Pediatric Neurosurgery, Lurie Children's Hospital and Northwestern University Feinberg School of Medicine, Chicago, Illinois

CORMAC O. MAHER, MD
Department of Neurosurgery, University of Michigan, Ann Arbor, Michigan

FRANCESCO T. MANGANO, DO
Department of Neurological Surgery, Mary Jane and Bob Tritsch Professor of Neurosurgery and Pediatrics, Division Chief, Pediatric Neurosurgery, Cincinnati Children's Hospital Medical Center, University of Cincinnati College of Medicine, Cincinnati, Ohio

JONATHAN MARTIN, MD, FAAP, FACS, FANS
Paul M. Kanev Chair of Pediatric Neurosurgery, Division of Neurosurgery, Connecticut Children's, Associate Professor, Department of Surgery, University of Connecticut School of Medicine, Hartford, Connecticut

SAMUEL G. McCLUGAGE III, MD
Department of Neurosurgery, Baylor College of Medicine, Department of Surgery, Division of Pediatric Neurosurgery, Texas Children's Hospital, Houston, Texas

ALAA MONTASER, MD, PhD
Department of Neurosurgery, Boston Children's Hospital, Harvard Medical School, Boston, Massachusetts

WHITNEY E. MUHLESTEIN, MD
Department of Neurosurgery, University of Michigan, Ann Arbor, Michigan

TOBA N. NIAZI, MD
Miller School of Medicine, University of Miami, Division of Pediatric Neurosurgery, Brain Institute, Nicklaus Children's Hospital, Miami, Florida

GREG OLAVARRIA, MD, FAANS, FAAP
Assistant Professor, UCF College of Medicine, Pediatric Neurosurgery, Arnold Palmer Hospital for Children, Orlando, Florida

SMRUTI K. PATEL, MD
Fellow, Pediatric Neurosurgery, Cincinnati Children's Hospital Medical Center, Cincinnati, Ohio

ROBERT C. PEDERSEN, MD
Department of Pediatrics, Hawaii Permanente Medical Group, Honolulu, Hawaii

MARTIN G. PIAZZA, MD
Department of Neurological Surgery, The University of North Carolina at Chapel Hill, Chapel Hill, North Carolina

REBECCA A. REYNOLDS, MD
Department of Neurosurgery, Vanderbilt University Medical Center, Medical Center North, Nashville, Tennessee

BRANDON G. ROCQUE, MD, MS
Associate Professor, Division of Pediatric Neurosurgery, Department of Neurosurgery, Children's of Alabama, The University of Alabama at Birmingham, Birmingham, Alabama

VERONICA J. ROOKS, MD
Department of Radiology, Tripler Army Medical Center, Honolulu, Hawaii

EDWARD R. SMITH, MD
Department of Neurosurgery, Boston Children's Hospital, Harvard Medical School, Boston, Massachusetts

JIGNESH TAILOR, MD, PhD
Carson-Spiro Fellow, Division of Pediatric Neurosurgery, Department of Neurosurgery, Johns Hopkins School of Medicine, Baltimore, Maryland

RABIA TARI, MD
Fellow, Pediatric Neurosurgery, Cincinnati Children's Hospital Medical Center, Cincinnati, Ohio

JONATHAN R. WOOD, MD
Department of Radiology, Tripler Army Medical Center, Honolulu, Hawaii

AARON M. YENGO-KAHN, MD
Department of Neurosurgery, Vanderbilt University Medical Center, Medical Center North, Nashville, Tennessee

MOHAMED A. ZAAZOUE, MD
Department of Neurological Surgery, Indiana University School of Medicine, Indianapolis, Indiana

Contents

Foreword: Pediatric Neurosurgery in Primary Care xv

Bonita F. Stanton

Preface: Pediatric Neurosurgery in Primary Care xvii

Jonathan Martin and Greg Olavarria

Review of Pediatric Neurologic History and Age-Appropriate Neurologic Examination in the Office 707

Ashley T. Ashby and Alexandra D. Beier

The neurologic examination of an infant or child can be daunting, as they are unable to verbally communicate or follow directions. It starts with tailoring the pediatric neurologic history and examination to the child's specific age group. A good neurologic history obtained from the patient and parents is key to evaluating a pediatric patient. This article offers pearls on what information to ask the caregivers and patients, and salient aspects of a brief neurologic examination.

Neuroimaging for the Primary Care Provider: A Review of Modalities, Indications, and Pitfalls 715

Jonathan R. Wood, Robert C. Pedersen, and Veronica J. Rooks

When evaluating a child with a potential neurologic or neurodevelopmental disorder, identifying indications for imaging and the correct imaging modality to order can be challenging. This article provides an overview of computed tomography, MRI, ultrasonography, and radiography with an emphasis on indications for use, pitfalls to be avoided, and recent advances. A discussion of the appropriate use of ionizing radiation, intravenous contrast, and sedation is also provided.

Diagnosis and Management of Suture-Related Concerns of the Infant Skull 727

David S. Hersh, Markus J. Bookland, and Christopher D. Hughes

The cranial fontanelles and sutures have several benign variations, including most cases of "early" or "late" closure of the anterior fontanelle, bathrocephaly, overriding sutures, and benign metopic ridging. However, recognizing true craniosynostosis and referring the patient to a craniofacial specialist in a timely fashion are imperative, as minimally invasive options can be offered to most patients younger than 6 months of age. Gaining comfort with the physical examination of an infant with an abnormal head shape is best achieved through experience and pattern recognition and will frequently facilitate an accurate diagnosis without the need for ionizing radiation.

Pediatric Neurosurgery in Primary Care: Masses of the Scalp and Skull in Children 743

Randaline R. Barnett, Martin G. Piazza, and Scott W. Elton

There are a wide variety of scalp and skull lesions that can affect the pediatric population, many of which are first encountered by primary care physicians. The differential consists of a broad range of more common congenital lesions, sequelae of trauma, and vascular anomalies, to very rare neoplastic processes. It is important to understand signs and symptoms that may indicate whether a lesion may be benign versus life threatening, what imaging studies are appropriate and how to interpret them, and when to seek referrals to specialists.

Macrocephaly in the Primary Care Provider's Office **759**

Jean-Paul Bryant, Nicole E. Hernandez, and Toba N. Niazi

Macrocephaly is commonly encountered in the primary care provider's office. It is defined as an occipitofrontal circumference that is greater than 2 standard deviations above the mean for the child's given age. Macrocephaly is a nonspecific clinical finding that may be benign or require further evaluation. An algorithmic approach is useful for aiding in the clinical decision-making process to determine if further evaluation with neuroimaging is warranted. Abnormal findings may signify a harmful underlying cause, requiring referral to a genetic specialist or neurosurgeon.

Incidental Intracranial Cysts in Children **775**

Whitney E. Muhlestein and Cormac O. Maher

With increasing use of intracranial imaging, the diagnosis of benign intracranial cysts is becoming more frequent in the pediatric population. These lesions are usually incidentally discovered during the work-up of unrelated symptoms. Most do not require treatment and many do not even require imaging follow-up. When symptomatic, symptoms of these lesions are usually caused by local mass effect. Symptomatic lesions warrant neurosurgical evaluation, and may require surgical intervention in rare, well-selected cases. This article describes three common benign intracranial cysts found in the pediatric population: arachnoid cysts, choroid cysts, and pineal cysts.

Chiari Malformation in Children **783**

Gregory W. Albert

Chiari malformation type 1 (CM1) is often found incidentally. However, patients with symptoms or signs referable to CM1 or an associated syrinx will likely benefit from surgical intervention. Patients who are not symptomatic from CM1 at presentation are unlikely to become symptomatic at follow-up.

Pediatric Hydrocephalus and the Primary Care Provider **793**

Smruti K. Patel, Rabia Tari, and Francesco T. Mangano

Hydrocephalus is a pathologic condition that results in the disruption of normal cerebrospinal fluid flow dynamics often characterized by an increase in intracranial pressure resulting in an abnormal dilation of the ventricles. The goal of this article was to provide the necessary background information to understand the pathophysiology related to hydrocephalus, recognize the presenting signs and symptoms of hydrocephalus, identify when to initiate a workup with further studies, and understand the management of pediatric patients with a new and preexisting diagnosis of hydrocephalus.

Brain and Spinal Cord Tumors in Children **811**

Jignesh Tailor and Eric M. Jackson

This article provides general principles of managing children with central nervous system tumors. The distribution, diagnostic work-up, and key principles of treatment are reviewed, and special circumstances that may be encountered by pediatricians in the community are discussed.

Intracranial Vascular Abnormalities in Children **825**

Alaa Montaser and Edward R. Smith

Intracranial vascular abnormalities rarely are encountered in primary care. Many of the pathologies are occult and prognosis varies widely between inconsequential variants of anatomy to acutely life-threatening conditions. Consequently, there often is a great deal of anxiety associated with any potential diagnosis. This article reviews anatomic intracranial vascular lesions, including vascular malformations (arteriovenous malformations/arteriovenous fistulae and cavernous malformations), structural arteriopathies (aneurysms and moyamoya), and common developmental anomalies of the vasculature. The focus includes a general overview of anatomy, pathology, epidemiology, and key aspects of evaluation for the primary care provider and a review of common questions encountered in practice.

Epilepsy Surgery in Children **845**

Luis E. Bello-Espinosa and Greg Olavarria

Epilepsy in children continues to present a major medical and economic burden on society. Left untreated, seizures can present the risk of sudden death and severe cognitive impairment. It is understood that primary care providers having concerns about abnormal movements or behaviors in children will make a prompt referral to a trusted pediatric neurologist. The authors present a brief introduction to seizure types, classification, and management with particular focus on what surgery for epilepsy can offer. Improved seizure control and its attendant improvements in quality of life can be achieved with timely referral and intervention.

Mild Traumatic Brain Injury in Children **857**

Aaron M. Yengo-Kahn, Rebecca A. Reynolds, and Christopher M. Bonfield

Mild traumatic brain injury accounts for an estimated 4.8 million cases of pediatric traumatic brain injuries worldwide every year. In the United States, 70% of mild traumatic brain injury cases are due to sports and recreational injuries. Early diagnosis, especially in active children, is critical to preventing recurrent injuries. Management is guided by graded protocols for returning to school and activity. Ninety percent of children recover within 1 month of injury. Promising research has shown that early referral to specialty concussion care and multidisciplinary treatment with physical and occupational therapy may shorten recovery time and improve neurologic outcomes.

Cervical Spine Injury in Children and Adolescents 875

Andrew Jea, Ahmed Belal, Mohamed A. Zaazoue, and Jonathan Martin

Complaints related to the neck are common following mild pediatric trauma. Although significant cervical spine injuries are most often seen and evaluated in the emergency room or inpatient setting, the primary care provider is faced with the evaluation of lower acuity complaints. We provide a review to assist with the efficient evaluation of these patients to facilitate decisions regarding return to play, the need for imaging, and need for referral to subspecialty providers.

Cutaneous Stigmata of the Spine: A Review of Indications for Imaging and Referral 895

Mandana Behbahani, Sandi K. Lam, and Robin Bowman

Cutaneous stigmata of the midline spine are a common question in pediatrics. They are known to be related to a higher likelihood of underlying dysraphic spinal abnormalities. Clear understanding of different types of cutaneous stigmata and correlating dysraphic findings can aid in appropriate imaging workup and timely management of patient pathology. In this article, the authors review midline spinal cutaneous findings in the pediatric population with occult spinal dysraphism.

Caring for the Child with Spina Bifida 915

Brandon G. Rocque, Betsy D. Hopson, and Jeffrey P. Blount

Care for a child with spina bifida can be complex, requiring multiple specialists. Neurosurgical care centers around the initial closure or repair of the spinal defect, followed by management of hydrocephalus, symptoms of the Chiari 2 malformation, and tethered cord. This article reviews definitions and types of spina bifida, considerations surrounding the initial treatment, including fetal surgery, and the ongoing neurosurgical management of common comorbid conditions. The role of interdisciplinary care is stressed, as well as the importance of coordinated transition to adult care at an appropriate age and developmental stage.

Review of Tone Management for the Primary Care Provider 929

Samuel G. McClugage III and David F. Bauer

Movement disorders in a pediatric population represent a spectrum of secondary functional deficits affecting ease of care, ambulation, and activities of daily living. Cerebral palsy represents the most common form of movement disorder seen in the pediatric population. Several medical and surgical options exist in the treatment of pediatric spasticity and dystonia, which can have profound effects on the functionality of these patients. Given the complex medical and surgical problems in these patients, children are well served by a multidisciplinary team of practitioners, including physical therapists, physical medicine and rehabilitation physicians, and surgeons.

PEDIATRIC CLINICS OF NORTH AMERICA

FORTHCOMING ISSUES

October 2021
Covid-19 in Children
Elizabeth Secord and Eric John McGrath, *Editors*

December 2021
Pediatric Gastroenterology
Harpreet Hall, *Editor*

February 2022
International Aspects of Pediatric Infectious Diseases
Chokechai Rongkavilit and Fouzia Naeem, *Editors*

RECENT ISSUES

June 2021
Integrated Behavioral Health in Pediatric Practice
Roger Apple, Cheryl Adele Dickson, Maria Demma I. Cabral, Editors

April 2021
Ending the War Against Children: The Rights of Children to Live Free of Violence
Danielle Laraque-Arena, Bonita F. Stanton, Editors

February 2021
Pulmonary Manifestations of Pediatric Diseases
Nelson L. Turcios, Editor

Foreword

Pediatric Neurosurgery in Primary Care

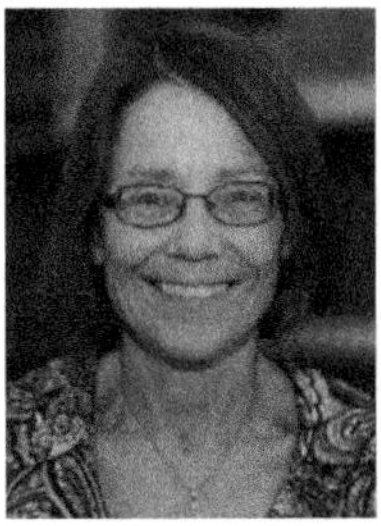

Bonita F. Stanton, MD
Consulting Editor

Among the estimated 2297 pediatric neurosurgeons in practice globally, the vast majority (86%) work in high-income and upper-middle-income countries. By contrast, an estimated 330 pediatric neurosurgeons serve the 1.2 billion children living in low-income and lower-middle-income countries.[1] While especially true for pediatric care providers in countries with limited resources, it is very important for all physicians serving children to understand how much they might be able to accomplish in their offices and/or with readily available diagnostic tests. Typically, these would be ordered in partnership with a pediatric neurosurgeon, but depending on their availability, could be ordered even before involving the limited number of pediatric neurosurgeons in some parts of the world.

The purpose of this issue of *Pediatric Clinics of North America*, edited by 2 pediatric neurosurgeons (Drs Martin and Olavarria), is to describe the presenting symptoms and physical characteristics of a child with a potential neurologic defect and to advise regarding potential diagnostic studies that the primary physician could conduct and/or order. Particularly striking is Drs Martin and Olavarria's simple statement in their Introduction that, "*Our goal is to partner with you to make each topic accessible and actionable within your practice setting.*"

The articulation of a desire to partner with a child's primary care provider is important for all pediatric specialists, but especially so among physicians whose primary training was not in pediatrics. In such instances, the child's primary care pediatrician may be aware of a broader differential diagnosis than might a highly trained specialist from another field. Likewise, for the follow-up after a major intervention such as brain surgery, the pediatrician may well be the first professional to see a potentially disturbing trend in the child's postsurgical recovery and/or growth or development. The articles in this issue of *Pediatric Clinics of North America* could be very helpful either to allay a parent's anxiety or to recognize a potentially disturbing deviation from a normal

Pediatr Clin N Am 68 (2021) xv–xvi
https://doi.org/10.1016/j.pcl.2021.05.001
0031-3955/21/© 2021 Published by Elsevier Inc.

postoperative course. It is worth noting that after graduating from medical school, a pediatrician will have received a minimum of 3 years of general pediatrics training, and a pediatric neurologist will have received an additional 3 years of pediatric neurology training. By contrast, a pediatric neurosurgeon will have received 7 to 8 years of neurosurgical training after graduating from medical school, followed by a 1-year pediatric neurosurgical fellowship.[2] In summary, the neurosurgeon, especially during his or her early years of serving as an attending, would not be expected to be a talented infant or child attending, and likewise, the pediatrician would not be expected to be familiar with or comfortable performing surgical procedures. But what would work well for a child's best interest would be a pediatric-neurosurgical team.

This is a wonderful issue that, read carefully, should greatly increase the pediatrician's capacity as a diagnostician and clinician regarding childhood neurologic disorders and offer the pediatrician a greater understanding as to the differential diagnosis and surgical options recommended by the neurosurgeon. As such, the pediatrician may be of enormous help to the afflicted child's parents.

Bonita F. Stanton, MD
Hackensack Meridian
School of Medicine
Academic Enterprise
Hackensack Meridian Health
123 Metro Boulevard
Nutley, NJ 07110, USA

E-mail address:
bonita.stanton@hmhn.org

REFERENCES

1. Dewan MC, Baticulon RE, Rattani A, et al. Pediatric neurosurgical work force, access to care, equipment and training needs worldwide. Neurosurg Focus 2015; 45(4):E13.
2. Carbonell WS. What is the procedure of becoming a pediatric neurosurgeon, how long does it take and how much is the salary in the USA? Available at: https://www.quora.com/What-is-the-procedure-of-becoming-a-pediatric-neurosurgeon-how-long-does-it-take-and-how-much-is-the-salary-in-the-USA. Accessed May 13, 2021.

Preface

Pediatric Neurosurgery in Primary Care

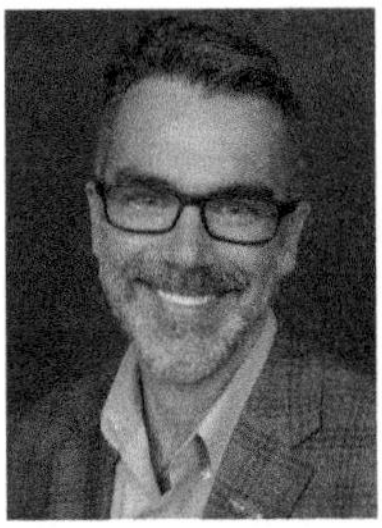

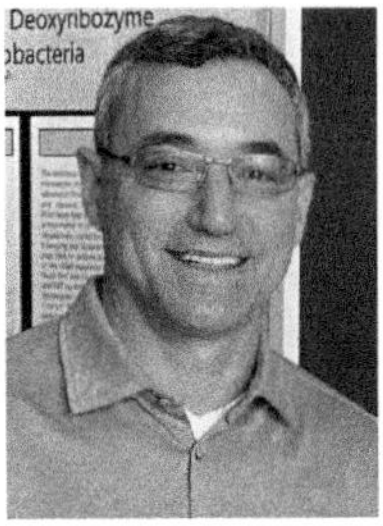

Jonathan Martin, MD, FAAP, FACS, FANS   Greg Olavarria, MD, FAANS, FAAP
Editors

Alone we do so little; together, we can do so much.

—Helen Keller

Nothing in life is to be feared, it is only to be understood. Now is the time to understand more, so that we may fear less.

—Marie Curie

Colleagues,

We would like to welcome you to this issue of *Pediatric Clinics of North America* dedicated to topics in pediatric neurosurgery. Our discipline carries with it a rather ominous reputation as a highly complex and nuanced field, employing advanced imaging modalities and surgical technology that can inspire both awe and trepidation to the uninitiated. While the number of children who require neurosurgical intervention is small, the average primary care pediatrician sees children on a daily basis with historical or physical findings that may prompt concern (or even anxiety) from the provider, family, or both! Pediatric neurosurgeons are frequently asked to speak on topics such as head size, head shape, and lumbar skin findings. When to image? When to refer?

Our group has endeavored to create for you a collection of articles that are practical, informative, and accessible to the nonsurgical provider. Our goal is to partner with you to make each topic accessible and actionable within your practice setting.

The first articles focus on patient assessment to include the neurologic examination of the child and diagnostic imaging studies pertinent to the nervous system. The former has not changed in many years and still is the most important part of the assessment of any child. The latter is a field constantly changing; while imaging provides abundant information to the provider of both anatomy and function, it does so at financial cost

Pediatr Clin N Am 68 (2021) xvii–xix
https://doi.org/10.1016/j.pcl.2021.04.019
0031-3955/21/© 2021 Published by Elsevier Inc.

to the family, and with potential exposures (radiation and sedation) that must be carefully considered.

The next articles provide information on common concerns in the office setting: head shape, the cranial sutures, skull lesions, and head size, and how to manage abnormal head growth. The ubiquity of imaging availability has made the findings of cysts and Chiari malformations commonplace. We hope to guide the reader in matching symptoms with imaging findings and help to determine when to refer the child to a specialist.

Subsequent articles delve into more specialized areas of neurosurgery: hydrocephalus and shunts, tumors of the brain and spine, vascular malformations, and epilepsy. These articles inform, with a goal to allow the pediatrician to partner with the neurosurgeon to share information and reassure families regarding these diagnoses.

Management of traumatic injury to the brain and spine follows, covering the spectrum of concussion to more severe injuries. Mild traumatic brain and cervical spine injuries are commonplace in primary care practice, and the structured discussion of this topic will be a welcome reference to any pediatrician.

The final articles deal with cutaneous lumbar stigmata, tethered cord disorders, and spina bifida. These articles cover an incredibly broad spectrum from primary care topics, such as when to image or refer for lumbar cutaneous findings, to a review of the MOMS fetal myelomeningocele study and the recent development of centers for fetal surgery in our field. We end with tone abnormalities in children, spasticity management, both nonsurgical and surgical.

This issue would not have been possible without the effort and support of many. The editors would like to thank our contributing authors for their work on this issue of *Pediatric Clinics of North America*. We also thank our consultant pediatricians, Drs Jack Lavalette and Alix Casler, who held us accountable to making the articles both useful and accessible to an audience of primary care providers. We appreciate the efforts of Ms Elsa Martin and Ms Liza Rooks, who contributed illustrations that strengthened several articles and made this issue a true family affair. Finally, we thank Dr Joseph H. Piatt Jr for his enormous contribution to the first issue of this journal in 2004. The original issue inspired us, and we hope to update and expand on the concepts from that. It is our hope that the articles forthcoming illuminate the basic concepts of pediatric neurosurgery in an easy-to-reference manner, and, as the first issue did, dampen the anxiety that accompanies an actual (or possible) neurosurgical diagnosis. Enjoy!

Sincerely,

Jonathan Martin, MD, FAAP, FACS, FANS
Pediatric Neurosurgery
Connecticut Children's
Department of Surgery
University of Connecticut School of Medicine
282 Washington Street
Hartford, CT 06106, USA

Greg Olavarria, MD, FAANS, FAAP
Pediatric Neurosurgery
Arnold Palmer Hospital for Children
100 West Gore Street
Orlando, Florida 32806 USA

E-mail addresses:
Jmartin03@connecticutchildrens.org (J. Martin)
Gregory.olavarria@gmail.com (G. Olavarria)

Review of Pediatric Neurologic History and Age-Appropriate Neurologic Examination in the Office

Ashley T. Ashby, PA-C, MPAS[a], Alexandra D. Beier, DO[b,*]

KEYWORDS

• Pediatric • Neurologic examination • Developmental milestones

KEY POINTS

- A good deal of information can be gleaned from simple observation of the child and listening to the parent's history.
- A detailed history and examination can avoid unnecessary and costly imaging.
- Acute change from baseline neurologic functioning, loss of milestones, or declining school performance warrant appropriate evaluation.

There is nothing more deceptive than an obvious fact.

—Sherlock Holmes

HISTORY

A good history can often provide an early diagnosis. Ask about past medical history and medications. A chief neurologic complaint should be identified including onset, location, duration of symptoms, associated symptoms, severity, quality of symptoms, and alleviating/aggravating factors. If there are concerns for neurologic disease processes, it must be determined if these findings are static (due to perinatal or congenital insults, trauma or cerebrovascular accident), progressive (degenerative disease process), intermittent (possible seizures), or saltatory (exacerbation and partial recovery, indicating demyelinating and vascular processes).[1] Previously tried interventions are also important. Inquiring about family history of neurologic disorders is also essential,

[a] Lucy Gooding Pediatric Neurosurgery Center, Wolfson Children's Hospital, 836 Prudential Drive, Suite 1205, Jacksonville, FL 32207, USA; [b] Pediatric Epilepsy Program, Division of Pediatric Neurosurgery, University of Florida Health Jacksonville, Lucy Gooding Pediatric Neurosurgery Center, Wolfson Children's Hospital, 836 Prudential Drive, Suite 1205, Jacksonville, FL 32207, USA
* Corresponding author.
E-mail address: Alexandra.Beier@jax.ufl.edu

Pediatr Clin N Am 68 (2021) 707–714
https://doi.org/10.1016/j.pcl.2021.04.001

as is the child's social environment. Prior hospitalizations and surgeries should be noted.

History-Taking: Neonates and Infants

Key portions of the history include birth history. Data to collect include estimated gestational age at delivery, mode of delivery, delivery complications, and if the baby left the hospital with mother or required a longer stay. Developmental history is also important. There is some variability in timing of reaching milestones between individuals, but the following may prompt further investigation: inability to hold an object by 5 months, not reaching for objects by 6 months, inability to sit unassisted by 12 months, not pointing to objects by 18 months, and delay in walking past 18 months (boys) or 2 years (girls).[2] Up until age 2 years, correcting for gestational age is essential in milestones and examination. Other valuable portions of the history include what the family has observed: asymmetric movements, gaze limitations, feeding difficulties, sleeping schedule, irritability/ability to be consoled. Early hand dominance (before 18 months) can suggest a hemiparesis.

History-Taking: Age 1 to 5 Years

Regression of milestones in this age group should raise concern. Ask about headaches, their timing, location, associated symptoms, and alleviating/exacerbating factors. Vomiting can be associated with a host of pediatric disease processes; however, headache with vomiting is concerning, especially nocturnal or early morning emesis.[3] In this age group, as they are beginning to ambulate, they often fall. However, worsening trips and falls should raise concern. In addition, in this age group, toilet training is occurring. Inquire about toileting habits, accidents, and infections, as regression with these functions can indicate spinal cord pathology.

Clinics Care Points: Concerning Clinical Features of Headache

- Nocturnal awakening with headache or headache in morning with vomiting
- Absence of family history of migraine
- Change in typical headache pattern or worsening over time

History-Taking: Age 6 Years and Older

A child in this age group can express his or her own symptoms. In addition to the aforementioned history, inquire about school performance. A sudden or even gradual decline in academic performance is a concerning finding. For example, a child with a ventriculoperitoneal shunt may only have worsening school performance as a symptom of shunt malfunction. Specific to the adolescent population, particularly athletes or those with large body mass index, low back pain can be a common complaint. The prevalence increased with age (6% at age 10 years, 18% at age 14–16 years) until it matches adulthood at 18 years old. Unfortunately, studies show that greater than 80% will not have an identifiable diagnosis at 1 year.[4,5] The most common associated diagnoses for low back pain are strain/spasm, scoliosis, degenerative disk disease, and disc herniation. Concerning symptomatology (red flags) include night pain, pain with bowel-bladder complaints, radicular symptoms, saddle paresthesias, back pain with fever/weight loss, and neurologic deficit.

Clinics Care Points: History

1. Birth history and correcting for gestational age is key to the infant history.
2. Milestone regression and premature hand dominance can suggest a neurologic disorder.

3. School performance provides a window into the child's cognitive functioning.

NEUROLOGIC EXAMINATION

The key components of the neurologic examination include mental status, cranial nerves, motor and sensory systems, cerebellar function, and reflexes. In children, additional focus on the supporting structures of the head and spine are also essential. Formal developmental assessments (ie, the Bayley Scale for Infant and Toddler Development) can be ordered to supplement the neurologic examination.

First and foremost, observe the patient and their interactions with their environment regardless of age. A lot can be gained from the pediatric patient by just watching their facial and extremity movements. Examine the child's skin, for neurocutaneous disorders can present with skin lesions, that is, cafe au lait spots of neurofibromatosis. The lumbar spine may show signs of dysraphism, that is, dimples above the gluteal crease or hair tufts (covered elsewhere in this volume). Assess if child is well nourished or not.

Components of the neurologic examination

- Mental status
- Cranial nerves
- Motor examination
- Sensory examination
- Cerebellar function
- Reflex examination
- Supporting structures

Examination: Neonates and Infants

Accounting for gestational age, the older infant will spend more time awake and visually fixate on objects or faces. Sunset sign or limited upgaze, as well as a full, tense fontanelle, can be signs of raised intracranial pressure. The quality of cry should be noted. Head circumference is a vital sign. In general, an infant's head circumference grows by 2 cm per month from 0 to 3 months and 1 cm per month from 3 to 6 months.[1] Correlate with the rate of weight gain and height (head shape and size concerns such as plagiocephaly or synostosis are covered in other chapters in this volume) (**Fig. 1**). A basic cranial nerve assessment includes pupillary reactivity and blink response. Allowing the infant to suck usually induces eye opening. Suck and swallow, as well as facial symmetry can assess facial motor function and lower cranial nerves. Hearing is assessed by response to noise or startle. Assess for spontaneous and stimulus-induced movements and symmetry. Tone in extremities should be noted, as well as muscle bulk. Babinski reflex usually disappears by 1 year of age, and other reflexes such as the Moro or the asymmetric tonic neck reflex (ATNR) can bring out a hemiparesis or brachial plexus palsy if asymmetric (**Fig. 2**). The persistence of these reflexes beyond 6 months is also abnormal. The parachute reflex (**Fig. 3**) appears around 6 months of age, and its absence can signal delayed ability to ambulate. In general, the infant should lift the head at 2 months, reach and grasp at 4 months, sit unsupported by 7 months, pull to stand by 9 or 10 months, and walk by 12 to 15 months.

Clinics Care Points: Infant Examination

1. Ensure proper technique is being performed for head circumference measurement and chart with height and weight.

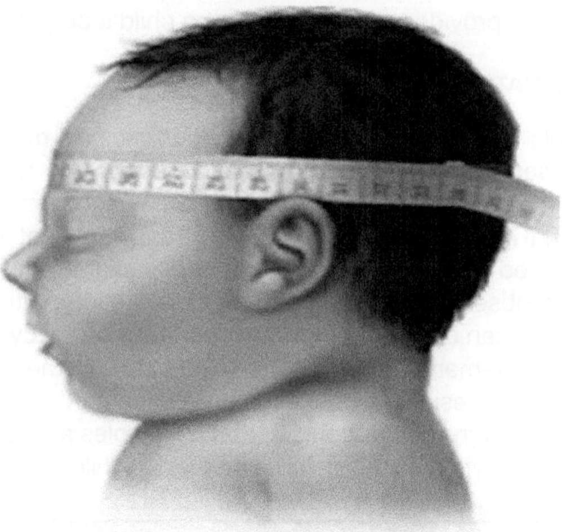

Fig. 1. Proper technique in measuring head circumference. The tape measure should rest above the eyebrows, above the ears, and around the occiput. The measuring tape should be parallel to the floor and should be pulled snug (courtesy Google images). (Contributed by Creative Commons, Ashley Arbuckle, (CC BY 2.0).)

2. Increasing head circumference, a tense fontanelle, and sunsetting eyes can be signs of raised intracranial pressure.
3. Examine the spine for dimples, hair tufts, and lipomas that could indicate spinal dysraphism.
4. The assessment of primitive reflexes can bring out a neurologic deficit.

Examination: Age 1 to 5 Years

The formal examination of the child starts with observation. Watching the child play with a toy gives a window into manual dexterity, coordination, and handedness. Note mental status, converse with the older child, observe spontaneous movements, measure head

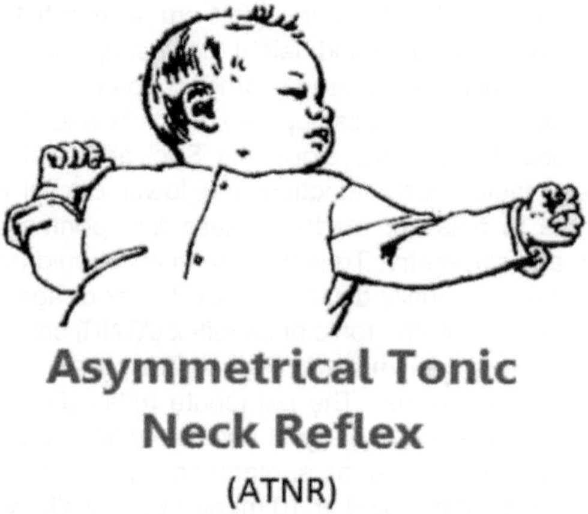

Fig. 2. Demonstration of the ATNR, the asymmetric tonic neck reflex; when the head is turned (here to the left) the left arm extends out and the right arm flexes. Asymmetry or persistence of some primitive reflexes can signal a neurologic deficit (courtesy Google images). (Contributed by Creative Commons, Ashley Arbuckle, (CC BY 2.0).)

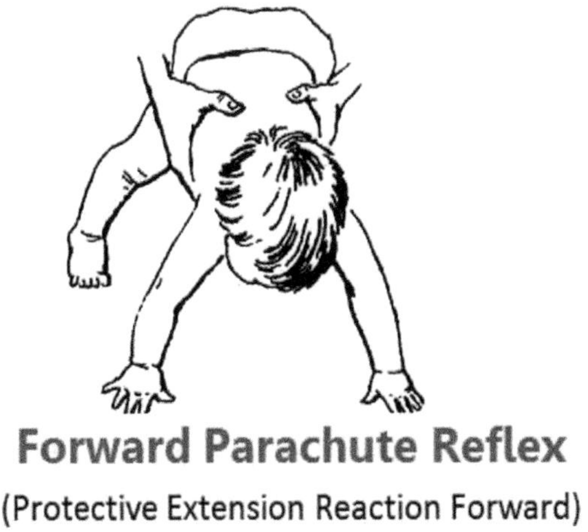

Fig. 3. Infant in the parachute reflex position. This primitive reflex develops later in infancy (around 6 months), and its absence can signal delayed walking. It is elicited by holding the infant face down and rapidly lowering the infant, causing the infant to extend out the arms (courtesy Bing Microsoft images).

circumference, and examine for skin lesions. Perhaps leave the more invasive parts of the examination for the end (fundoscopy or reflexes). A more detailed cranial nerve examination can be done at this age. Assess pupil size and reactivity, conjugate extraocular movements, and look for ptosis. Again, limitation of upgaze can signify raised intracranial pressure. Note facial asymmetry, and remember, a central seventh nerve palsy spares the forehead wrinkling and eye closure (bilateral innervation of upper face).

Assess movements for symmetry and have the child get up from the floor to measure leg power. Assess proprioception (**Fig. 4**). Check the child's tone, and note scissoring of the legs is a sign of spasticity. Observe gait and perform a Romberg test (feet together standing, eyes closed, this tests proprioception in the lower extremities). Attempt finger to nose testing for coordination, and children older than 3 years can

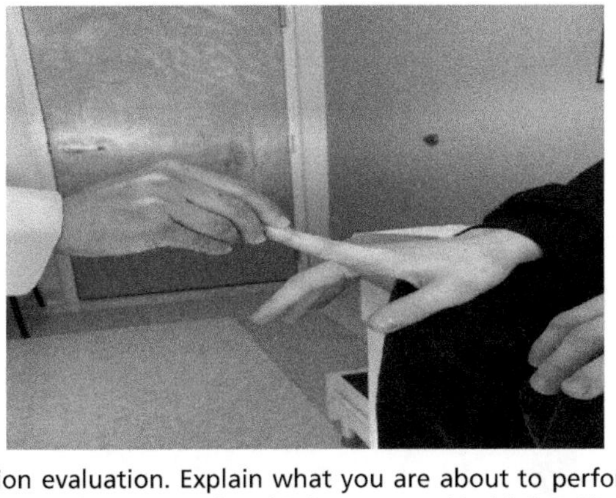

Fig. 4. Proprioception evaluation. Explain what you are about to perform and what "up" and "down" mean. Have the patient close his/her eyes and hold the side of the index finger (or big toe) and move it up and down a few times and then hold it in one position. Ask the patient if the finger (toe) is "up" or "down."

usually stand on one foot. Check deep tendon biceps, knee, and ankle reflexes. Decreased or exaggerated reflexes alone are not pathologic but should be noted in context of other parts of the examination.

Clinics Care Points: Examination 1 to 5 Years

1. Normal or abnormal development can be assessed at this age, and playing with a toy can be very informative
2. Start with less intrusive parts of the examination and leave the more threatening parts for the end

Examination: Age 6 Years and Older

The examination of the older child is similar to that of the preschool child. The patient can express their symptoms and concerns at this age; engage them in conversation to assess language and mentation. Again, the examination should proceed sequentially, with mental status, cranial nerve examination, sensorimotor function, cerebellar function/coordination, and reflexes. Visual acuity, visual fields, and extraocular movements as well can be more clearly assessed. Cranial nerve function can be tested in more detail, and motor function can be assessed using a 5-point scale (0 = no movement, 1 = minimal, 2 = movement with gravity eliminated, 3 = movement against gravity but against little resistance, 4 = against some resistance, 5 = normal power). Pronator drift, looking for subtle weakness, is easy to assess (**Fig. 5**). Finger to nose testing should be done, along with gait assessment and Romberg (proprioception). In the older age group, reflexes are easier to elicit in a more cooperative patient, and a Hoffman reflex can be done (**Fig. 6**).

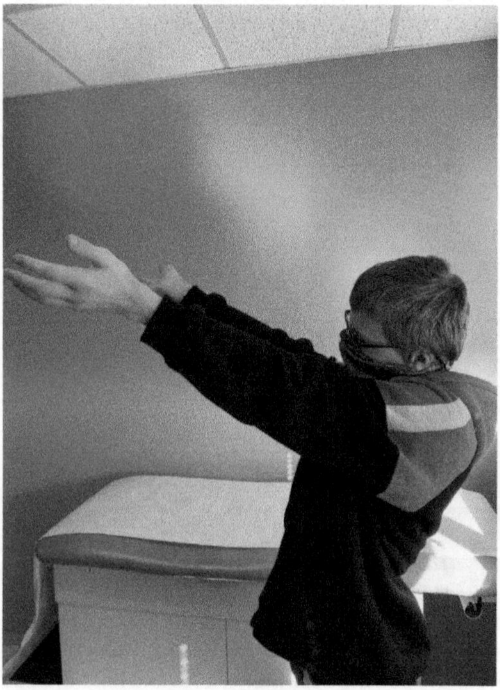

Fig. 5. Assessment of pronator drift. Child is holding out arms supine in extension and asked to close his or her eyes. It can elicit subtle weakness.

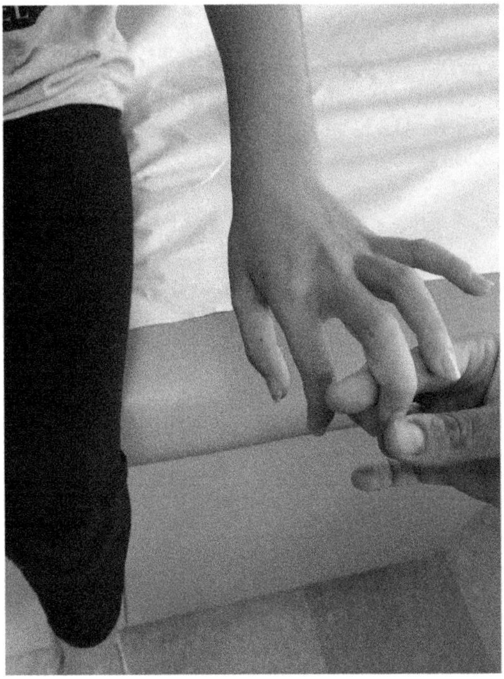

Fig. 6. The Hoffman reflex. With a relaxed patient's hand, loosely hold the patient's middle finger and flick the fingernail downward. Flexion of the thumb or index finger is considered an abnormal response and can indicate an upper motor neuron disorder or myelopathy of the spinal cord.

Medical research council motor grading scale
0: no movement
1: trace movement, muscular contraction palpable
2: movement to include through range of motion with gravity eliminated
3: movement through full range of motion against gravity
4: movement against resistance
5: full power

DISCLOSURE

The authors have nothing to disclose.

REFERENCES

1. Painter M, Yang M. Neurological examination of the newborn, infant and child. In: Albright A, Pollack I, Adelson P, editors. Principles and practice of pediatric neurosurgery. New York: Thieme; 2008. p. 31–42.
2. Hughes H, Kahl L. The harriette lane handbook: a manual for pediatric house officers. 21st edition. Philadelphia: Elsevier; 2018.

3. Dooley J. The evaluation and management of paediatric headaches. Paediatr Child Healt 2009;14(1):24–30.
4. MacDonald J, Stuart E, Rodenberg R. Musculoskeletal low back pain in school-aged children: a review. Jama Pediatr 2017;171(3):280.
5. Yang S, Werner BC, Singla A, et al. Low back pain in adolescents. J Pediatr Orthoped 2017;37(5):344–7.

Neuroimaging for the Primary Care Provider

A Review of Modalities, Indications, and Pitfalls

Jonathan R. Wood, MD[a,*], Robert C. Pedersen, MD[b],
Veronica J. Rooks, MD[a]

KEYWORDS

• Computed tomography • Magnetic resonance imaging • Ultrasound • Radiation
• Contrast • Sedation

KEY POINTS

- Familiarity with ultrasonography, computed tomography (CT), and magnetic resonance imaging (MRI) is imperative to ordering the correct examination to appropriately answer a clinical question.
- Continuous advancements in computed tomography and MRI have led to decreased sedation time and ionizing radiation dose.
- The risks and benefits of ionizing radiation, intravenous contrast, and sedation must be carefully evaluated before an imaging examination is ordered to ensure benefit to the child while minimizing risk.

INTRODUCTION

The most commonly used techniques for pediatric neuroimaging (computed tomography, MRI, ultrasound, and radiography) each have advantages, disadvantages, and appropriate indications. When ordering an imaging study, providers must weigh the diagnostic utility of the examination with concerns regarding sedation, ionizing radiation, availability, convenience, and cost. A basic familiarity of these techniques is essential for the pediatrician, to ensure appropriate patient care and to answer the clinical question while decreasing risk to the patient.

DISCUSSION

Ultrasound

Ultrasound uses a handheld probe that contains vibrating crystals that emit ultrasonic pressure waves into soft tissue and receive the reflecting pressure waves to create an

[a] Department of Radiology, Tripler Army Medical Center, 1 Jarrett White Road, MCHK-DR, Honolulu, HI 96859, USA; [b] Department of Pediatrics, Hawaii Permanente Medical Group, 2828 Paa Street, Honolulu, HI 96819, USA
* Corresponding author.
E-mail address: jonathan.r.wood.mil@mail.mil

Pediatr Clin N Am 68 (2021) 715–725
https://doi.org/10.1016/j.pcl.2021.04.014
0031-3955/21/Published by Elsevier Inc.

image.[1] Ultrasound can be easily performed at the bedside with small computers, including commercially available transducers that can be connected to smartphones. Ultrasound is appealing because of its excellent soft tissue contrast, allowing different structures to be delineated and evaluated. Other advantages of ultrasound include its lack of harmful ionizing radiation, its relative low cost, and it is less intimidating compared with MRI or CT. Advantages and disadvantages of ultrasound are listed in **Table 1**. An example of a spine ultrasound is shown in **Fig. 1**.

Indications

Ultrasonography of the brain is limited to infants who still have an open anterior fontanelle. A cranial ultrasound is the imaging modality of choice for those thought to be at high risk for hydrocephalus or with enlarging head circumference, as it will provide a good view of the ventricular system.[2] There are some limitations, such as poor visualization of the posterior fossa and significant interoperator variability. In addition, findings of early ischemia may not be apparent on ultrasound. Ultrasound of the spine can also be used to evaluate for dysraphism and signs of a tethered spinal cord. Ossified posterior elements preclude transmission of the ultrasound waves, which limits evaluation of the spinal cord and is therefore limited to infants less than 4 to 6 months of age.

Recent advances

Point-of-care ultrasound has become more prevalent with the advent of handheld ultrasound devices, which have the potential to be used in a clinical setting. Ultrasound technology has advanced, allowing for improved image quality with higher-resolution images. Other recent advances have been in the area of artificial intelligence to help the medical ultrasound technologist capture standard views of anatomy and decrease interoperator variability.[3]

An exciting new advancement has been the development of contrast-enhanced ultrasound (CEUS). Ultrasound contrast is an intravenous agent composed of microbubbles of gas, stabilized by a phospholipid membrane, that appear echogenic (bright) with ultrasound. CEUS allows for dynamic evaluation of contrast enhancement, potentially at the bedside. There is active research in using CEUS to evaluate cerebral perfusion in neonates. Potential clinical applications include evaluation of hypoxic ischemic injury, intracranial hemorrhage, hydrocephalus, and focal central nervous system (CNS) lesions.[4,5]

Pitfalls

The accuracy of ultrasound examination is greatly influenced by the skill and experience of the medical sonographer. The examination is dependent on accurate images

Table 1
Ultrasound

Advantages	Disadvantages
No ionizing radiation	Highly dependent on sonographer skill
Sedation not necessary	Ultrasound cannot pass through dense air or bone
Real-time examination yielding dynamic information	
Can detect blood flow without contrast	

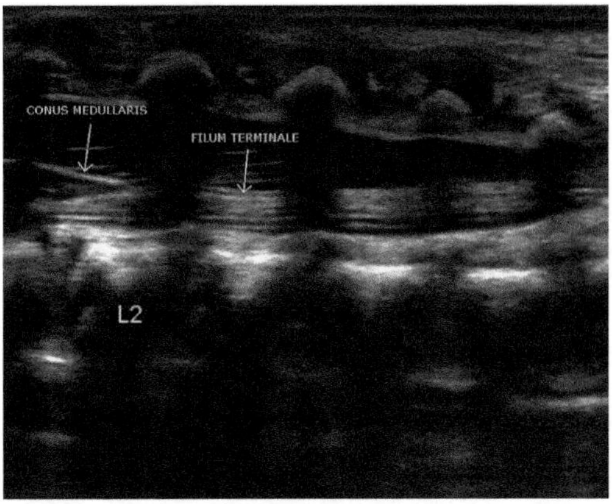

Fig. 1. Ultrasound of an infant spine demonstrates a normal appearance of the conus medullaris and cauda equina.

being obtained with standard views. Ultrasound machine settings must be appropriately set to optimize the examination and to reduce artifacts. In addition, a sonographer must have the knowledge to recognize potential pathologic condition from normal anatomy. Pediatricians should be aware that an open dialogue with their local radiologist is essential when ordering an unfamiliar or uncommon ultrasound, to ensure it can be performed adequately.

Computed Tomography

CT was first introduced in the 1970s, and since then, its use has exploded because of its cost-effectiveness, availability, and accuracy.[6] CT is acquired as a gantry, containing an x-ray generator and detector, rotates around the patient. Multiple sequential images can be compiled that create a scan of a volume of tissue, such as a patient's head or the entire body. These images can be displayed various ways to accentuate different body tissues, from the osseous structures to the differences between gray and white matter in the brain. Advantages and disadvantages of CT are listed in **Table 2**. Examples of CT images are shown in **Figs. 2** and **3**.

Indications

CT is the "go-to" modality in the acute setting to screen for lesions that might warrant neurosurgical intervention (hemorrhage, hydrocephalus, edema or mass effect, tumor) or admission for closer monitoring (head trauma, fracture, extra-axial hemorrhage). CT

Table 2
Computed tomography

Advantages	Disadvantages
Fast; sedation usually not required	Ionizing radiation
Detailed evaluation of osseous structures	Poor soft tissue contrast
Sensitive for detection of hemorrhage	No dynamic information without multiple scans
	Requires intravenous contrast to detect blood flow

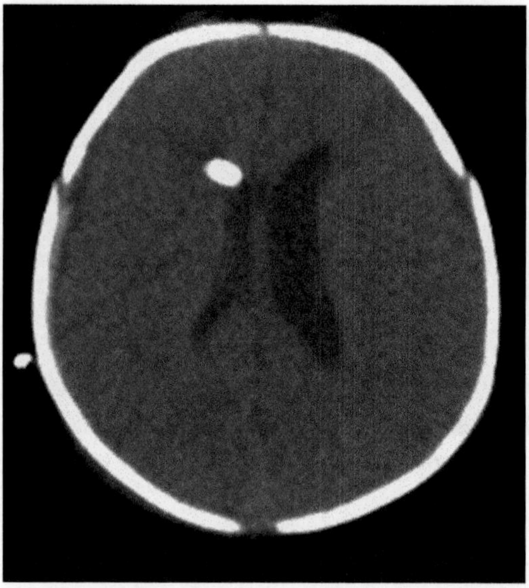

Fig. 2. CT of an infant head with a right frontal approach extraventricular drain in the right frontal horn.

is readily available and quick, so sedation can usually be avoided. CT is the preferred modality to evaluate for intracranial hemorrhage, as it is more sensitive than MRI or ultrasound for detecting acute blood products. In the setting of trauma, 3-dimensional models of the calvarium can be quickly created to demonstrate a fracture that may be subtle on radiographs and easily overlooked with ultrasound or MRI. Temporal

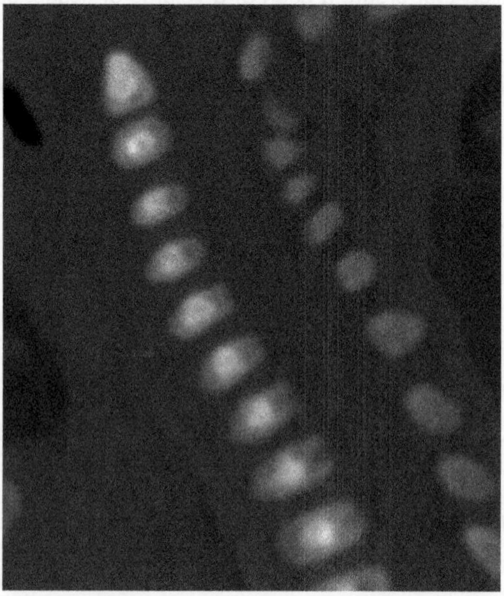

Fig. 3. CT of an infant spine after trauma shows normal alignment and no fractures.

bone fractures, spinal fractures, and facial fractures are all more easily seen with CT, making it the preferred modality in the setting of trauma.

Recent advances

In the past decade, CT technology has rapidly advanced, which has allowed images to be obtained with ever-decreasing ionizing radiation dose and compensating for patient motion. Recent advances in CT techniques and technology have led to a reduction in ionizing radiation dose with noncontrast head CT between 22% and 43%.[7–9]

There have been other recent advances that reduce motion artifacts. Ultrahigh-pitch CT and ultrawide detector arrays have significantly decreased the time needed to perform a CT, resulting in significantly reduced motion. A single-axial acquisition with a 16-cm field of view can scan a pediatric head with a single rotation of the gantry in less than a second.[10]

Pitfalls

The most significant disadvantage of CT is the dose the patient receives from ionizing radiation. Pediatric patients are more susceptible to the harmful effects of ionizing radiation when compared with adults due at least in part to their longer lifespans and more rapidly replicating DNA. Clinical decision-making tools have been developed, such as the Pediatric Emergency Care Applied Research Network rules, to help clinicians determine when a CT is indicated.[11] Despite the risks of ionizing radiation, missing an intracranial hemorrhage or a fracture may lead to significant morbidity and possible mortality for the patient. Pediatricians should be reassured that a CT is likely indicated when the benefits outweigh the risks of ionizing radiation, and the information obtained from the examination will influence patient management. When frequent follow-up examinations are needed, such as in children with ventriculoperitoneal shunts, fast MRIs can be performed to be spare the child excessive ionizing radiation.

Magnetic Resonance Imaging

MRI uses strong magnetic fields and radiofrequency pulses to image the patient and is attractive for the use in pediatric imaging because of its lack of ionizing radiation. MRI provides excellent soft tissue contrast compared with CT and creates detailed images of the CNS, which can differentiate white matter from the gray matter. MRI is the only imaging modality that can evaluate for metabolites, such as lactate, and visualize cerebrospinal fluid flow. MRI can visualize ischemia with minutes of onset, whereas CT can take hours to become apparent. MRI can create images that accentuate various details of the soft tissue, such as edema, fat content, blood products, and cellular swelling from ischemia. MRI has many disadvantages. MRI examinations are expensive compared with CT and ultrasound. MRI examinations may take over an hour to perform and require sedation for certain pediatric patients, especially those under the age of 6 years. Many medical devices may also not be compatible with MRI, such as cochlear implants, pacemakers, vagus nerve stimulators for epilepsy, and magnet-controlled growing rods sometimes used in children with scoliosis. Advantages and disadvantages of MRI are listed in **Table 3**. An example of a quick brain MRI is shown in **Fig. 4**.

Indications

In general, CT is the preferred imaging modality in the setting of acute trauma or when urgent surgical intervention may be required. MRI is frequently used for follow-up examinations. Some patients also require frequent imaging, such as children with ventriculoperitoneal shunts. Cumulative exposure from recurrent CT scanning over a child's

Table 3
Magnetic resonance imaging

Advantages	Disadvantages
No ionizing radiation	Sedation may be necessary
Excellent soft tissue contrast	Expensive
Limited dynamic information	Many medical devices are not MRI compatible
	Less sensitive than CT for calvarial fractures

lifetime have many proposing a fast-brain MRI or even axial diffusion-weighted imaging as an alternative to CT when ruling out shunt malfunction, as these modalities are quick enough to avoid sedation and adequately assess ventricle size.[12,13] Other indications for brain MRI are not limited to but can include the workup of seizures, cerebral palsy, developmental delay, infection, tumor, stroke, vasculopathy, and metabolic disorders.

Recent advances

MRI is a rapidly developing tool to image the CNS. New techniques are continually being created or refined to improve pediatric imaging to shorten scan times and increase the variety of pathologic conditions that can be evaluated, such as abnormalities with cerebral perfusion, the brachial and lumbar plexus, and biochemical characterization of tumors.[14–17]

Pitfalls

Extreme care must be taken for those children with programmable shunts, as the settings may be changed during the MRI because of the changing magnetic field. Radiographic examination after the MRI may be necessary, depending on the device, and

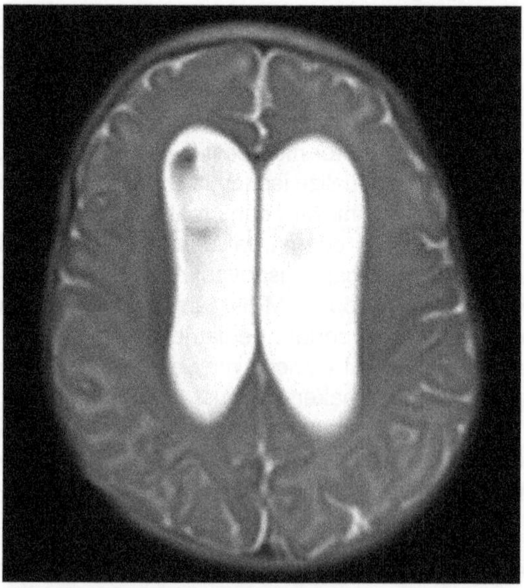

Fig. 4. MRI of an infant head using a quick brain HASTE protocol without sedation demonstrates ventriculomegaly. This MRI technique can be used in children who require multiple follow-up examinations to decrease exposure to ionizing radiation.

will require neurosurgery staff to reprogram the device immediately following the MRI if the flow settings were changed.[18,19] Other medical devices, such as vagus nerve stimulators and pacemakers, may not be MRI compatible or need to be turned off before the examination. Metal can cause distortion artifact with MRI. Children with metal in their body, such as braces or spinal fixation hardware, may have limited evaluation depending on the amount of metal adjacent to the area being examined as well as the available techniques the MR technologist has at their disposal to reduce the artifacts.

Radiography

Radiography is the preferred technique to evaluate osseous structures or medical devices. The child suspected of having a shunt problem may require a shunt series to verify continuity of the shunt tubing. The exact protocol and images may vary from different institutions, although in general includes radiographs along the entire course of the shunt tubing, from the head to the pelvis.

Radiography of the cervical spine is an option for pediatric patients in the setting of trauma who are alert and have a low-risk mechanism of injury, normal neurologic examination, and no distracting injuries.[20] Follow-up CT and MRI of the cervical spine can be used to problem solve in select cases. Radiography may not be indicated at all if the child meets certain clinical criteria.

Radiography is the preferred choice for imaging abnormal head shape when a diagnosis can not be established with confidence based on physical examination alone. In these circumstances, a 4-view skull series of the major calvarial sutures (metopic, bilateral coronal, sagittal, and bilateral lambdoid) can be considered. Ultrasound can also be used only if there is expertise available and the child is less than 12 months old.[21,22] Imaging is not needed for characteristic findings of positional plagiocephaly, frequently caused by infants sleeping on their backs, as this does not represent premature closure of a suture or craniosynostosis.[23]

IONIZING RADIATION RISK IN PEDIATRIC MEDICAL IMAGING

A common concern among parents and clinicians is the harmful effect of ionizing radiation from radiographic and CT studies. The lay press has extensively portrayed ionizing radiation, particularly regarding CT, as harmful to children, and this has contributed to a fear of radiation among many parents and clinicians.[24] The deleterious effects of ionizing radiation used in medical imaging is a debated topic, and continuous research is ongoing. The traditional approach to assessing risk from exposure to ionizing radiation has been the use of the linear-no-threshold model, which assumes that there is no safe level of radiation that does not promote carcinogenesis, that the effects of radiation are cumulative over time, and that injury from radiation shows a direct or linear correlation with dose. The data used to extrapolate harm from ionizing radiation have been traditionally extrapolated from atomic bomb survivors. It is accepted that, although the model is imperfect, it is the most conservative model and is the most prudent to use for policy decisions.

Within the past 10 years, multiple epidemiologic studies have been performed to help determine the biological risks from medical imaging. Pearce and colleagues[25] performed a retrospective cohort study in patients younger than 22 years of age, without previous cancer diagnoses, who had at least 1 CT examination in England, Wales, or Scotland between 1985 and 2002. They analyzed 178,604 individuals for risk of developing leukemia and 176,587 for risk of developing a brain tumor. They estimated approximately 1 excess case of leukemia and 1 excess case of brain tumor for every 10,000 head CT examinations performed.

The utilization of CT for pediatric patients has decreased over the past decade, and CT protocols continue to be improved to deliver better-quality images with less dose. Radiography is a much lower dose compared with CT and may offer accurate assessment, such as when evaluating for craniosynostosis or cervical spine fracture in the setting of trauma. Effective dose from a skull radiograph is approximately 0.01 to 0.04 mSv, whereas head CT effective dose may range from 0.2 to 2 mSv.[26,27] As long as medical imaging is appropriately selected and used only when it may alter management, parents and clinicians should be reassured when a CT examination is performed that the benefits outweigh the risks for the health of the child.

CONTRAST USE IN NEUROIMAGING

Over the past 5 years, multiple studies have shown that the gadolinium molecule used in the standard MRI contrast agents can cross the blood-brain barrier and deposit in the CNS, with a propensity to deposit in the basal ganglia and dentate nucleus. Stanescu and colleagues[28] demonstrated that elemental gadolinium is found in CNS tissue after administration of single as well as multiple doses of gadolinium-based contrast agents. It is important to note that there have been no demonstrated adverse outcomes from this gadolinium retention at this time. However, given the ongoing research and uncertainty regarding gadolinium retention, it is best to administer gadolinium judiciously. MRI is better able to distinguish multiple soft tissue types, when compared with CT, and contrast is frequently not needed. Indications for gadolinium use are, in general, limited to neoplasm, infection, inflammation, and demyelinating/dysmyelinating disease. Parents and clinicians should be reassured about the use of MRI contrast when the benefits outweigh the potential harm.

BALANCING SEDATION WITH IMAGING

Imaging optimization for an individual child in a specific clinical context is a balance between the relative risk and the benefit of an imaging study. If the question can be answered with ultrasound, it should be the first choice, as no sedation is required. However, both CT and MRI provide invaluable diagnostic benefit to many patients. There is ongoing debate whether a child should undergo CT without sedation versus MRI with anesthesia for a given clinical indication. The ability of modern CT scanners to reduce and eliminate the need for anesthesia in many children adds a measure of safety to CT that might not be possible with MRI for the same indication.[24]

Anesthesia risk stratification is dependent on multiple factors, not all of which are known at this time. Three large-scale studies (GAS, PANDA, and MASK) on anesthesia and exposure of infants and children showed no difference in cognitive function between children exposed to a single anesthesia exposure.[29–32] A single exposure to general anesthesia in young children does not have detectable risks of long-term neurocognitive injury as measured by neuropsychological testing. These findings are consistent with both previous studies in humans and preclinical studies, which support a dose-response relationship between general anesthesia exposure and adverse cellular outcomes and is reassuring for most young children who experience only a single short exposure to general anesthesia.[33,34]

The potential for cumulative anesthetic neurotoxicity in the neonate, young infant, and fetus is a pressing question facing the field of pediatric and fetal anesthesia in which more research is warranted. The very rapid development of the fetal brain potentially makes this the patient group most vulnerable to neurotoxicity from anesthesia.[34] Because most MRI studies in young children require sedation or general anesthesia, and sedation is no safer than general anesthesia, clinicians should be familiar with the risks in order to best discuss parental concerns.[35] Families differ regarding the information desired, and an individualized approach by discussing risks of anesthesia in general terms is warranted. A consensus statement can be found at: http://smarttots.org/about/consensus-statement/ that recommends a conversation involving all members of the family and care team regarding timing of procedures and anesthesia be held. If parents and older children do ask about sedation risks, it is best to emphasize how the test result will directly alter the child's treatment plan as well as provide reassurance that a single, short exposure of general anesthesia does not appear to increase the risk of an adverse neurodevelopmental outcome.[36] Regardless of what the future demonstrates about correlations between early exposure to anesthesia and neurotoxicity as well as neurodevelopmental and cognitive impairments, it is prudent that anesthesia exposure, like unnecessary radiation, be avoided.[35]

SUMMARY

Ordering neuroimaging for a specific patient is a shared decision involving the referring provider, pediatric neurologist, pediatric radiologist, pediatric anesthesiologist, and the child's family. As technologies evolve, the choice of which imaging study to perform in a given clinical circumstance must carefully balance the benefits with the risks in order to help guide clinical management, always keeping patient safety a priority.

Clinics Care Points

- Ultrasound is the go-to initial imaging modality for concerns about spinal dysraphism, tethered cord, or enlarging head circumference in a neonate.
- Radiography of the cervical spine is the initial modality of choice for pediatric patients in the setting of trauma who are alert, and have a low-risk mechanism of injury, normal neurologic examination, and no distracting injuries. Computed tomography and MRI can then be used to problem solve select cases.
- When frequent follow-up head computed tomography examinations are needed, such as in children with ventriculoperitoneal shunts, fast MRIs can be performed to be spare the child excessive ionizing radiation.
- Extreme care must be taken when ordering an MRI in children with programmable shunts, as the shunt settings may be changed during the MRI. Radiographic examination should be performed after the MRI to ensure the settings remain unchanged.
- The use of ionizing radiation, intravenous contrast, and sedation should be discussed with parents and caregivers, and risk and benefits should be weighed, ensuring the information obtained from the examination will influence patient management.

DISCLOSURE

The authors have no commercial or financial conflicts of interest to disclose. The views expressed in this article are those of the authors and do not reflect the official policy or position of the Department of the Army, Department of Defense, or the US Government.

REFERENCES

1. Arshadi R, Cobbold R. A pioneer in the development of modern ultrasound: Robert William Boyle (1883-1955). Ultrasound Med Biol 2007;33(1):3–14.
2. Orru E, Calloni SF, Tekes A, et al. The child with macrocephaly: differential diagnosis and neuroimaging findings. AJR Am J Roentgenol 2018;210(4):848–59.
3. Davis A, Billick K, Horton K, et al. Artificial intelligence and echocardiography: a primer for cardiac sonographers [published online ahead of print June 11, 2020]. J Am Soc Echocardiogr 2020. https://doi.org/10.1016/j.echo.2020.04.025.
4. Hwang M. Introduction to contrast-enhanced ultrasound of the brain in neonates and infants: current understanding and future potential. Pediatr Radiol 2019; 49(2):254–62.
5. Knieling F, Ruffer A, Cesnejevar R, et al. Transfontanellar contrast-enhanced ultrasound for monitoring brain perfusion during neonatal heart surgery. Circ Cardiovasc Imaging 2020;13(3):e010073.
6. Nagayama Y, Oda S, Nakaura T, et al. Radiation dose reduction at pediatric CT: use of low tube voltage and iterative reconstruction. Radiographics 2018;38(5): 1421–40.
7. Southard RN, Bardo DME, Temkit MH, et al. Comparison of iterative model reconstruction versus filtered back-projection in pediatric emergency head CT: dose, image quality, and image-reconstruction time. AJNR Am J Neuroradiol 2019; 40(5):866–71.
8. Ren Q, Dewan SK, Li M, et al. Comparison of adaptive statistical iterative and filtered back projection reconstruction techniques in brain CT. Eur J Radiol 2012;81(10):2597–601.
9. Mirro AE, Brady SL, Kaufman RA. Full dose-reduction potential of statistical iterative reconstruction for head T protocols in a predominantly pediatric population. AJNR Am J Neuroradiol 2016;37(7):119–205.
10. Gottumukkal RV, Kalra MK, Tabari A, et al. Advanced CT techniques for decreasing radiation dose, reducing sedation requirements, and optimizing image quality in children. Radiographics 2019;39(3):206–726.
11. Kuppermann N, Holmes JF, Dayan PS, et al. Identification of children at very low risk of clinically-important brain injuries after head trauma: a prospective cohort study. Lancet 2009;374(9696):1160–70.
12. Tekes A, Senglaub SS, Ahn ES, et al. Ultrafast brain MRI can be used for indications beyond shunted hydrocephalus in pediatric patients. Am J Neuroradiol 2018;39(8):1515–8.
13. Gunes A, Oncel IH, Gunes SO, et al. Use of computed tomography and diffusion weighted imaging in children with ventricular shunt. Childs Nerv Syst 2019;35(3): 477–86.
14. Krishnamurthy R, Wang DJJ, Cervantes B, et al. Recent advances in pediatric brain, spine, and neuromuscular magnetic resonance imaging techniques. Pediatr Neurol 2019;96:7–23.
15. Hamilton J, Franson D, Seiberlich N. Recent advances in parallel imaging for MRI. Prog Nucl Magn Reson Spectrosc 2017;101:71–95.
16. Jaspan ON, Fleysher R, Lipton ML. Compressed sensing MRI: a review of the clinical literature. Br J Radiol 2015;88(1056):20150487.
17. European Society of Radiology (ESR). Magnetic resonance fingerprinting – a promising new approach to obtain standardized imaging biomarkers from MRI. Insights Imaging 2015;6(2):163–5.

18. Sivaganesan A, Krishnamurthy R, Sahni D, et al. Neuroimaging of ventriculoperitoneal shunt complications in children. Pediatr Radiol 2012;42(9):1029–46.
19. Inoue T, Kuzu Y, Ogasawara K, et al. Effect of 3-Tesla magnetic resonance imaging on various pressure programmable shunt valves. J Neurosurg 2005;103(2 Suppl):163–5.
20. McAllister A, Nagaraj U, Radhakrishnan R. Emergent imaging of pediatric cervical spine trauma. Radiographics 2019;39(4):1126–42.
21. Badve CA, Mallikarjunappa KM, Iyer RS, et al. Craniosynostosis: imaging review and primer on computed tomography. Pediatr Radiol 2013;43(6):728.
22. Massimi L, Bianchi F, Frassanito P, et al. Imaging in craniosynostosis: when and what? Childs Nerv Syst 2019;35:2055–69.
23. Proisy M, Bruneau B, Riffaud L. How ultrasonography can contribute to diagnosis of craniosynostosis. Neurochirurgie 2019;65:228–31.
24. Callahan MJ, MacDougall RD, Bixby SD, et al. Ionizing radiation from computed tomography versus anesthesia for magnetic resonance imaging in infants and children: patient safety considerations. Pediatr Radiol 2018;48(1):21–30.
25. Pearce MS, Salotti JA, Little MP, et al. Radiation exposure from CT scans in childhood and subsequent risk of leukaemia and brain tumours: a retrospective cohort study. Lancet 2012;380(9840):499–505.
26. Kim HK, Roh GH, Lee IW. Craniosynostosis: updates in radiologic diagnoses. J Korean Neurosurg Soc 2016;59(3):219–26.
27. Matthews J, Forsythe A, Brady Z, et al. Cancer risk in 680,000 people exposed to computed tomography scans in childhood or adolescence: data linkage study of 11 million Australians. BMJ 2013;346:f2360.
28. Stanescu AL, Shaw DW, Murata N, et al. Brain tissue gadolinium retention in pediatric patients after contrast-enhanced magnetic resonance exams: pathological confirmation. Pediatr Radiol 2020;50(3):388–96.
29. Davidson AJ, Disma N, de Graaff JC, et al, GAS Consortium. Neurodevelopmental outcome at 2 years of age after general anaesthesia and awake-regional anaesthesia in infancy (GAS): an international multicentre, randomised controlled trial. Lancet 2016;387(10015):239250.
30. Terushkin V, Brauer J, Bernstein L, et al. Effect of general anesthesia on neurodevelopmental abnormalities in children undergoing treatment of vascular anomalies with laser surgery: a retrospective review. Derm Surg 2017;43(4):534–40.
31. Sun LS, Li G, Miller TL, et al. Association between a single general anesthesia exposure before age 36 months and neurocognitive outcomes in later childhood. JAMA 2016;315(21):2312–20.
32. Rosenblatt A, Kremer M, Swanson B, et al. Anesthesia exposure in the young child and long-term cognition: an integrated review. AANA J 2019;87(3):231–42.
33. Shi Y, Hu D, Rodgers EL, et al. Epidemiology of general anesthesia prior to age 3 in a population-based birth cohort. Paediatr Anaesth 2018;28(6):513–9.
34. O'Leary JD. Human studies of anesthesia-related neurotoxicity in children: a narrative review of recent additions to the clinical literature. Clin Perinatol 2019; 46(4):637–45.
35. Barton K, Nickerson JP, Higgins T, et al. Pediatric anesthesia and neurotoxicity: what the radiologist needs to know. Pediatr Radiol 2018;48(1):31–6.
36. Bjur KA, Payne ET, Nemergut ME, et al. Anesthetic-related neurotoxicity and neuroimaging in children: a call for conversation. J Child Neurol 2017;32(6):594–602.

Diagnosis and Management of Suture-Related Concerns of the Infant Skull

David S. Hersh, MD[a,*], Markus J. Bookland, MD[a],
Christopher D. Hughes, MD, MPH[b,c]

KEYWORDS

- Cranial sutures • Anterior fontanelle • Plagiocephaly • Craniosynostosis
- Bathrocephaly

KEY POINTS

- Anterior fontanelle closure between 5 months and 24 months of age can be considered "normal." Early closure can be related to craniosynostosis or microcephaly, whereas delayed closure can occur because of intracranial hypertension, hypothyroidism, or malnutrition.
- Positional plagiocephaly is a common diagnosis and can be differentiated from lambdoid craniosynostosis with a careful physical examination.
- Early referral of patients with craniosynostosis to a craniofacial specialist is critical, as minimally invasive options can be offered to most patients younger than 6 months of age.

THE CRANIAL FONTANELLES

Normal Development

The newborn neurocranium comprises a collection of expanding ossification centers. Rapid expansion of the intracranial contents during the first 2 years of life stretches the membranous folds within which the neurocranial plates float, maintaining separations between the developing bony plates in the form of cranial sutures and fontanelles.[1] Six fontanelles are typically present at birth (**Fig. 1**) and gradually close over the first 1 to 2 years of life (**Table 1**).[2,3]

[a] Division of Neurosurgery, Connecticut Children's, UCONN School of Medicine, 282 Washington Street, Hartford, CT 06106, USA; [b] Division of Plastic Surgery, Connecticut Children's, UCONN School of Medicine, 282 Washington Street, Hartford, CT 06106, USA; [c] Division of Craniofacial Surgery, Connecticut Children's, UCONN School of Medicine, 282 Washington Street, Hartford, CT 06106, USA
* Corresponding author.
E-mail address: dhersh@connecticutchildrens.org

Pediatr Clin N Am 68 (2021) 727–742
https://doi.org/10.1016/j.pcl.2021.04.002
0031-3955/21/

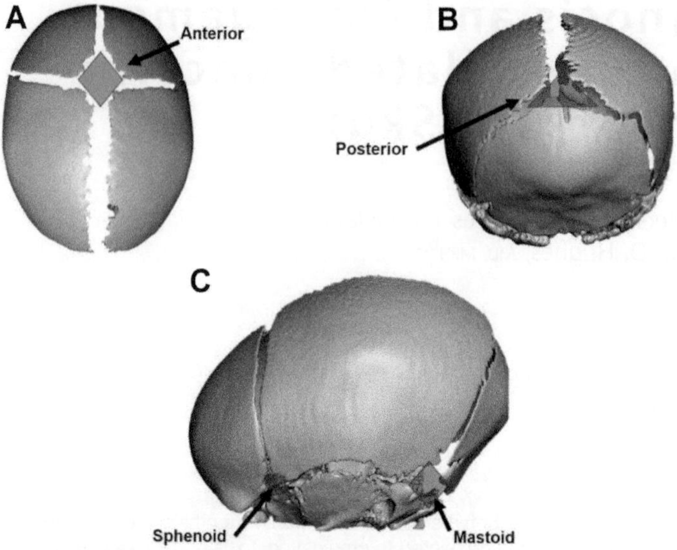

Fig. 1. Six fontanelles are present at birth. (*A*) The anterior fontanelle. (*B*) The posterior fontanelle. (*C*) The sphenoid and mastoid fontanelles (which are present bilaterally).

Examination of the Anterior Fontanelle

The anterior fontanelle is the largest, most persistent, and most easily palpated of the fontanelles. The anterior fontanelle should be examined in both the upright and the recumbent positions, noting changes in the fullness of the fontanelle. Palpation of the fontanelle in the upright and calm state should reveal a soft, mildly depressible fontanelle. The difference between a full and a normal anterior fontanelle is not always obvious, and this rather subjective examination finding becomes more reliable only with experience.

Shape

The anterior fontanelle should adopt a slightly elongated diamond shape (see **Fig. 1**A). However, the margins of the anterior fontanelle often provide more useful clinical information than the ballotable, central fontanelle. The newborn cranium is particularly distensible and plastic, allowing a great deal of expansion and contraction of the cranial plates, which can mask both high- and low-intracranial pressure by leaving the anterior fontanelle relatively flat and soft despite progressive, pathologic intracranial pressure changes. Widening of the anterior fontanelle's vertices and splaying of the metopic, coronal, and sagittal sutures can provide a reliable indication of increased

Table 1
Neonatal fontanelles

Fontanelle	Typical Age of Closure, mo
Anterior	12–18
Posterior	2
Mastoid (left and right)	12–18
Sphenoid (left and right)	6

intracranial pressure, even when the fontanelle itself is not bulging. In a cohort of 483 infants, the average width of a normal cranial suture immediately adjacent to the margin of the anterior fontanelle was 5 mm at birth, 2.4 mm at 1 month of age, and 1.3 mm until 12 months of age.[4] Therefore, if the examining provider can easily lay the width of his or her finger within the proximal cranial sutures along the margin of the anterior fontanelle, the sutures can be considered to be abnormally widened. Conversely, an asymmetrical obliteration of one or more of the corners of the anterior fontanelle can indicate craniosynostosis along the adjacent suture line. For example, in patients with metopic craniosynostosis, the anterior fontanelle may take on a triangular shape, rather than its typical diamond shape (**Fig. 2**).

Size

There is little evidence that the size of the anterior fontanelle has clinical relevance. The anterior fontanelle of a newborn can range in size from 0.6 cm to 3.6 cm, and ethnic differences have been described.[3,5,6] The size of the anterior fontanelle does not follow a linear relationship with patient age, and smaller or larger anterior fontanelles do not correlate with early or late closure of the cranial vault.[7] More significant than the size of the anterior fontanelle is the relative size of the gaps between the cranial plates. A particularly enlarged anterior fontanelle, in conjunction with symmetrically widened sutures, strongly suggests a state of elevated intracranial pressure, nutritional deficiencies, or congenital metabolic disorders.

Auscultation

Auscultation of the anterior fontanelle can be considered if the patient has other findings commonly associated with intracranial arteriovenous anomalies, such as heart failure or macrocephaly.[3] The superior sagittal sinus, a major venous outflow for the

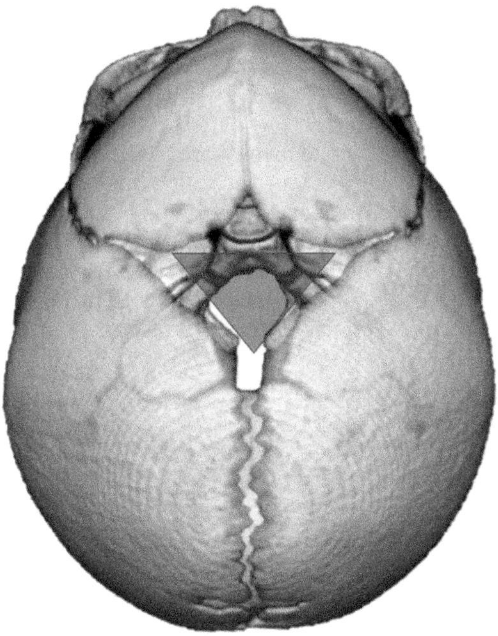

Fig. 2. The anterior fontanelle may have a triangular shape in patients with metopic craniosynostosis.

cerebrum, runs immediately beneath the anterior fontanelle in the midline. The presence of a bruit may indicate an aberrant arteriovenous shunt leading to increased flow and pressure within the underlying venous sinus. The presence of a bruit can be found in vein of Galen malformations, dural arteriovenous fistulas, and true arteriovenous malformations.

Closure of the Anterior Fontanelle

"Normal" closure

The rate at which the anterior fontanelle decreases in size and the age at which it ultimately closes are markedly variable. In general, anterior fontanelle closure between 5 months and 24 months of age can be considered "normal." The prevalence of anterior fontanelle closure increases from 5% at 5 months of age to 88% at 20 months. Radiographically, the prevalence of anterior fontanelle closure surpasses 50% at 16 months of age, whereas it surpasses 50% at only 12 months of age when using the "fingertip cutoff" technique to assess the anterior fontanelle at the bedside. Notably, 10% of normal infants may continue to have a patent anterior fontanelle between 20 and 24 months of age.[7,8]

Early closure

There are several potential causes for early closure of the anterior fontanelle (**Box 1**). Craniosynostosis must be considered in any infant with closure of the anterior fontanelle before 4 months of age, as the time to presentation to a craniofacial specialist can have a dramatic impact on therapeutic options and neurodevelopmental outcomes.[9,10] If craniosynostosis is suspected because of early closure of the anterior fontanelle or partial obliteration of the fontanelle, the patient should be inspected for ridging along the cranial sutures and/or abnormalities in cranial or facial symmetry. Under these circumstances, the patient should be referred to a pediatric neurosurgeon or to a craniofacial specialist for further evaluation.[11–13]

Pan-synostosis of the cranial sutures, causing impaired cranial growth and subsequent elevated intracranial pressure owing to craniocerebral disproportion, is exceedingly rare. The cranial volume of the newborn is driven by cerebral expansion, and even in cases of nonsyndromic craniosynostosis, this mechanism typically allows the head circumference to continue to follow normalized growth curves.[14] Syndromic multisuture craniosynostosis is the exception to this rule, but the diagnosis of these forms of craniosynostosis rarely hinges on the status of the anterior fontanelle, given the involvement of multiple organ systems.

In some cases, early closure of the anterior fontanelle will result from microcephaly and can be seen in the setting of perinatal infections or cerebral ischemia, whereby there is insufficient cerebral expansion to drive calvarial growth. Although this can

Box 1
Differential diagnosis of early anterior fontanelle closure

- Craniosynostosis
- Microcephaly
  - Perinatal cerebral ischemia
  - Intracranial infection
  - Traumatic brain injury
  - Congenital disorders
  - Perinatal spinal fluid shunting
- Hyperthyroidism

have dramatic implications for neurodevelopment, it is rarely associated with elevated intracranial pressure and typically does not have a surgical solution, unlike craniosynostosis. Microcephaly can be differentiated from syndromic craniosynostosis by the frequent involvement of the midface and skeletal system (particularly the hands and feet) in patients with syndromic craniosynostosis.

Late closure

The key factors to consider when evaluating a patient with late closure of the anterior fontanelle are the rate of change in the head circumference and the rate of neurodevelopmental progress. A persistent anterior fontanelle can often be observed so long as the head circumference continues to track along the patient's growth curve and the patient continues to meet expected milestones. Patients who fail to meet these criteria are at higher risk of elevated intracranial pressure, hypothyroidism, or malnutrition (**Box 2**).

POSITIONAL DEFORMATION OF THE SKULL

Prevalence

Positional deformation of the soft infant skull, also known as positional molding, can result from external forces that are applied in utero, or more commonly postnatally. These external forces may produce plagiocephaly, which is a unilateral flattening of the posterior aspect of the head, or brachycephaly, whereby the skull is wide and flat bilaterally. The prevalence of both conditions has increased dramatically since 1992, when the American Academy of Pediatrics Task Force on Infant Positioning and SIDS initiated the "Back to Sleep" campaign to reduce the incidence of sudden infant death syndrome.[15] Estimates of the prevalence of positional plagiocephaly are age dependent but range from ~20% to almost 50% in otherwise healthy infants.[16,17] Less commonly, one may encounter positional dolichocephaly-elongation and narrowing of the skull; this particular shape can be seen in hospitalized infants who are frequently turned from side to side.

Diagnosis

Upon encountering a patient with unilateral posterior flattening of the skull, it is critical to differentiate positional plagiocephaly from premature fusion of the lambdoid suture. Although rare, with an estimated prevalence of 0.003%, lambdoid synostosis is a surgical diagnosis and should be expeditiously referred to a craniofacial specialist. Imaging is rarely required, and the diagnosis is typically confirmed with a thorough physical examination. A bird's-eye view demonstrates a "parallelogram" shape in patients with

Box 2
Differential diagnosis of late anterior fontanelle closure

- Familial macrocephaly
- Down syndrome
- Achondroplasia
- Elevated intracranial pressure
  - Hydrocephalus
  - Traumatic brain injury
  - Brain tumor
- Hypothyroidism
- Rickets

positional plagiocephaly; external forces on the back of the head cause that side to shift anteriorly, resulting in ipsilateral advancement of the ear and prominence of the forehead. In contrast, a "trapezoid" shape characterizes patients with lambdoid synostosis: prominence of the forehead is *contralateral* to the flattened occipital region. When viewed from the back, positional plagiocephaly is associated with ears that are at the same horizontal level, indicating a level skull base, whereas the patient with lambdoid synostosis will have a tilted skull base, with inferior displacement of the ipsilateral ear and mastoid (**Fig. 3**).[18] In addition to differences on physical examination, the natural history of these 2 conditions diverges: whereas positional plagiocephaly typically improves over time, craniosynostosis often leads to a head shape that becomes more asymmetric over time, as the remainder of the skull continues to grow. Nevertheless, the authors do not recommend a period of observation for the patient with suspected lambdoid synostosis; rather, an immediate referral to a craniofacial specialist should be arranged.

Several anthropomorphic measurements have been used to describe the severity of positional/deformational changes, including the cranial vault asymmetry, diagonal difference, transcranial difference, and transcranial diameter.[19] Most commonly, plagiocephaly is described using the cranial vault asymmetry index (**Fig. 4**A). Brachycephaly,

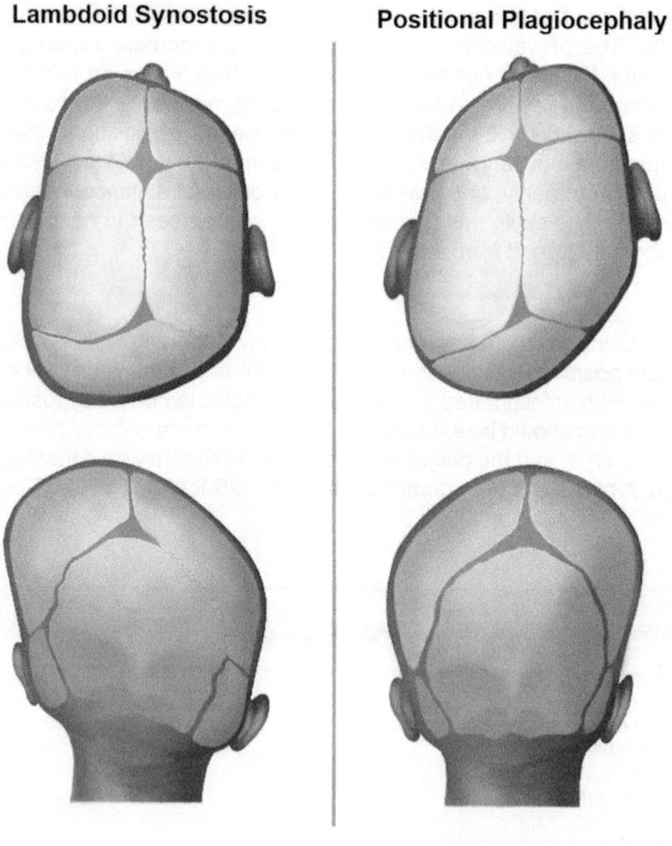

Fig. 3. Differentiating lambdoid synostosis from positional plagiocephaly on physical examination.

on the other hand, is described using the cephalic index (**Fig. 4**B). A more detailed severity scale has been developed by Children's Healthcare of Atlanta and describes a 5-level classification scale to help guide treatment decisions (**Fig. 5**).[20]

Counseling

Parents often present with a great deal of anxiety surrounding the diagnosis of plagiocephaly or brachycephaly. The authors reassure parents that positional deformation of the skull is a common diagnosis, and that current evidence supports that its implications are *cosmetic*. Studies that have associated positional plagiocephaly with a higher rate of developmental delay have significant methodological limitations that confound the results.[21,22] In particular, supine positioning during infancy has been correlated with motor delays that tend to resolve by 18 months of age, with no effect on long-term outcomes.[23] Supine positioning may therefore be an important confounder in studies of plagiocephaly that focus on short-term developmental outcomes. To date, there is no strong evidence to support a link between plagiocephaly and developmental delay.[19]

Evidence-Based Treatment Guidelines

In 2016, the Congress of Neurological Surgeons published a "Systematic Review and Evidence-Based Guidelines for the Management of Patients with Positional Plagiocephaly."[24] Guidelines related to repositioning, physical therapy, and the use of helmet therapy are detailed in **Table 2**. Repositioning education is recommended for all patients, whereas physical therapy is an option for infants 7 weeks of age or older, particularly those with torticollis and/or those who have failed repositioning therapy. Helmet therapy is recommended for patients with persistent moderate to severe plagiocephaly after a course of repositioning and physical therapy *or* presenting at an advanced age (6 months of age or older).

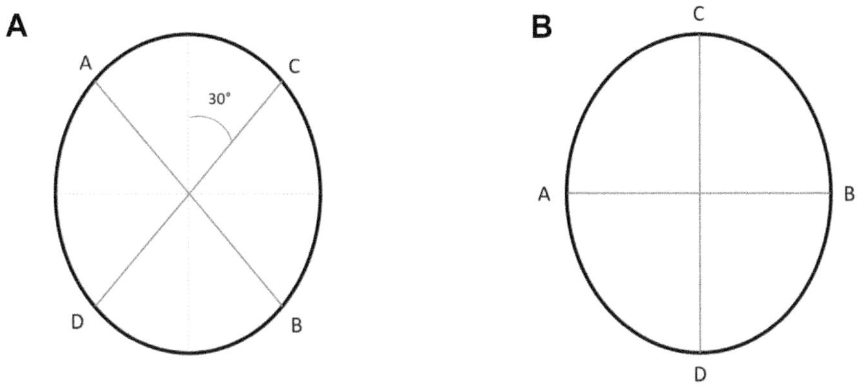

Cranial Vault Asymmetry Index (CVAI)

$$\frac{AB - CD}{AB \text{ or } CD \text{ (whichever is greater)}} \times 100$$

Cephalic Index (CI)

$$\frac{AB \text{ (width)}}{CD \text{ (length)}} \times 100$$

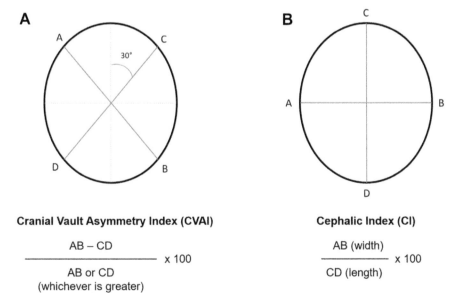

Fig. 4. The (*A*) cranial vault asymmetric index and (*B*) cephalic index.

Level	Clinical Presentation	Recommendation	CVAI
1	• All symmetry within normal limits	No treatment required	<3.50
2	• Minimal asymmetry in one posterior quadrant • No secondary changes	Repositioning program	3.5 to 6.25
3	• Two quadrant involvement • Moderate to severe posterior quadrant flattening • Minimal ear shift and/or anterior involvement	Conservative treatment: Repositioning program cranial remolding orthosis (based on age and history)	6.25 to 8.75
4	• Two or three quadrant involvement • Severe posterior quadrant involvement • Moderate ear shift • Anterior involvement including noticeable orbit asymmetry	Conservative treatment: cranial remolding orthosis	8.75 to 11.0
5	• Three or four quadrant involvement • Severe posterior quadrant flattening • Severe ear shift • Anterior involvement including orbit and cheek asymmetry	Conservative treatment: cranial remolding orthosis	>11.0

Fig. 5. Children's Healthcare of Atlanta plagiocephaly severity scale. (*From* Holowka et al. Plagiocephaly severity scale to aid in clinical treatment recommendations. *J Craniofac Surg*. 2017;28(3):717-722, with permission from Wolters Kluwer Health, Inc.)

Table 2
Congress of Neurological Surgeons evidence-based guidelines for the treatment of pediatric positional plagiocephaly

Guideline	Strength of Recommendation
Repositioning	
• Repositioning is an effective treatment for deformational plagiocephaly, but is inferior to physical therapy and to use of a helmet	Level I: high clinical certainty (inferior to physical therapy); level II: moderate clinical certainty (inferior to helmet)
Physical Therapy	
• Physical therapy is recommended over repositioning education alone for reducing prevalence of infantile positional plagiocephaly in infants 7 wk of age or older	Level I: high clinical certainty
• Physical therapy is as effective for the treatment of positional plagiocephaly as a positioning pillow, but physical therapy is recommended over the use of a positioning pillow to ensure a safe sleeping environment, in compliance with American Academy of Pediatrics recommendations	Level II: moderate clinical certainty
Helmet Therapy	
• Helmet therapy is recommended for infants with persistent moderate to severe plagiocephaly after a course of conservative treatment (repositioning and/or physical therapy)	Level II: uncertain clinical certainty
• Helmet therapy is recommended for infants with moderate to severe plagiocephaly presenting at an advanced age	Level II: uncertain clinical certainty

CRANIOSYNOSTOSIS

Background

Craniosynostosis refers to the premature fusion of one or more of the calvarial sutures. Estimates suggest an incidence of 1 in 1700 live births.[12] Craniosynostosis can be isolated or can occur in the context of a genetic mutation, with alterations in the FGFR or TWIST genes being the most common.[25] Craniosynostosis results in stereotypical abnormal head shapes because of Virchow's law, which states that brain-directed skull growth occurs perpendicular to each of the cranial sutures.[26] This process does not occur at synostotic sutures, and compensatory growth in the opposite direction results in predictable alterations in skull morphology.

Diagnosis

Physical examination

The clinical examination can be remarkably accurate in diagnosing craniosynostosis.[11] Although sutural ridging alone may not be diagnostic of an underlying premature fusion, it should prompt a careful assessment for specific, characteristic head shapes (**Fig. 6**, **Table 3**).

Imaging

A computed tomographic (CT) scan with a 3-dimensional (3D) reconstruction remains the gold standard for diagnosing craniosynostosis and may be particularly useful in cases of syndromic craniosynostosis, when multiple sutures are often involved. In such cases, a CT scan may also provide information regarding signs of intracranial hypertension. However, increasing recognition of the long-term risks of cumulative ionizing radiation has prompted many pediatric providers to minimize the use of CT scans.[27] Skull radiographs are sometimes used, but also involve ionizing radiation. Some centers have begun to use ultrasonography of the cranial sutures when the physical examination findings are equivocal (**Fig. 7**).[28] The type of imaging modality can be left up to the consulting specialist.

Multidisciplinary Approach

Children with suspected craniosynostosis are best treated in the context of a multidisciplinary craniofacial team. Effective teams use input from neurosurgeons, plastic

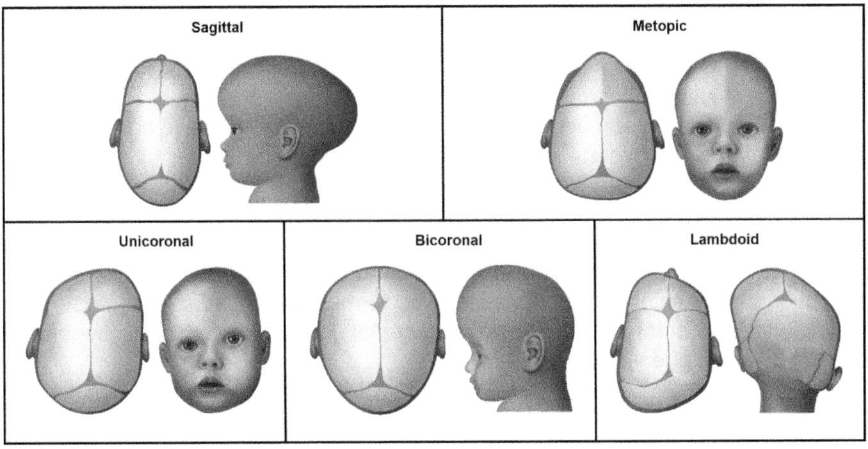

Fig. 6. The characteristic features of (*A*) sagittal, (*B*) metopic, (*C*) coronal, (*D*) bilateral coronal, and (*E*) lambdoid synostosis.

Table 3
Phenotypic features of craniosynostosis

Involved Suture	Phenotype	Description
Sagittal	• Elongated, narrow head • Frontal bossing • Parietal narrowing • Tapered, prominent occiput • Anteriorly displaced vertex	• Scaphocephaly • Dolichocephaly
Metopic	• Narrow forehead • Hypotelorism • Pterional "pinching" • Prominent midline ridge	• Trigonocephaly
Coronal	• Ipsilateral forehead recession • Elevation of the ipsilateral orbit (Harlequin eye) • Contralateral frontal bossing • Deviation of nasal root to the affected side (variable)	Not applicable (N/A)
Bilateral coronal	• Short, wide head • Recession of the midface and orbits bilaterally • Proptosis • Bilateral frontal bossing • Increased skull height	• Brachycephaly • Turricephaly
Lambdoid	• Ipsilateral flattening of the occiput • Posterior and inferior displacement of the ipsilateral mastoid and ear • Contralateral frontal bossing • Trapezoid" appearance on vertex view	N/A

surgeons, developmental pediatricians, ophthalmologists, speech and language pathologists, oral and maxillofacial surgeons, orthodontists, pediatric dentists, otolaryngologists, and social workers to formulate a comprehensive management plan for the patient.

Surgical Management

Indications

Surgical intervention allows for the correction of the phenotypic deformity associated with craniosynostosis. For many surgeons, the cosmetic and social impact of the abnormal head shape represents the primary indication for operative correction.[29,30] However, intracranial hypertension has been documented in up to 15% to 20% of cases of single-suture craniosynostosis, and even higher rates have been noted among patients with syndromic craniosynostosis because of craniocerebral disproportion, upper airway obstruction, and/or cerebral venous congestion.[31,32] Developmental delays have also been described among patients with craniosynostosis,[33] and although it remains rare in nonsyndromic forms, surgical intervention has been recommended by some to mitigate developmental delays that may occur secondary to intracranial hypertension.

Technique

There is no clear consensus on the optimal operative treatment of craniosynostosis. Although open operations have historically been the standard of care, many centers are now embracing endoscopic-guided suturectomy with adjuvant helmet therapy

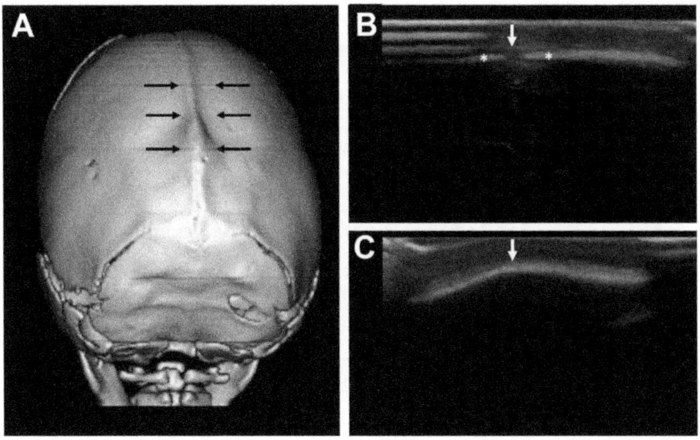

Fig. 7. (*A*) A CT scan with a 3D reconstruction obtained by an outside facility demonstrating sagittal synostosis (*black arrows*) in a 1-day-old girl. (*B*) Ultrasound of the sagittal suture demonstrating a hypoechoic gap (*white arrow*) between the parietal bones (*asterisks*), representing a patent suture in a 3-month-old girl. (*C*) Ultrasound of the sagittal suture demonstrating closure of the suture (*white arrow*) in a 3-month-old girl with scaphocephaly.

as an initial treatment option.[34] This minimally invasive approach "releases" the synostotic suture, facilitating subsequent remodeling over the next several months as the skull grows, guided by a cranial orthosis. Several large institutional and multicenter studies have found that minimally invasive suturectomy is associated with shorter operative times, less blood loss, fewer transfusions, and shorter hospital stays compared with open remodeling procedures (**Table 4**).[35,36] However, because of the reliance on subsequent skull growth, optimal outcomes have been observed when minimally invasive surgery is performed in children less than 4 months of age, and age greater than 6 months is generally considered a relative contraindication.[37]

Follow-up

Multidisciplinary care becomes especially important postoperatively. Surveillance is required in order to assess for delayed intracranial hypertension, restenosis of the synostotic suture, and secondary craniosynostosis of other sutures.[31,38] The patient's head circumference should be monitored, and serial funduscopic examinations by an ophthalmologist are performed to assess for papilledema. Cosmetic outcomes and neurodevelopmental milestones should also be tracked.

NONSYNOSTOTIC ABNORMALITIES

Bathrocephaly

Bathrocephaly refers to a prominent, midline, symmetric protuberance over the occipital bone (**Fig. 8**) and is a common reason for referral to a craniofacial specialist, although its true prevalence is unknown.[39] Although sagittal synostosis also features occipital bulging, the presence or absence of dolichocephaly confirms the appropriate diagnosis. In isolation, bathrocephaly is considered a normal variant without clinical significance and does not require additional imaging.

Overriding Sutures

In isolation, ridging along the cranial sutures is an often unreliable indicator of craniosynostosis. Some degree of overlapping of the sutures is common shortly after birth,

Table 4
Minimally invasive suturectomy versus open reconstruction

	Minimally Invasive Suturectomy	Open Reconstruction
Surgical philosophy	Minimal bone removal, skull remodeling is directed by brain growth	Maximal correction at time of surgery
Incision	1 vs 2 small (2–3 cm) incisions behind hairline	Bicoronal incision ("ear to ear")
Age	<6 mo of age, ideally <4 mo of age	6+ mo
Postoperative helmet	Yes	No
Transfusion rate	Low	High
Hospital stay	1–2 d	3–5 d (on average)
Neurocognitive benefit	Research ongoing	Research ongoing

when compression by the birth canal causes the bony plates of the cranium to overlap at the suture line. Persistent ridging should prompt a careful examination of the anterior fontanelle and the infant's head shape.

Benign Metopic Ridging

The metopic suture is the only cranial suture to close normally during infancy, typically between 3 and 9 months of age.[40,41] Therefore, imaging that demonstrates closure of the metopic suture during this timeframe is *not* necessarily indicative of craniosynostosis. Further complicating the situation, physiologic closure of the metopic suture often produces a noticeable midline ridge along the suture. A benign finding that often remodels with time, metopic ridging is often confused with metopic craniosynostosis. Imaging is not required, and a careful physical examination should instead be performed, with a particular emphasis on assessing the relationship between the lateral

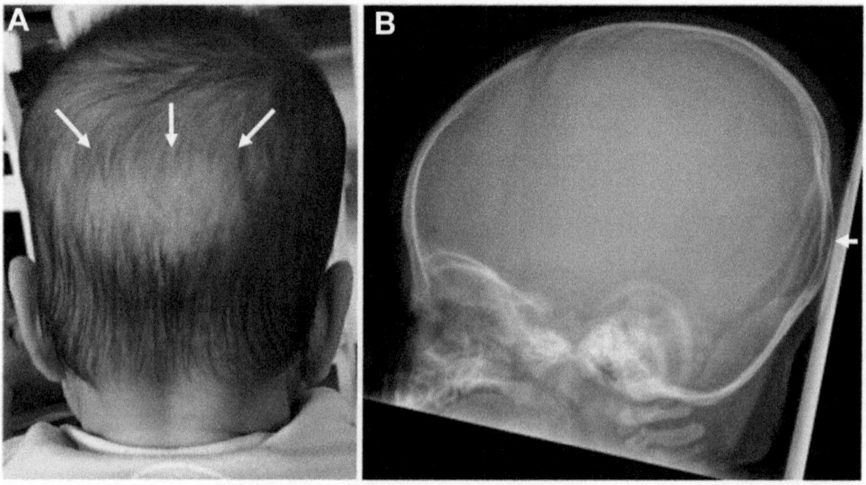

Fig. 8. (*A*) Clinical photograph and (*B*) lateral skull radiograph demonstrating bathrocephaly (*arrows*). Note that radiographs are not necessary for diagnosing bathrocephaly, but in this case, had been obtained before the referral.

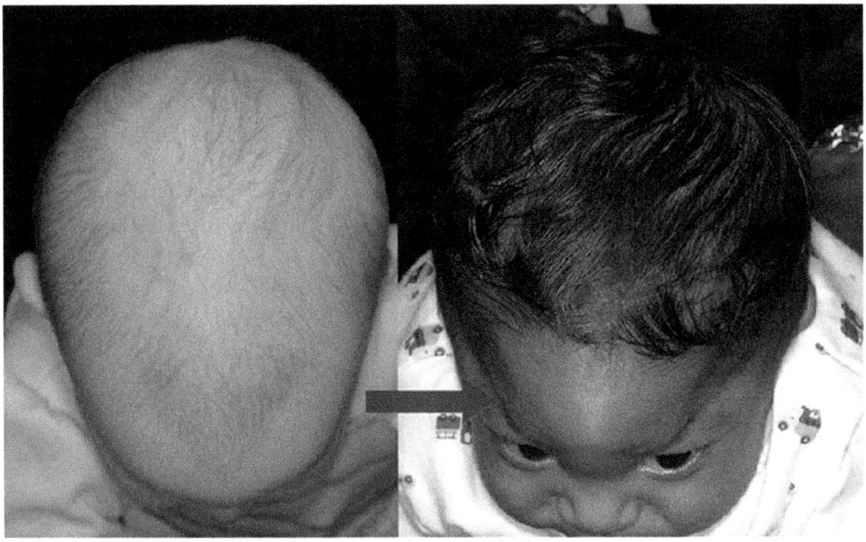

Fig. 9. The relationship of forehead shape and superior orbital rim in metopic ridge (MR) and metopic craniosynostosis (MCS). In MR (*left*), the forehead is rounded and protects the superolateral orbital rim, obscuring the orbit in this top-down view. In MCS (*right*), the frontal bone is straight and exposes the globe, revealing the superolateral orbital rim (*arrow*) in this top-down view. (*From* Birgfield et al. Making the diagnosis: metopic ridge versus metopic craniosynostosis. *J Craniofac Surg.* 2013;24(1):178-185, with permission from Wolters Kluwer Health, Inc.)

orbit and frontal bone, which will appear "pinched" in cases of true metopic craniosynostosis (**Fig. 9**).[42] Patients with benign metopic ridging are more likely to have had a normal head shape in early infancy, with development of the ridge after several months (upon physiologic closure of the metopic suture). Conversely, patients with metopic craniosynostosis are more likely to demonstrate an abnormal head shape at birth that does not improve over time.[4] Notably, patients with benign metopic ridging should not undergo surgical intervention.

SUMMARY

A thorough understanding of the normal anatomy and development of the cranial fontanelles and sutures is critical. Numerous conditions represent benign variations of what is typically considered "normal," including most cases of "early" or "late" closure of the anterior fontanelle, bathrocephaly, overriding sutures, and benign metopic ridging. However, recognizing true craniosynostosis and referring the patient to a craniofacial specialist in a timely fashion are imperative, as minimally invasive options can be offered to most patients younger than 6 months of age. Gaining comfort with the physical examination of an infant with an abnormal head shape is best achieved through experience and pattern recognition and will frequently facilitate an accurate diagnosis without the need for ionizing radiation.

CLINICS CARE POINTS

- A cranial suture is abnormally widened if you can easily lay the width of your finger within the proximal portion of the suture along the margin of the anterior fontanelle.

- In general, anterior fontanelle closure between 5 months and 24 months of age can be considered "normal." Craniosynostosis must be considered in any infant with closure of the anterior fontanelle before 4 months of age.
- Positional plagiocephaly and lambdoid synostosis can be differentiated on physical examination: a bird's-eye view demonstrates a "parallelogram" shape in patients with positional plagiocephaly versus a "trapezoid" shape in patients with lambdoid synostosis. Lambdoid synostosis is also associated with skull-base changes that produce inferior displacement of the ipsilateral ear and mastoid when viewed from behind.
- Recognition of true craniosynostosis and referral to a craniofacial specialist in a timely fashion are imperative, as minimally invasive options can be offered to most patients younger than 6 months of age.

REFERENCES

1. Enlow D. Normal craniofacial growth. In: Cohen MM Jr, RE M, editors. Craniosynostosis: diagnosis, evaluation, and management. 2nd edition. New York: Oxford University Press; 2000. p. 35–47.
2. Chemke J, Robinson A. The third fontanelle. J Pediatr 1969;75(4):617–22.
3. Kiesler J, Ricer R. The abnormal fontanel. Am Fam Physician 2003;67(12): 2547–52.
4. Mitchell LA, Kitley CA, Armitage TL, et al. Normal sagittal and coronal suture widths by using CT imaging. AJNR Am J Neuroradiol 2011;32(10):1801–5.
5. Chang BF, Hung KL. [Measurements of anterior fontanels]. Zhonghua Min Guo Xiao Er Ke Yi Xue Hui Za Zhi 1990;31(5):307–12 [in Chinese].
6. Jackson GL, Hoyer A, Longenecker L, et al. Anterior fontanel size in term and late preterm Hispanic neonates: description of normative values and an alternative measurement method. Am J Perinatol 2010;27(4):307–12.
7. Duc G, Largo RH. Anterior fontanel: size and closure in term and preterm infants. Pediatrics 1986;78(5):904–8.
8. Pindrik J, Ye X, Ji BG, et al. Anterior fontanelle closure and size in full-term children based on head computed tomography. Clin Pediatr (Phila) 2014;53(12): 1149–57.
9. Bellew M, Mandela RJ, Chumas PD. Impact of age at surgery on neurodevelopmental outcomes in sagittal synostosis. J Neurosurg Pediatr 2019;1–8. https://doi.org/10.3171/2018.8.PEDS18186.
10. Proctor MR. Endoscopic craniosynostosis repair. Transl Pediatr 2014;3(3): 247–58.
11. Fearon JA, Singh DJ, Beals SP, et al. The diagnosis and treatment of single-sutural synostoses: are computed tomographic scans necessary? Plast Reconstr Surg 2007;120(5):1327–31.
12. Fearon JA. Evidence-based medicine: craniosynostosis. Plast Reconstr Surg 2014;133(5):1261–75.
13. Pogliani L, Zuccotti GV, Furlanetto M, et al. Cranial ultrasound is a reliable first step imaging in children with suspected craniosynostosis. Childs Nerv Syst 2017;33(9):1545–52.
14. Sgouros S. Skull vault growth in craniosynostosis. Childs Nerv Syst 2005;21(10): 861–70.
15. American Academy of Pediatrics AAP Task Force on Infant Positioning and SIDS: positioning and SIDS. Pediatrics 1992;89(6 Pt 1):1120–6.

16. Hutchison BL, Hutchison LA, Thompson JM, et al. Plagiocephaly and brachycephaly in the first two years of life: a prospective cohort study. Pediatrics 2004;114(4):970–80.
17. Mawji A, Vollman AR, Hatfield J, et al. The incidence of positional plagiocephaly: a cohort study. Pediatrics 2013;132(2):298–304.
18. Cunningham ML, Heike CL. Evaluation of the infant with an abnormal skull shape. Curr Opin Pediatr 2007;19(6):645–51.
19. Robinson S, Proctor M. Diagnosis and management of deformational plagiocephaly. J Neurosurg Pediatr 2009;3(4):284–95.
20. Holowka MA, Reisner A, Giavedoni B, et al. Plagiocephaly severity scale to aid in clinical treatment recommendations. J Craniofac Surg 2017;28(3):717–22.
21. Panchal J, Amirsheybani H, Gurwitch R, et al. Neurodevelopment in children with single-suture craniosynostosis and plagiocephaly without synostosis. Plast Reconstr Surg 2001;108(6):1492–8 [discussion: 1499-–500].
22. Collett B, Breiger D, King D, et al. Neurodevelopmental implications of "deformational" plagiocephaly. J Dev Behav Pediatr 2005;26(5):379–89.
23. Davis BE, Moon RY, Sachs HC, et al. Effects of sleep position on infant motor development. Pediatrics 1998;102(5):1135–40.
24. Flannery AM, Tamber MS, Mazzola C, et al. Congress of Neurological Surgeons Systematic Review and Evidence-Based Guidelines for the management of patients with positional plagiocephaly: executive summary. Neurosurgery 2016; 79(5):623–4.
25. Melville H, Wang Y, Taub PJ, et al. Genetic basis of potential therapeutic strategies for craniosynostosis. Am J Med Genet A 2010;152A(12):3007–15.
26. Persing JA, Jane JA, Shaffrey M. Virchow and the pathogenesis of craniosynostosis: a translation of his original work. Plast Reconstr Surg 1989;83(4):738–42.
27. Pearce MS, Salotti JA, Little MP, et al. Radiation exposure from CT scans in childhood and subsequent risk of leukaemia and brain tumours: a retrospective cohort study. Lancet 2012;380(9840):499–505.
28. Rozovsky K, Udjus K, Wilson N, et al. Cranial ultrasound as a first-line imaging examination for craniosynostosis. Pediatrics 2016;137(2):e20152230.
29. Doumit GD, Papay FA, Moores N, et al. Management of sagittal synostosis: a solution to equipoise. J Craniofac Surg 2014;25(4):1260–5.
30. Anolik RA, Allori AC, Pourtaheri N, et al. Objective assessment of the interfrontal angle for severity grading and operative decision-making in metopic synostosis. Plast Reconstr Surg 2016;137(5):1548–55.
31. Lam S, Wagner KM, Middlebrook E, et al. Delayed intracranial hypertension after surgery for nonsyndromic craniosynostosis. Surg Neurol Int 2015;6:187.
32. Tamburrini G, Caldarelli M, Massimi L, et al. Intracranial pressure monitoring in children with single suture and complex craniosynostosis: a review. Childs Nerv Syst 2005;21(10):913–21.
33. Speltz ML, Kapp-Simon K, Collett B, et al. Neurodevelopment of infants with single-suture craniosynostosis: presurgery comparisons with case-matched controls. Plast Reconstr Surg 2007;119(6):1874–81.
34. Rottgers SA, Lohani S, Proctor MR. Outcomes of endoscopic suturectomy with postoperative helmet therapy in bilateral coronal craniosynostosis. J Neurosurg Pediatr 2016;18(3):281–6.
35. Isaac KV, MacKinnon S, Dagi LR, et al. Nonsyndromic unilateral coronal synostosis: a comparison of fronto-orbital advancement and endoscopic suturectomy. Plast Reconstr Surg 2019;143(3):838–48.

36. Thompson DR, Zurakowski D, Haberkern CM, et al. Endoscopic versus open repair for craniosynostosis in infants using propensity score matching to compare outcomes: a multicenter study from the pediatric craniofacial collaborative group. Anesth Analg 2018;126(3):968–75.
37. Berry-Candelario J, Ridgway EB, Grondin RT, et al. Endoscope-assisted strip craniectomy and postoperative helmet therapy for treatment of craniosynostosis. Neurosurg Focus 2011;31(2):E5.
38. Yarbrough CK, Smyth MD, Holekamp TF, et al. Delayed synostoses of uninvolved sutures after surgical treatment of nonsyndromic craniosynostosis. J Craniofac Surg 2014;25(1):119–23.
39. Gallagher ER, Evans KN, Hing AV, et al. Bathrocephaly: a head shape associated with a persistent mendosal suture. Cleft Palate Craniofac J 2013;50(1):104–8.
40. Weinzweig J, Kirschner RE, Farley A, et al. Metopic synostosis: defining the temporal sequence of normal suture fusion and differentiating it from synostosis on the basis of computed tomography images. Plast Reconstr Surg 2003;112(5): 1211–8.
41. Vu HL, Panchal J, Parker EE, et al. The timing of physiologic closure of the metopic suture: a review of 159 patients using reconstructed 3D CT scans of the craniofacial region. J Craniofac Surg 2001;12(6):527–32.
42. Birgfeld CB, Saltzman BS, Hing AV, et al. Making the diagnosis: metopic ridge versus metopic craniosynostosis. J Craniofac Surg 2013;24(1):178–85.

Pediatric Neurosurgery in Primary Care

Masses of the Scalp and Skull in Children

Randaline R. Barnett, MD[1], Martin G. Piazza, MD[1],
Scott W. Elton, MD*

KEYWORDS

- Scalp lesion • Skull lesion • Extracranial lesion • Pediatric

KEY POINTS

- Most scalp and skull masses are benign and can be worked up on an outpatient basis unless red flag symptoms are present that require more urgent workup, such as rapid growth of a lesion, neurologic deficits, infectious symptoms, or a lesion discovered in the context of a syndrome or known history of malignancy.
- Ultrasound is an inexpensive and readily available imaging modality to start with in most cases.
- Computed tomography imaging is optimal for workup and further characterization of skull masses, as this provides the best method for evaluating bony lesions.
- MR imaging is optimal for workup and further characterization of soft tissue lesions in addition to evaluating significant anatomic structures that may affect surgical planning.
- When in doubt, referral to a pediatric neurosurgeon for further evaluation and workup is beneficial for timely diagnosis, and if necessary, surgical intervention.

CONGENITAL

Dermoid and Epidermoid Cysts

Dermoid and epidermoid cysts are non-neoplastic ectodermal inclusion cysts lined by epithelium, each containing different contents, typically presenting in the first 4 decades of life and more commonly found in male individuals (**Table 1**).[1] Dermoids can be composed of tissue derived from ectoderm, including hair, sebaceous and sweat glands, and squamous epithelium, whereas epidermoids are made of only squamous epithelium.[1] Both types of cysts arise from pouches of ectoderm that either become trapped or from failure of the surface ectoderm to separate from the

Department of Neurological Surgery, University of North Carolina, Chapel Hill, NC 27514, USA
[1] Present address: 170 Manning Drive, Campus Box 7060, Chapel Hill, NC 27599.
* Corresponding author. Department of Neurological Surgery, University of North Carolina, 170 Manning Drive, Campus Box 7060, Chapel Hill, NC 27599.
E-mail address: Scott.Elton@med.unc.edu

Pediatr Clin N Am 68 (2021) 743–757
https://doi.org/10.1016/j.pcl.2021.04.003 pediatric.theclinics.com
0031-3955/21/

Table 1
Summary of scalp and skull lesions with referral information

Category of Lesion	Types of Lesions	What Needs to Be Referred?
Congenital	• Dermoid and epidermoid cysts • Encephalocele • Parietal/biparietal foramina • Fibrous dysplasia	• Dermoid/epidermoid cysts, encephaloceles, and fibrous dysplasia should be referred for surgical evaluation. • Parietal foramina are benign unless the defects are large. Refer for surgical evaluation if persistently enlarged.
Traumatic	• Cephalohematoma • Subgaleal hematoma • Leptomeningeal cyst	• Cephalohematoma and subgaleal hematomas are nonoperative in most cases. • Skull fractures should be followed for development of a leptomeningeal cyst. If this occurs, surgery is required to repair the defect.
Vascular	• Scalp/intraosseous hemangioma • Scalp arteriovenous malformation (AVM) • Venous malformation • Sinus pericranii • Venous lakes	• Most scalp hemangiomas will regress without intervention. • Intraosseous hemangiomas should be referred for surgical evaluation. • Scalp AVMs can be followed with imaging over time, but intervention is indicated for cosmesis, headache and tinnitus, and hemorrhage prevention. • Small venous malformations can be watched, but larger ones should be referred for surgical evaluation. • Sinus pericranii should be referred for surgical evaluation. • Venous lakes are benign and do not necessitate a referral.
Infectious	• Pott puffy tumor • Osteomyelitis	• Pott puffy tumor can lead to life-threatening complications and should be seen emergently for a surgical evaluation. • Osteomyelitis is generally treated with a prolonged course of antibiotics unless there is intracranial involvement or a skull defect.
Neoplastic	• Eosinophilic granuloma • Neurofibroma • Osteoma • Osteoid osteoma • Osteoblastoma • Osteosarcoma • Lipoma • Rhabdomyosarcoma • Metastatic disease	• All neoplasms should be referred for a surgical evaluation to discuss observation, surgery for diagnosis/management, and other multidisciplinary care options if necessary.

neuroectoderm during fetal development.[1] They also can occur at any age in the subcutaneous tissues or the spinal canal as a result of traumatic or iatrogenic implantation that causes surface skin elements to track into deeper tissue.[1] They are commonly located in the orbit, the soft tissues of the scalp, the cancellous bone of the skull, and intracranially in the middle and posterior fossae.[1,2]

Epidermoids are often found in lateral regions of the skull, frequently in association with the coronal or lambdoid sutures.[1] They can occur within the diploic space of the skull, usually in the temporal or parietal bones.[1] They can be located in the subcutaneous tissues but are usually covered by intact skin without a fistulous tract.[1]

Dermoid cysts are most commonly found in the midline, but they are also the most common orbital tumors in children, located at sites of embryologic fusion such as the zygomaticofrontal and frontoethmoidal sutures or in the lateral lacrimal fossa when off midline. Dermoid cysts can be associated with spinal dysraphism and have a fistulous sinus tract extending intradurally with associated risk of cerebrospinal fluid leak and meningitis.[1]

Both epidermoid and dermoid cysts grow larger over time as cutaneous elements accumulate within them.[1] Epidermoids have a thin squamous lining, and the cysts contain debris, mostly keratin and some cholesterol, from desquamation of their squamous epithelial lining.[1] Dermoid cysts have a thicker epithelial lining and contain lipid material, derived from sebaceous secretions, and they may contain hair.[1]

The typical presentation of these lesions is presence early in infancy, and subsequent development or enlargement of a painless, well-circumscribed, subcutaneous palpable mass on the head.[3] If in the scalp, it will be mobile and rubbery on palpation, whereas if it is located within the skull, it will feel immobile and hard.[2] Imaging is not necessary for most of these lesions, as they have a prototypical location and appearance, but ultrasound is a useful, noninvasive, and widely available modality to begin evaluating these lesions (**Fig. 1**). MRI is recommended if there is concern for a sinus tract that extends intracranially (if occipital and midline for example, or cerebrospinal fluid (CSF) is leaking from a pinhole site), if the lesion appears solid or concerning for a malignant process, or there is concern for vascularity within or near the mass noted on ultrasound[2] (**Fig. 2**). Both lesions have the potential to progressively expand, erode through the skull, and produce mass effect on the brain, so it is recommended that early surgical resection be performed to prevent a more extensive surgery in the future.[4] Recurrence is rare following complete resection.[3]

Encephaloceles

An encephalocele is a term that describes intracranial contents herniating through a defect in the skull.[5–7] Most of them occur in the occipital region and are often

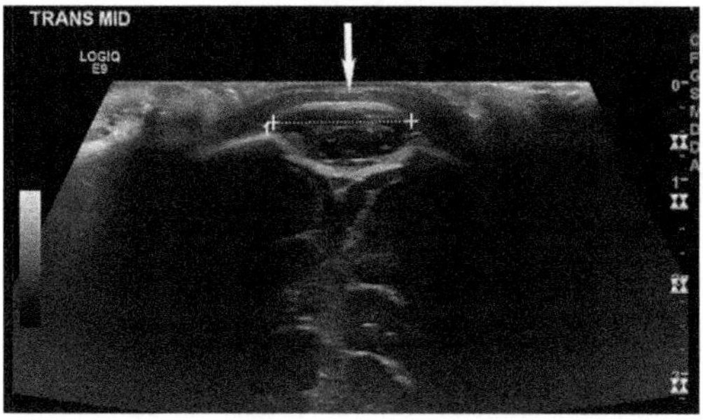

Fig. 1. Dermoid of anterior fontanelle (*arrow*), cranial ultrasound.

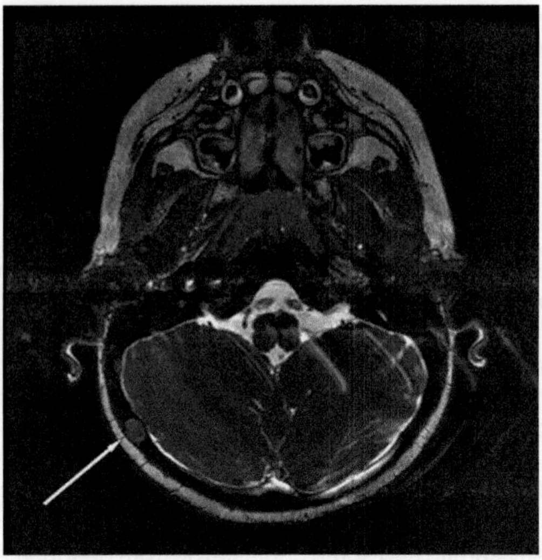

Fig. 2. Intradiploic dermoid (*arrow*). MRI, T2-weighted image.

associated with significant intracranial abnormalities (**Figs. 3** and **4**).[5] Hydrocephalus is commonly associated with large encephaloceles, and on physical examination, they are often soft, fluctuant, translucent, and nontender.

These children should be referred to a tertiary center for MRI and evaluation. Encephaloceles are typically treated with surgical resection and cranial repair. Given that the ventricular anatomy is often distorted, it is important to follow for signs and symptoms of hydrocephalus after resection.

Parietal/Biparietal Foramina

Parietal/biparietal foramina occur as the result of abnormal calvarial ossification during fetal development.[6,8] This is inherited in an autosomal dominant fashion with high

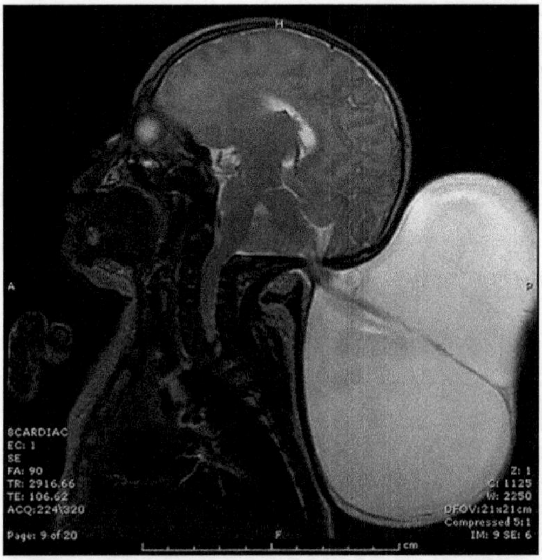

Fig. 3. Occipital encephalocele, sagittal T2 MRI. Note small defect with herniation of cerebellar tissue into large fluid-filled sac.

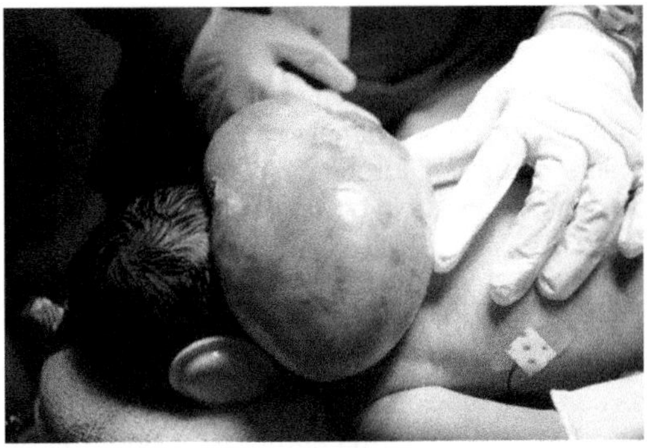

Fig. 4. Same child, large occipital encephalocele.

penetrance.[8] At birth, there may be one large midline or bilateral skull defect with the brain parenchyma covered by only the dura, pericranium, and scalp.[6] The defects usually close during childhood but leave behind symmetric foramina within the parietal bones.[6,8] On physical examination, the defects are palpable soft areas behind the skull apex that are symmetric across the midline.[8] These foramina are usually asymptomatic and thought to be benign; however, they can be associated with intracranial venous abnormalities that can predispose patients to epilepsy.[6,8] Computed tomography (CT) imaging is optimal for assessing the bony anatomy, and MRI can be obtained to evaluate for venous anomalies.[6,8] Parietal/biparietal foramina generally do not require intervention unless the size of the defect poses a risk to the underlying brain parenchyma, and in such cases cranioplasty may be considered.[6] It is recommended that children with large defects avoid activities and contact sports that may pose risk of injury, and seek neurosurgery evaluation.

Fibrous Dysplasia

Fibrous dysplasia is a slow, indolent condition that affects 1 or multiple bones in which normal bone and marrow are replaced by fibrous tissue and disorganized woven bone.[9] It can be a part of McCune-Albright syndrome, a triad of polyostotic fibrous dysplasia, café-au-lait spots, and endocrinopathies.[10] The most commonly involved bones are the craniofacial bones, specifically the zygomatic-maxillary complex, proximal femur, and ribs.[9] Fibrous dysplasia involves the craniofacial region in 90% of cases and the anterior skull base in more than 95% of cases.[9] Presenting signs and symptoms, such as facial deformity, vision changes, hearing impairment, nasal congestion, pain, and paresthesia can vary depending on the location of the fibrous dysplasia.[9] Most patients are asymptomatic and present after facial asymmetry is noticed.[9]

Growth of monostotic and polyostotic forms of fibrous dysplasia lesions taper off as patients enter puberty.[9] These lesions can be managed conservatively with observation. Rarely, lesions may exhibit more rapid growth, cortical bone expansion, and displacement of adjacent vital structures, such as the optic nerve, globe, auditory canal, and nasal passageways.[9] In this scenario, surgical resection and reconstruction are recommended to prevent functional deficits from mass effect, which may result in blindness, hearing loss, or airway obstruction.[9]

The growth of lesions in McCune-Albright syndrome also tends to slow down as children approach puberty, but the overall severity of bone expansion and deformity is more prominent than in other types.[9] Studies have shown that patients with poorly controlled growth hormone excess have more severe deformities and symptoms. For this reason, it is recommended that growth hormone excess be aggressively managed in patients with polyostotic fibrous dysplasia and McCune-Albright syndrome.[9]

CT imaging with bone windows is optimal to assess the extent of bony involvement and adjacent anatomic structures. Fibrous dysplasia is characterized by exhibiting a "ground-glass" appearance with a thin cortex and without defined borders[9] (**Fig. 5**).

Clinics Care Points

- Midline occipital and spinal dermal sinus tracts can be associated with deep dermoid lesions, MRI is indicated, and these present a risk of meningitis.
- Encephaloceles can be associated with cerebral anomalies and hydrocephalus .
- Fibrous dysplasia has various forms and can cause facial deformity; referral is recommended.

TRAUMATIC

Cephalohematoma

Cephalohematomas occur in 1% to 2% of neonates and are characterized as hemorrhage between the pericranium and the skull.[2] This occurs as the result of birth-related trauma in cases of vacuum-assisted or forceps-assisted delivery and sometimes spontaneously from prolonged labor.[2] Because the pericranium is adherent to the sutures of the skull, a cephalohematoma will typically not cross suture lines. Ultrasound imaging will show a subperiosteal hemorrhage with moderate echogenicity and typically underlying normal-appearing brain parenchyma.[2] They typically increase in size for a few days following birth,[5,11] soften over time, and usually are absorbed within 1 month, although large cephalohematomas may take longer.[11] If they do not absorb within that time, the hematoma may begin to calcify as a result of the elevated periosteum.[2,11] Expectant and conservative management is appropriate. These hematomas can initially look disfiguring and concerning to patients' caregivers; however, over time, the skull will remodel and smooth out, requiring no intervention.[11] Surgery is generally not performed unless they remain disfiguring or become infected.

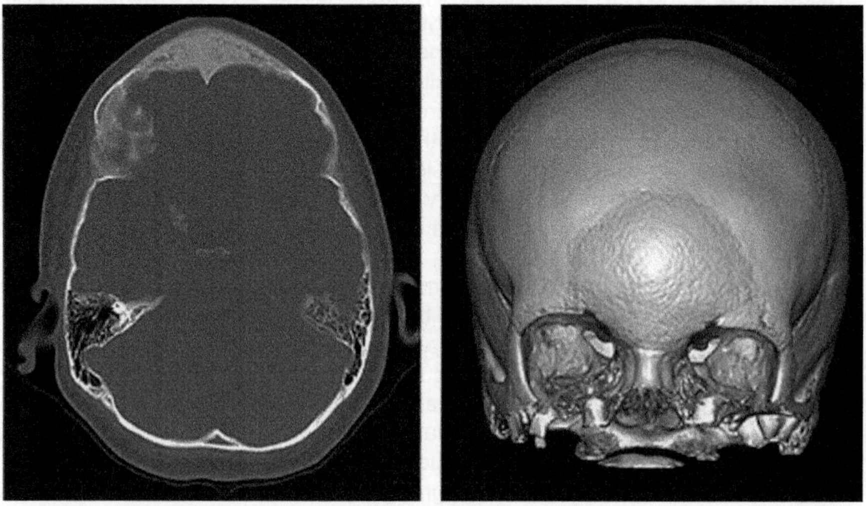

Fig. 5. Fibrous dysplasia, CT scan with 3-dimensional reconstruction. Left image, axial CT, note the "ground-glass" appearance of the lesion in the frontal bone.

Subgaleal Hematoma

A subgaleal hematoma occurs when there is bleeding from emissary veins within the space between the pericranium and the galea aponeurotica.[2,12] It can be associated with a skull fracture. Because the hemorrhage is not limited by the pericranium as in a cephalohematoma, it can spread across suture lines within the subgaleal space. This allows for the hematoma to become life threatening, as this space can hold up to 260 mL of blood, leading to severe hypovolemia in neonates.[2,12] Moderate to severe subgaleal hemorrhages can occur in 1.5 per 10,000 births.[2,12] Physical examination findings will include a boggy, fluctuant scalp mass with increasing head circumference. If a large hemorrhage occurs, infants will exhibit pallor, hypotonia, and tachycardia.[2]

Ultrasound imaging is useful for determining the size of the hematoma, contents and characteristics of the fluid collection, and whether there is an underlying fracture or other abnormality.[2] It will demonstrate moderate echogenicity in acute hemorrhages.[2] As the hematoma ages and resolves, it will become less echogenic.[2]

There is no specific treatment for subgaleal hematomas other than supportive care with close monitoring in intensive care and resuscitation.[12] Subgaleal hematomas will typically resolve over a period of 2 to 3 weeks.[12]

Leptomeningeal Cysts

A leptomeningeal cyst is a rare complication that occurs in 0.05% to 1.6% of pediatric skull fractures, usually within the first year of life, and is often referred to as a "growing skull fracture." It is thought that a tear in the dura allows for brain and CSF pulsations to result in progressive enlargement of the fracture.[13,14] Because brain volume increases rapidly in infancy, the pulsations of brain and CSF during the maximum period of brain growth will lead to herniation of brain and leptomeningeal contents through the dural laceration, causing enlargement of the skull fracture.[15] Growing skull fractures can develop in children as late as 1.9 years of age, and timing to diagnosis can range from 20 to 125 days post injury.[14]

Skull fractures are often initially diagnosed with skull radiographs or CT imaging following head trauma (**Fig. 6**). A growing skull fracture can be diagnosed clinically based on physical examination through palpation of a skull defect and associated soft, pulsatile mass within the defect. These are often evident within 4 to 8 weeks post injury. MRI imaging can be helpful in confirmation to determine if there are nearby vascular structures involved, especially if the fracture is located near a venous sinus.

Growing skull fractures can be corrected only with surgical intervention, and early surgery once the lesion is identified is recommended to repair the dural defect and keep brain tissue from herniating into the defect.

Clinics Care Points

- Cephalohematomas and subgaleal hematomas can be differentiated by the ability to cross cranial suture lines.
- Consider a leptomeningeal cyst in an infant with history of trauma and soft pulsatile mass at fracture site.

VASCULAR LESIONS

Scalp and Intraosseous Hemangiomas

Hemangiomas are the most common tumor in infancy, occurring in 1% to 2% of the population.[5] These lesions are benign tumors that arise from the endothelium and undergo cellular proliferation and enlargement during the first year of life.[5] Cutaneous hemangiomas typically regress throughout childhood.[5] They can be located superficially in the scalp with a reddish appearance or deep with a flesh-colored or blueish appearance.[5] They may become darker or blush with Valsalva maneuvers, such as crying or straining (**Fig. 7**).

Intraosseous cavernous hemangiomas represent 0.7% of primary bone tumors[3] and 1% to 5% of calvarial tumors in the pediatric population.[6] They are most commonly found in the frontal and parietal bones[3,16,17] and have a female predilection.[3] Patients may present with immobile lumps on the head and headaches in addition to neurologic symptoms, depending on the location, if there is intracranial extension.[16,17] Intraosseous hemangiomas do not spontaneously involute unlike cutaneous hemangiomas.[17]

Hemangiomas can be a component of a rare syndrome known as PHACE Syndrome, in which there are large segmental or plaquelike hemangiomas located within the scalp and face, which can be associated with other extracutaneous manifestations.[5] Most patients will have one other clinical finding in addition to the hemangiomas, the most common being posterior fossa and arterial abnormalities including Dandy-Walker malformation, ipsilateral cerebellar hypoplasia, and cerebellar vermian hypoplasia with cortical dysgenesis.[5]

Most cutaneous hemangiomas can be managed clinically without imaging unless neurologic symptoms arise or if they are associated with other congenital anomalies,[5] and in those instances, a referral should be made to a geneticist, pediatric neurosurgeon, or craniofacial surgeon, and possibly oncologist for further evaluation. Most cutaneous hemangiomas regress over time and do not require intervention.[18] Those that are located in regions that may affect vital structures and functions, such as vision, can be treated initially with medications such as beta blockers or steroids.[18] If medication fails, laser therapy, sclerotherapy, or surgery is considered.[18]

Intraosseous hemangiomas, if found incidentally or suspected, should be referred to a pediatric neurosurgeon for further evaluation and appropriate imaging. These do not spontaneously regress. Surgical resection with normal bony margins is thus recommended to address the mass effect and repair deformity.[17,19] If completely

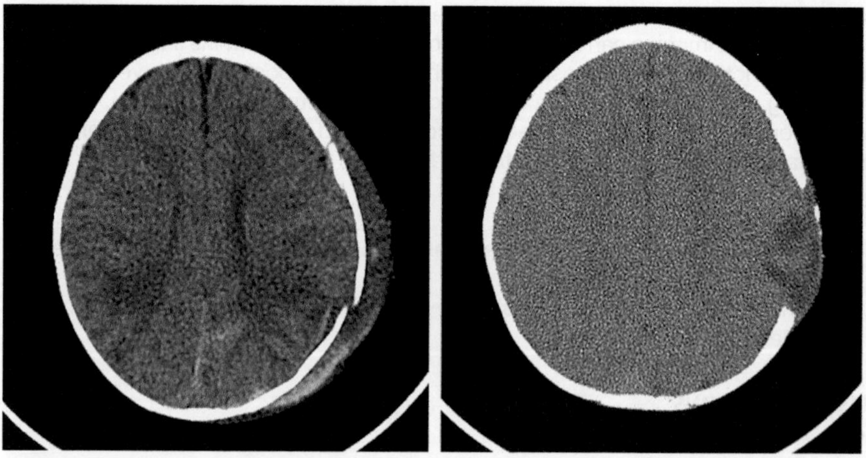

Fig. 6. Leptomeningeal cyst, CT scan. Note the left image, linear fracture immediately post-trauma, left parietal. Right image, 3 months later, note the loss of bone and herniation of cerebral tissue.

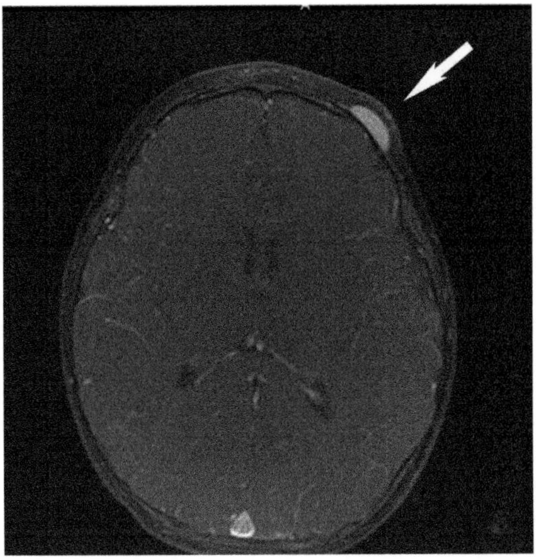

Fig. 7. Scalp hemangioma (*arrow*), MRI, T1-weighted image with contrast. Note the brightly enhancing lesion, left frontal. Clinically, lesion would change color with straining.

resected, recurrence is rare.[17] Preoperative embolization can be considered to reduce blood loss.[19] Skull base lesions and residual tumors also can be treated with radiation, although this must be carefully weighed against the long-term risk.[17]

Scalp Arteriovenous Malformations

Also referred to as cirsoid aneurysms, scalp arteriovenous malformations (AVMs) are located within the subcutaneous fatty layer of the scalp with feeding arteries that come from vessels that normally vascularize the scalp and are drained by enlarged, tortuous veins that can have variceal dilation.[20] Patients most commonly present with scalp swelling that gradually increases in size over time and can experience more rapid enlargement during periods of puberty, menstruation, and pregnancy.[20] Scalp AVMs may also cause pain, throbbing headaches, and bruits.[20] These lesions, although uncommon, have been known to hemorrhage as a result of large, untreated lesions and trauma.[20] Scalp necrosis and high-output cardiac failure also can be associated with larger lesions.[20]

Scalp AVMs are usually diagnosed clinically but can be further worked up with an MRI and MR angiography in addition to digital subtraction angiography.[20] These lesions can be observed with surveillance imaging over time, but intervention is indicated for cosmetic purposes, headache and tinnitus, and hemorrhage prevention.[20] Surgical resection, ligation of the arterial feeders, endovascular embolization, sclerotherapy, and electrothrombosis are all treatment options that can be considered.[20]

Venous Malformations

Venous malformations represent a wide variety of congenital venous lesions, with 40% of cases occurring in the head and neck.[5,6] Patients present with a soft, nonpulsatile bluish-colored mass.[6] These are best evaluated with an MRI, often showing up as hyperintense on T2 with internal septation and varying degrees of enhancement.[5,6] Clots can be seen, which show up as flow signal voids.[5,6] Most venous malformations are treated with a combination of sclerotherapy and surgery.[5,6] Small lesions can be watched expectantly.

Sinus Pericranii

Sinus pericranii are abnormal veins that are located within the scalp, most commonly in the frontal and parietal regions, and communicate with the intracranial venous sinuses.[5] These abnormal veins are typically found in isolation but can be associated with other conditions such as craniosynostosis and intracranial venous anomalies, including dural sinus hypoplasia.[21] These are thought to be congenital in nature.[5]

Patients are usually asymptomatic and present with a soft tissue mass that becomes enlarged with crying, Valsalva maneuver, and supine positioning.[21] The soft tissue mass may be associated with red or blue skin discoloration.[21] When symptoms do arise, patients often report headache, nausea, dizziness, vertigo, and local pain.[21] Severe complications include increased intracranial pressure, bradypnea, bradycardia, ataxia, hearing loss, epileptic seizures, air embolism, and cardiac failure due to hemorrhagic or thrombotic complications, changes in blood flow and metabolism, or head trauma, but these are rare.[21]

When suspected, we recommend referral to a pediatric neurosurgeon for imaging and consideration of possible embolization, surgery, or observation.

Venous Lakes

Venous lakes are enlarged emissary veins that pass through the skull connecting external scalp veins with the dural venous sinuses intracranially.[6] The channels they travel within appear as serpiginous or linear lucent spaces with sclerotic borders that extend through the skull and can be mistaken for suture lines or fractures.[6] Venous lakes are often found incidentally and are benign vascular structures that require no treatment. They are of importance when planning for intracranial surgery, as significant blood loss can occur when a venous lake is breached.

Clinics Care Points

- A variety of vascular lesions affect the scalp and skull. Referral is essential to better define the anatomy involved and determine the need for intervention.

INFECTIOUS LESIONS

Pott Puffy Tumor

Pott puffy tumor is a subperiosteal abscess involving the frontal bone with adjacent osteomyelitis as the result of a frontal sinus infection that spreads contiguously through the wall of the sinus or through hematogenous spread via the veins that drain sinus mucosa.[5,6] The most common organisms involved are streptococci, staphylococci, and anaerobic bacteria.[5,6] The infection can travel intracranially through a network of veins draining the frontal sinus leading to epidural abscesses, subdural empyema, meningitis, brain abscesses, and venous sinus thromboses.[5,6]

Imaging workup often includes a CT of brain and sinuses to assess the extent of bony erosion from osteomyelitis in addition to an MRI with contrast to evaluate for intracranial extension. MRI may show dural enhancement, extra-axial fluid, and cerebritis and/or brain abscess. Within the tissue of the scalp, a fluid collection may be seen with contrast enhancement peripherally.[5,6]

Treatment includes surgical drainage and removal of infected tissue, sometimes including bone, followed by initiation of long-term antibiotic therapy.[5,6] Cranioplasty for removed or eroded bone can be done once the antibiotic course has been completed and there is no further concern for active infection.

Osteomyelitis

Osteomyelitis of the skull in children is most commonly caused by complications of a traumatic or iatrogenic nature.[6] It also can develop secondary to ear or sinus infections, as with Pott puffy tumor, involving the parietotemporal and frontal bones.[6] Less common causes include contiguous spread from an infected scalp wound caused by the use of forceps as well as devices for intrauterine monitoring.[6] Children may present with nonspecific constitutional symptoms, including fever, chills, lethargy, fussiness, and general malaise. Physical examination findings may include erythema, swelling, and localized pain.

CT with contrast is useful for evaluating subcutaneous soft tissue enhancement and the degree of bony erosion.[6] MRI with contrast can be obtained for evaluation of potential intracranial involvement.[6] Skull osteomyelitis alone is typically treated with a prolonged course of antibiotics and does not require surgery unless there is intracranial involvement and/or a skull defect secondary to bony erosion.[6] In this case, a cranioplasty is necessary following resolution of the infection.

Clinics Care Points

- Pott puffy tumor and osteomyelitis require urgent referral for appropriate imaging and antibiotic therapy. With intracranial involvement, they can become a neurosurgical emergency if left untreated.

NEOPLASTIC LESIONS

Eosinophilic Granuloma

Eosinophilic granuloma (EG) is a type of lesion that belongs to a benign subset of Langerhans cell histiocytosis. EG is characterized by single or multiple skeletal lesions that primarily affect children, adolescents, and young adults and accounts for 2.4% to 12.0% of calvarial masses.[22,23] EG most commonly affects the skull, mandible, spine, ribs, and long bones. Patients will often present with inflammatory symptoms, including localized pain at the site of involvement in addition to swelling, fever, and sometimes leukocytosis.[22,24] On physical examination, an EG lesion is often noted to be soft, tender, and swollen. The underlying bone may be absent if eroded completely or may feel as if it gives way. This can be confirmed with skull radiographs, which show a punched out lytic lesion with nonsclerotic well-defined borders or the "hole within a hole" sign, in which a beveled edge can be appreciated due to a greater involvement of the inner table of the skull than the outer table.[2,5,6,23,25–27] If there is concern for EG based on radiographs or physical examination, a referral to a pediatric neurosurgeon should be facilitated.

Neurofibroma

As a clinical manifestation of Neurofibromatosis Type 1 (NF-1), a neurofibroma is one of the most common neurogenic tumors, arising from the endoneurium of nerves.[2] NF-1 is autosomal dominant and affects 1 in 3500 people, leading to the development of neurofibromas throughout the body that can be cutaneous, subcutaneous, deep, or plexiform.[2] A plexiform neurofibroma is unique in that it involves multiple nerves and can extend into surrounding structures in the context of NF-1.[2] They are often associated with large overlying cutaneous pigmented lesions.[10] Given that plexiform neurofibromas can undergo malignant degeneration, these lesions should be monitored with close follow-up by an NF-1 specialist. Most neurofibromas can be conservatively managed with observation over time. If a neurofibroma is causing disfigurement, pain, or neurologic symptoms or if it experiences growth or morphologic changes, the patient should be referred for an evaluation to a surgeon with expertise in removing neurofibromas.

Rare Neoplastic Lesions

Osteoma

Osteomas are the most common benign bony tumor in adults but are rarely seen in children, usually presenting as an asymptomatic painless lump or found incidentally on imaging studies.[6,28] Depending on their size and location, they can cause painless swelling, facial asymmetry, exophthalmos, proptosis, ptosis, diplopia, lid swelling, amaurosis fugax, and symptoms secondary to obstruction of the nasal and paranasal sinuses, such as nasal discharge, sinusitis, and development of mucoceles.[28] Osteomas, when asymptomatic, can be managed by observation. Surgical resection is reserved for symptomatic lesions.

Osteoid osteoma

An osteoid osteoma is another benign bone tumor that is more commonly seen in children and young adults with a predilection for male individuals.[28] This lesion is typically small in size (1 to 2 cm in diameter), has limited growth potential, and presents with severe localized pain, often worse nocturnally and relieved with nonsteroidal anti-inflammatory drugs.[28] Osteoid osteomas are uncommon in craniofacial bones, but rarely, they usually affect the mandible.[28] In recent years, percutaneous radiofrequency ablation has become the most common form of management.[28]

Osteoblastoma

Osteoblastoma is a bone-forming neoplasm, occurring mostly in young adults with a predilection for male individuals.[28] It accounts for nearly 1% of primary bone tumors, and 10% to 15% of these lesions occur with the craniofacial bones, most commonly the mandible.[28] It appears histologically the same as osteoid osteoma, but it is larger in size, lacks significant reactive sclerosis, and has no nerve fibers compared with osteoid osteoma.[28] Osteoblastoma usually does not cause the characteristic nocturnal pain of osteoid osteoma.[28] Osteoblastoma usually presents with a painful mass, and craniofacial lesions may be associated with headache, tooth impaction, and epistaxis.[28] Osteoblastoma is treated with surgical resection.[28]

Osteosarcoma

Osteosarcoma is the most common malignant bony neoplasm, primarily affecting the long bones, but also can occasionally involve the craniofacial region, most commonly arising in the medullary region of the mandible or maxilla.[28] It is larger than an osteoid osteoma, has poorly defined margins on imaging studies, and histologically has more cytologic atypia and mitoses.[28] Presentation depends on its size, growth pattern, and location, but most patients develop swelling and pain in addition to paresthesia, loosening or loss of teeth, toothaches, bleeding, and nasal obstruction.[28] Workup may include an elevated serum alkaline phosphatase. Imaging characteristics include a destructive lesion with ill-defined borders and may or may not involve the adjacent soft tissue.[28] Osteosarcomas are treated with radical surgery with or without adjuvant chemotherapy and/or radiation therapy.[28]

Lipoma

A lipoma is a benign tumor composed of mature adipocytes.[6] Lipomas are usually found in the subcutaneous tissues and present as a soft painless mass. Lipomas of the bone are rare, and there are only a few reported cases of intraosseous lipomas involving this skull.[29] On radiographs, intraosseous lipomas are radiolucent and well circumscribed with occasional dilatation of the medullary bone.[29] These appear well defined on imaging with signal characteristics of fat on CT and MRI.[30] Most lipomas do not require any intervention. If a lipoma is causing pain or a cosmetic issue, surgical resection is reasonable. If there is any concern for malignancy, a biopsy and/or resection is recommended for confirmation of diagnosis.

Rhabdomyosarcoma

Rhabdomyosarcoma is the most common soft tissue sarcoma in children,[5,6] with approximately one-third of pediatric cases occurring in the head and neck.[5] They are more common in male individuals, and two-thirds of cases are diagnosed in children younger than 6 years.[5] Presentation depends on the size and location of the tumor. It is important to note that rhabdomyosarcomas can be difficult to differentiate from other soft tissue lesions based on physical examination alone.[5] If there are concerns, a referral should be placed to a pediatric neurosurgeon or craniofacial surgeon.

Metastatic disease: neuroblastoma and Ewing sarcoma

Metastatic disease also can affect the scalp and the skull, although extremely rare. Metastatic neuroblastoma is the third most common malignancy in children.[6,31] Neuroblastoma, an embryonal neuroendocrine tumor that arises from neural crest progenitor cells,[32] typically starts in the adrenal gland or along the sympathetic chain,[31] and can metastasize to the calvaria, orbit, and skull base[5,6,31]; 25% of children with neuroblastoma have skull metastases.[31] Neuroblastoma is the most common malignant metastasis to the skull in children and can involve the dura.[6,31] Metastases that involve the dura very rarely involve the brain parenchyma.[31]

Ewing sarcoma is a highly malignant small round blue cell tumor[33] and is the second most common primary bone cancer in children.[6] Primary involvement of the skull is rare, but metastases from Ewing sarcoma to the skull are more common.[6] Children usually present with localized pain and swelling.[6,33] Imaging characteristics include a poorly defined lytic lesion with an aggressive appearance, extension into the bordering soft tissues, and intense heterogeneous enhancement.[6]

Children with metastatic lesions with involvement of the scalp, skull, or brain should be managed at a tertiary center by oncologists, radiation oncologists, and pediatric neurosurgeons.

Clinics Care Points

- A variety of tumors can involve the skull and soft tissues of the head and neck. EG and neurofibroma lesions can be part of a larger systemic disease process, and referral to a specialized center is recommended.

DISCLOSURE

The authors do not have any commercial or financial conflicts of interest.

REFERENCES

1. Smirniotopoulos JG, Chiechi MV. Teratomas, dermoids, and epidermoids of the head and neck. Radiographics 1995;15(6):1437–55.
2. Bansal AG, Oudsema R, Masseaux JA, et al. US of pediatric superficial masses of the head and neck. Radiographics 2018;38(4):1239–63.
3. Gibson SE, Prayson RA. Primary skull lesions in the pediatric population: a 25-year experience. Arch Pathol Lab Med 2007;131(5):761–6.
4. Khalid S, Ruge J. Considerations in the management of congenital cranial dermoid cysts. J Neurosurg Pediatr 2017;20(1):30–4.

5. Moron FE, Morriss MC, Jones JJ, et al. Lumps and bumps on the head in children: use of CT and MR imaging in solving the clinical diagnostic dilemma. Radiographics 2004;24(6):1655–74.
6. Choudhary G, Udayasankar U, Saade C, et al. A systematic approach in the diagnosis of paediatric skull lesions: what radiologists need to know. Pol J Radiol 2019;84:e92–111.
7. Younus M, Coode PE. Nasal glioma and encephalocele: two separate entities. Report of two cases. J Neurosurg 1986;64(3):516–9.
8. Mavrogiannis LA, Wilkie AOM. Enlarged parietal foramina. In: Adam MP, Ardinger HH, Pagon RA, et al, editors. GeneReviews. Seattle (WA): University of Washington, Seattle; 1993.
9. Lee JS, FitzGibbon EJ, Chen YR, et al. Clinical guidelines for the management of craniofacial fibrous dysplasia. Orphanet J Rare Dis 2012;7(Suppl 1):S2.
10. Ferner RE, Huson SM, Thomas N, et al. Guidelines for the diagnosis and management of individuals with neurofibromatosis 1. J Med Genet 2007;44(2):81–8.
11. Kaufman HH, Hochberg J, Anderson RP, et al. Treatment of calcified cephalohematoma. Neurosurgery 1993;32(6):1037–9 [discussion: 1039–40].
12. Davis DJ. Neonatal subgaleal hemorrhage: diagnosis and management. CMAJ 2001;164(10):1452–3.
13. Taveras JM, Ransohoff J. Leptomeningeal cysts of the brain following trauma with erosion of the skull; a study of seven cases treated by surgery. J Neurosurg 1953;10(3):233–41.
14. Northam W, Chandran A, Quinsey C, et al. Pediatric nonoperative skull fractures: delayed complications and factors associated with clinic and imaging utilization. J Neurosurg Pediatr 2019;1–9. https://doi.org/10.3171/2019.5.PEDS18739.
15. Khandelwal S, Sharma G, Gopal S, et al. Growing skull fractures/leptomeningeal cyst. Indian J Radiol Imaging 2002;12(4):485–6.
16. Nasrallah IM, Hayek R, Duhaime AC, et al. Cavernous hemangioma of the skull: surgical treatment without craniectomy. J Neurosurg Pediatr 2009;4(6):575–9.
17. Liu JK, Burger PC, Harnsberger HR, et al. Primary intraosseous skull base cavernous hemangioma: case report. Skull Base 2003;13(4):219–28.
18. Zheng JW, Zhang L, Zhou Q, et al. A practical guide to treatment of infantile hemangiomas of the head and neck. Int J Clin Exp Med 2013;6(10):851–60.
19. Vural M, Acikalin MF, Adapinar B, et al. Congenital cavernous hemangioma of the calvaria. Case report. J Neurosurg Pediatr 2009;3(1):41–5.
20. Fisher-Jeffes ND, Domingo Z, Madden M, et al. Arteriovenous malformations of the scalp. Neurosurgery 1995;36(4):656–60 [discussion: 660].
21. Pavanello M, Melloni I, Antichi E, et al. Sinus pericranii: diagnosis and management in 21 pediatric patients. J Neurosurg Pediatr 2015;15(1):60.
22. Ruge JR, Tomita T, Naidich TP, et al. Scalp and calvarial masses of infants and children. Neurosurgery 1988;22(6 Pt 1):1037–42.
23. Kim YJ, Jo KW. Rapid growing eosinophilic granuloma in skull after minor trauma. Korean J Neurotrauma 2015;11(1):22–5.
24. Rawlings CE 3rd, Wilkins RH. Solitary eosinophilic granuloma of the skull. Neurosurgery 1984;15(2):155–61.
25. David R, Oria RA, Kumar R, et al. Radiologic features of eosinophilic granuloma of bone. AJR Am J Roentgenol 1989;153(5):1021–6.
26. Stull MA, Kransdorf MJ, Devaney KO. Langerhans cell histiocytosis of bone. Radiographics 1992;12(4):801–23.
27. De Angulo G, Nair S, Lee V, et al. Nonoperative management of solitary eosinophilic granulomas of the calvaria. J Neurosurg Pediatr 2013;12(1):1–5.

28. Nielsen GP, Rosenberg AE. Update on bone forming tumors of the head and neck. Head Neck Pathol 2007;1(1):87–93.
29. Tomabechi M, Sako K, Daita G, et al. Lipoma involving the skull. Case report. J Neurosurg 1992;76(2):312.
30. Gaskin CM, Helms CA. Lipomas, lipoma variants, and well-differentiated liposarcomas (atypical lipomas): results of MRI evaluations of 126 consecutive fatty masses. AJR Am J Roentgenol 2004;182(3):733–9.
31. D'Ambrosio N, Lyo JK, Young RJ, et al. Imaging of metastatic CNS neuroblastoma. AJR Am J Roentgenol 2010;194(5):1223–9.
32. Mahapatra S, Challagundla KB. Cancer, neuroblastoma. In: StatPearls. Treasure Island (FL): StatPearls Publishing LLC; 2020.
33. Bhattacharjee S, Venkata SR, Uppin MS. Skull and spinal ewing's sarcoma in children: an institutional study. J Pediatr Neurosci 2018;13(4):392–7.

Macrocephaly in the Primary Care Provider's Office

Jean-Paul Bryant, MSc[a], Nicole E. Hernandez, MS[b], Toba N. Niazi, MD[a,b,*]

KEYWORDS

• Macrocephaly • Hydrocephalus • Megalencephaly • Ultrasound

KEY POINTS

- Macrocephaly is a common clinical finding that can result from benign or pathologic causes.
- Careful history and physical are important to distinguish between normal or deleterious etiologies.
- Neuroimaging may be necessary in evaluating a child with macrocephaly, with head ultrasound being the most appropriate initial study in a child with an open fontanelle.
- Immediate neurosurgical referral is warranted in a child with a rapidly enlarging head or signs demonstrating elevated intracranial pressure.

INTRODUCTION

Macrocephaly is a frequently encountered entity within the pediatric clinical practice, affecting approximately 2% to 5% of the population. It is diagnosed primarily in infants in whom head circumference is tracked diligently within the first year of life. Macrocephaly is defined as an occipitofrontal circumference (OFC) that is at least 2 standard deviations above normal, or 0.5 cm above the 97th percentile. The OFC extends from the most prominent part of the glabella to the most prominent posterior portion of the occipital region.[1] OFC, like other basic measures of children, is typically tracked along growth curves. This allows for the monitoring of development over time and also delineates the percentile that the child's OFC falls under in a given patient population. The causes of macrocephaly are broad, ranging from benign to severe, and require thoughtful evaluation.

OFC is used as a surrogate for the proper development of the skull and its contents, namely the cerebrum, cerebrospinal fluid (CSF) spaces, and cerebrovasculature. After the closing of the cranial sutures the head becomes a closed system in

[a] Miller School of Medicine, University of Miami, 1600 NW 10th Avenue #1140, Miami, FL 33136, USA; [b] Division of Pediatric Neurosurgery, Brain Institute, Nicklaus Children's Hospital, 3100 SW 62nd Avenue Suite 3109, Miami, FL 33155, USA
* Corresponding author.
E-mail address: Toba.niazi@nicklaushealth.org

Pediatr Clin N Am 68 (2021) 759–773
https://doi.org/10.1016/j.pcl.2021.04.004

which these 3 components are in dynamic volumetric equilibrium defined by the Monroe-Kellie Doctrine. If there is an increase in 1 component there will be an automatic reduction in 1 or both of the other components. Maladaptation due to cerebral pathology leads to nonadherence of this doctrine, resulting in an increase in intracranial pressure and potential for subsequent development of a brain herniation syndrome.

Infants and young children, however, represent a unique patient population in whom most of the intracranial sutures remain open until early childhood. Thereby, any increase in either the volume of the CSF, blood vessels, or brain will accommodate intracranial volumetric expansion by increasing the OFC. Children rarely present with symptoms indicative of a brain herniation syndrome, as open sutures can accommodate intracranial expansion of any of the 3 major components. Instead, children typically present with other signs and symptoms in conjunction with a rapidly increasing OFC.

As a result, macrocephaly is a nonspecific clinical finding without indication of the underlying etiology. The expansion of any of the cerebral contents could be the underlying causative factor, such as an increase in the intraventricular or extraventricular CSF spaces, increase in brain parenchyma, or increase of the intracranial blood volume. For this reason, a systematic approach consisting of a detailed clinical examination, measurement and tracking of OFC, and appropriate neuroimaging is important to assess the causative nature of the macrocephaly.

NORMAL AND ABNORMAL HEAD GROWTH CURVES

The landmark observational study conducted by Nellhaus[2] in 1968 provided the foundation for measuring the cranium in pediatric visits. Later, Weaver and Christian[3] noted the importance of comparing the OFC of the child to that of the parent when presenting to the pediatrician's office. Today, essential to the diagnosis of macrocephaly is a thorough understanding of normal and abnormal cranial growth. In most children, head circumference grows by approximately 2 cm per month at 0 to 3 months of age, 1 cm per month from 3 to 6 months of age, and 0.5 cm per month during the last 6 months of the traditional infancy period. Although the first year of life is characterized by rapid head growth, including an average 12 cm growth in OFC, after 1 year, cranial growth rate greatly slows. After the first year of life, head growth rate reduces to 1 cm every 6 months until the age of 3. From 3 to 5 years of age it is expected that the child's head will grow at a rate of 1 cm per year. The treating physician will observe that on average, pediatric patients will have a 5-cm total increase in head circumference from 1 to 5 years of age.[4] Although age is an important factor when evaluating for normal head growth, it is also essential to consider the sex of the patient as well as the head size of the same-sex parent. Previous studies by Nellhaus[2] in 1968 and Ounsted and colleagues[5] in 1986 highlighted sex differences, with the former citing that boys had a greater mean head circumference (~0.9 cm larger) than girls through 18 years of age. Within the past decade, Rollins and colleagues[6] expounded on these results, generating a set of sex-specific head circumference charts spanning from birth to 21 years of age. Some academic pediatric neurosurgical and genetic departments have completely adopted the use of the more recently produced Rollins graphs.[7] Further, they have begun to necessitate the presence of the same-sex parent to accurately compare the percentile of the parent's OFC with that of the child.[7]

There are several growth charts available for tracking OFC that are organized by the characteristics of each unique patient population. Familiarity with these charts and appropriate selection for tracking is imperative, as children can fall at drastically different percentiles based on the chart that is used. Some of the most commonly used growth charts for children consist of the following: the standard Centers for Disease Control (CDC) or World Health Organization (WHO) for boys and for girls (**Fig. 1**), head circumference for premature patients, head circumference for patients with trisomy 21, and the head circumference chart for patients with achondroplasia. If serial measurements cross 2 or more major percentile lines, or if the patient is younger than 6 months old and head size increases more than 2 cm in a month, further testing is warranted. When suspecting an abnormal OFC measurement, it is imperative to double check this finding.

Clinics Care Points

- Pediatricians should be familiar with appropriate growth charts and adjust curves when necessary depending on the child's associated clinical conditions.
- Pediatricians should consistently track the OFC of children with initial abnormal measurements.

> *Key components of physical examination:*
>
> - Head circumference measurement
> - Asses fullness of fontanelle in child when upright
> - Assess for separation of cranial sutures, particularly the sagittal suture
> - Assess for prominence of scalp veins
> - Assess extraocular motility

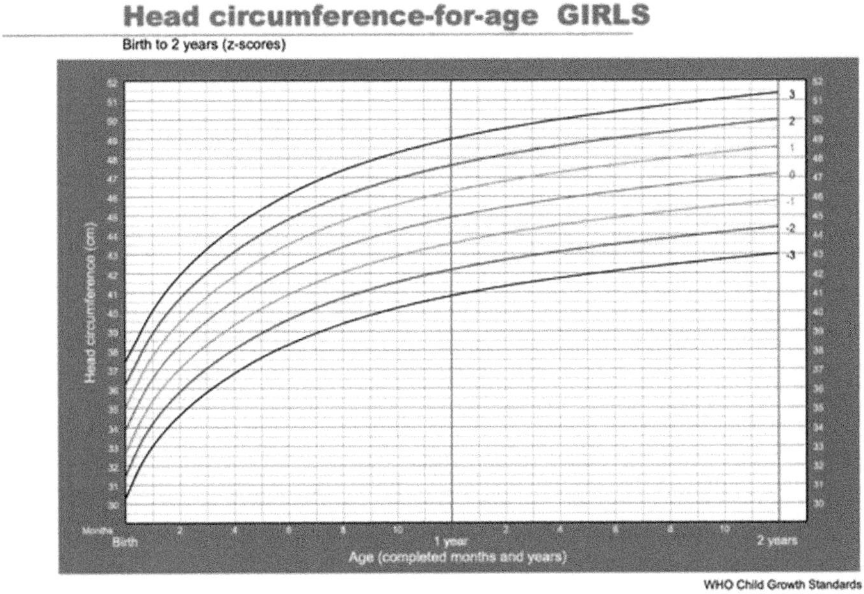

Fig. 1. WHO Growth Standards chart for girls from birth to age 2 years old.

HISTORY AND PHYSICAL

A detailed history should be taken on each patient with attention to the OFC measurement at birth and growth trajectory. A prior history of familial macrocephaly, neonatal or prenatal infection, or prematurity with or without intraventricular hemorrhage is essential to note. Serial OFC measurements should be taken in every office visit up to 24 to 36 months of age as an assessment of the child's head growth velocity.

Physical examination should consist of palpation of the fontanelles and cranial sutures. In addition, providers should note the child's general appearance, facial features, skin, and superficial cranial vessels. Evaluation of a macrocephalic patient also necessitates a complete neurologic examination. A wide, full, and firm fontanelle along with splayed cranial sutures and prominent scalp veins are signs of elevated intracranial pressure. These children warrant expeditious workup with an ultrasound or other cranial imaging and prompt referral to a neurosurgeon. A complete ophthalmologic examination is of the utmost importance in children. Because of the open sutures, infants and young children often do not have signs and symptoms of papilledema; however, they can present with impaired upgaze with the classic "sundowning" appearance that is pathognomonic for elevated intracranial pressure and warrants immediate neurosurgical assessment.

Ensuring that children are meeting their developmental milestones and not regressing is imperative when assessing a child with macrocephaly. Evaluation of nutrition and weight gain is also critical in these patients, as children who have benign macrocephaly will continue to gain weight and meet developmental milestones in a normal progression. A slight delay in motor skill development may be evident in benign familial macrocephaly; however, this is most often still within the normal developmental range.

The classic clinical presentation of a child with pathologic macrocephaly includes a rapidly increasing OFC, a bulging or tense fontanelle, splayed sutures, prominent scalp

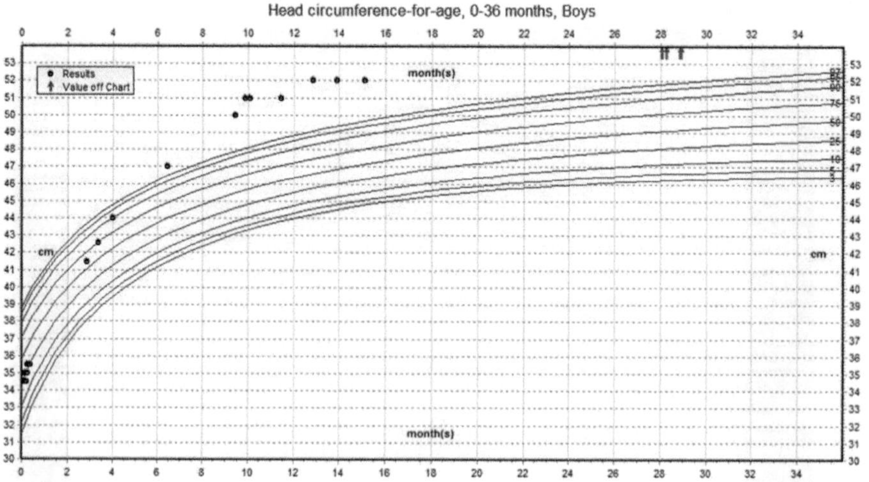

Fig. 2. Head circumference of a patient with untreated congenital hydrocephalus, graphed on the standard CDC growth chart for boys ages 0 to 36 months. This shows increasing head circumference disproportional for patient age. The patient began crossing percentiles at 3 months old and continued to do so until he was off the chart.

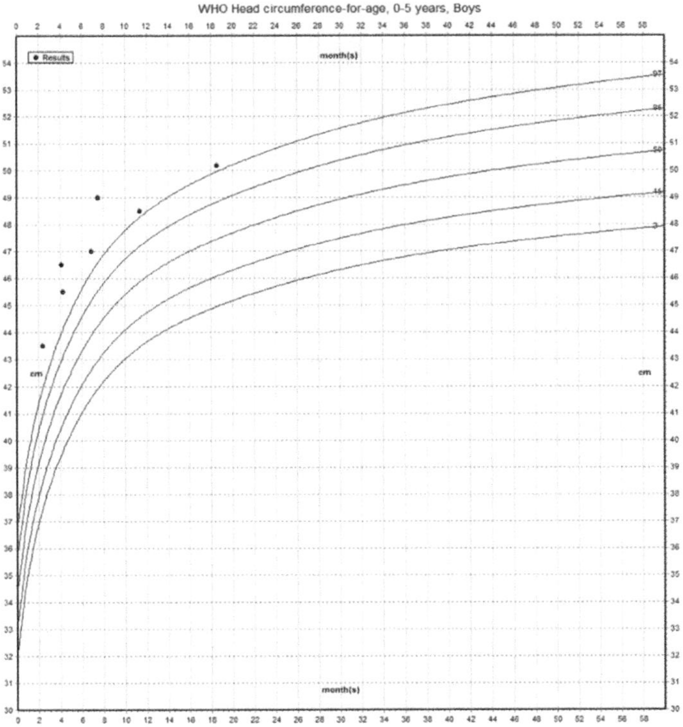

Fig. 3. Head circumference of a patient with familial macrocrania. Head circumference has always been above the 97% line and continues to follow his own trajectory parallel to the 97% line.

veins, sunsetting eyes with paralysis of upgaze with irritability, and failure to thrive. This requires urgent neurosurgical assessment (**Fig. 2**). It is important to distinguish between a child presenting with 1 of the preceding findings in conjunction with a rapidly increasing OFC or stable macrocephaly (**Fig. 3**). Parsing out these differences can aid in the decision-making process of the appropriate next step of clinical evaluation. It is helpful to have an algorithm for how to approach a patient with macrocephaly (**Fig. 4**).

Classic examination in the infant with pathologic macrocephaly

- Rapidly increasing head circumference
- Bulging/tense fontanelle
- Prominent scalp veins
- Paralysis of upgaze
- Failure to thrive

Clinics Care Points

- A detailed family history is critical to assessing a child with macrocephaly, with particular attention paid to abnormalities in parental cranial size.

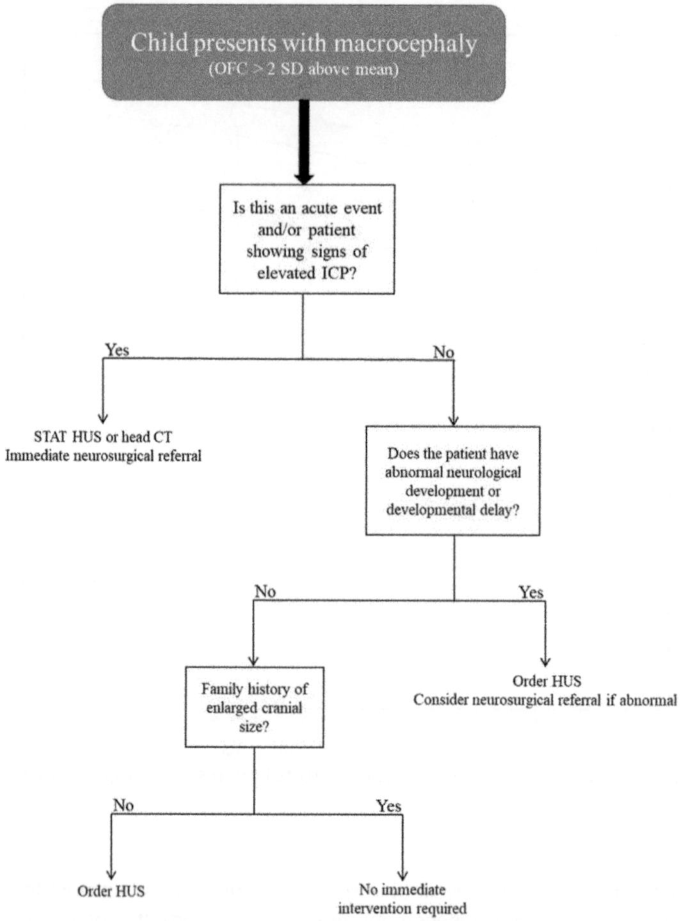

Fig. 4. Demonstration of an algorithm for the approach to the macrocephalic patient in the setting of a primary care provider's office. *Note: algorithm is applicable to infants with an open fontanelle.

- Pediatricians should immediately refer children to neurosurgery if displaying signs and symptoms of increased intracranial pressure.

IMAGING

Head imaging will be required to assess the underlying causative factors of the macrocephaly. The American Academy of Pediatrics Section on Neurosurgery recommends against obtaining CT or MRI scans in developmentally normal, clinically asymptomatic infants with macrocephaly (https://www.choosingwisely.org/societies/american-academy-of-pediatrics-section-on-neurological-surgery/). Retrospective studies have added to a growing body of literature determining when imaging is necessary and what studies are most appropriate to order.[8–13] If the anterior fontanelle is open, head ultrasound (HUS) is the most appropriate option in these children. This modality is noninvasive and cost-effective and is easily performed in an outpatient setting, as no sedation is required. HUS in children with an open anterior fontanelle allows for adequate visualization of most brain structures. A computed tomography (CT) scan can be performed; however, radiation exposure is typically avoided in children whenever possible. Ordering a head CT should be reserved for acute events, instances in which sedation is not possible, or HUS will not provide enough information. MRI can safely be performed, as this test does not expose children to radiation; however, it requires the child to remain still, which is often difficult, necessitating the use of sedation. Certain institutions have integrated a rapid MRI sequence, called a FAST MRI, that provides general information of the major fluid spaces of the brain. Attributable to the speed of this sequence, general anesthesia is not necessary.

Considering the advantages and disadvantages of each imaging study, the provider can develop an algorithm for selecting the proper modality (see **Fig. 4**). A reasonable approach is to potentially use HUS to screen infants initially with open fontanelles. If this study is abnormal or cannot adequately provide information of the underlying intracranial pathology, head CT or brain MRI should be ordered next.[9] If ordering a brain MRI, fast sequence MR can provide rapid evaluation of ventricular caliber and cranial anatomy while avoiding sedation or anesthetics. Full-brain MRI will likely require sedation but can provide high-resolution or volumetric sequences.[9]

Clinics Care Points

- Pediatricians can use HUS to assess macrocephaly in young children with open anterior fontanelles.
- There should be a high threshold for the use of head CT due to early radiation exposure in children.

BENIGN MACROCEPHALY

There are 2 causes of benign macrocephaly: benign familial macrocephaly (BFM) and benign enlargement of the subarachnoid space in infancy (BESSI). These 2 entities do not require any acute intervention and can be adequately assessed by brain ultrasound.

Benign Familial Macrocephaly

Children with BFM will usually have at least 1 parent with a history of macrocephalic features. If the patient is neurologically healthy, meeting developmental milestones, and has a family history of enlarged cranial size, then it is likely that the patient has this hereditary and benign cause of macrocephaly that does not require any treatment. Children with BFM are typically normocephalic at birth and subsequently, their OFC increases to surpass 2.0 SD by 1 year of age.[14] OFC typically stabilizes by approximately age 3 and remains in the upper percentiles thereafter. The inheritance pattern of BFM is unclear but has been proposed as autosomal dominant by several investigators.[15–18] Recognizing BFM in children is traditionally based on diagnostic criteria originally proposed by DeMyer.[16] The criteria include the following: absence of neurocutaneous, craniofacial, or somatic anomalies more closely associated with a syndrome, normal radiographic neuroimaging, and a first-degree relative with well-documented macrocephaly through multiple generations.[16] Clinically, these patients appear asymptomatic, with only a small percentage demonstrating developmental delay.

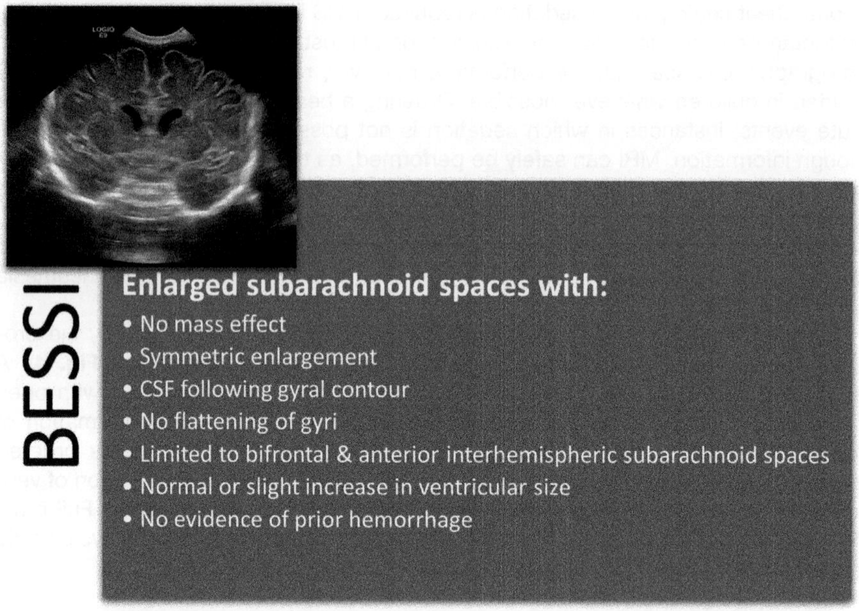

Fig. 5. Neuroimaging findings in a patient with BESSI and an HUS showing the characteristic enlargement of extra-axial spaces.

Benign Enlargement of the Subarachnoid Space in Infancy

BESSI is the most common cause of macrocephaly in infants, with an estimated prevalence as high as 75%. Children typically present as an outpatient with a rapidly increasing head circumference, crossing percentiles with macrocephaly and minimal to no motor and/or developmental decline. The OFC characteristically increases rapidly and then plateaus from 18 to 24 months of age and generally resolves by 2 to 3 years of age. The cause of this is unclear but some have postulated that this revolves around the impaired ability of the arachnoid granulations to reabsorb CSF.[19,20] Imaging usually reveals symmetric enlargement of the subarachnoid fluid spaces along the frontoparietal convexities and widening of the interhemispheric sulcus (**Fig. 5**). This may be in conjunction with mild supratentorial ventriculomegaly and oftentimes bridging veins are visible traversing the subarachnoid fluid spaces. Currently, there is no consensus on the definition of what exactly defines an "enlarged" subarachnoid space.

Clinics Care Points

- BFM should be suspected in a child with macrocephalic parents and a normal neurologic examination who is meeting developmental milestones.

PATHOLOGIC CAUSES OF MACROCEPHALY

Pathologic causes of macrocephaly are numerous and of varying etiology. In this section, we review the most common causes of macrocephaly that may present to the pediatrician's office.

Hydrocephalus

Hydrocephalus is a common cause of treatable macrocephaly, affecting approximately 1 in 1000 children. Patients who present with rapid increases in OFC and associated developmental or neurologic deficits with significant enlargement of the intraventricular spaces fit the diagnostic criteria for hydrocephalus. Ultrasound or other cranial imaging modalities show marked enlargement of the ventricular system with effacement of the gyri and sulci and obliteration of the subarachnoid fluid spaces. This can be an acute or chronic pathophysiological process in which acute obstruction warrants immediate attention and neurosurgical evaluation, as this can quickly become life-threatening if ventricular volume expansion followed by subsequent brain herniation were to occur. The reader is referred to the excellent chapter by Mangano and Patel 'Pediatric Hydrocephalus and the Primary Care Provider' in this issue for more detail.

Abusive Head Trauma

Abusive head trauma (AHT) usually occurs in the first year of life and is an important cause of long-term morbidity and mortality in children. These children do not always present in the acute phase of injury but instead can present in a delayed fashion with macrocephaly. Children with AHT commonly are found to have subdural hematomas (SDH) that are caused by injury to the bridging veins over the surface of the brain secondary to an acceleration/deceleration injury. The classic triad of SDH, retinal hemorrhage, and neurologic dysfunction is pathognomonic for AHT. However, a diagnosis of abusive head trauma does not require each of these findings to be present.[21] Generally, signs of overt trauma are lacking in these children or may be subtle. Repeated injuries can typically create layers of hemorrhage of different ages that is best seen on MRI of the brain. These different layers over time can create the appearance of subdural hygromas and this can progressively increase in size and contribute to increases in OFC across percentile lines.

Causes of macrocephaly

- Benign
  - Benign familial macrocephaly
  - Benign enlargement of the subarachnoid space in infancy
- Pathologic
  - Hydrocephalus
  - Abusive head trauma
  - Venous hypertension due to vascular disease
- Genetic/syndromic
  - Many, with achondroplasia the most common
- Metabolic

Vascular Abnormalities: Vein of Galen Malformation

Vein of Galen malformations (VOGM) are an unusual malformation of blood vessels within the central nervous system.[22,23] Children with a VOGM can present in a delayed fashion with macrocephaly if not acutely ill in the immediate perinatal period from cardiovascular compromise. These children may present with an audible cranial bruit that can be auscultated by placing a stethoscope over the fontanelle. There is typically an increased cerebrovascular blood volume with the development of venous congestion and venous intracranial hypertension.[24,25] If venous congestion persists, and subsequent hydrocephalus persists, this can lead to significant developmental abnormalities. The reader is referred to the excellent article by Smith and Montaser titled 'Intracranial vascular abnormalities in children' for more information on this topic.

Achondroplasia

Patients with achondroplasia have marked macrocephaly at birth that typically worsens in the first year of life. It is important to graph these children on the achondroplasia head circumference chart. These children typically have a large cranium with a hypoplastic skull base with associated frontal bossing and depression of the nasion. In these children, there is stenosis at the jugular venous outflow so there is associated intracranial venous hypertension with resultant ventriculomegaly. It is important to note that these children tend to have delayed motor developmental milestones and that they typically do not need to have the ventriculomegaly addressed. It is important in this patient population to have a low threshold for imaging if there is continued developmental delay past a 6-month window with associated bulbar signs and symptoms, as these children can tend to present with occipitocervical stenosis and compression at the occipitocervical junction.

GENETIC OR SYNDROMIC CAUSES OF MACROCEPHALY

Fragile X Syndrome

Fragile X syndrome is caused by trinucleotide repeat expansion and is the most common cause for mental disability in male individuals.[14] Affected children may present with a long face, prominent jaw, and large ears. These facial features may be absent in some, thus are not required for diagnosis. Similarly, macrocephaly is not always present; however, in infancy the OFC in children with Fragile X is greater than the mean. The usual pattern of OFC growth in children with Fragile X involves an accelerated growth rate that peaks at approximately 30 months of age but then returns to normal by 60 months.[26] Neuroimaging will likely be insignificant in these children. The diagnosis of Fragile X should be considered in the macrocephalic child with a family history of Fragile X who is showing signs of developmental delay in conjunction with the aforementioned facial features.

Neurofibromatosis Type 1

Neurofibromatosis Type 1 (NF1) is caused by a mutation in the *NF1* gene and has an estimated incidence of 1 in 2500 to 3000 individuals.[27] Diagnostic criteria for NF1 requires the presence of 2 of the following entities: inguinal or axillary freckling, neurofibromas, Lisch nodules, café-au-lait spots, optic pathway gliomas (OPGs), osseous lesions, or a first-degree relative with NF1. Macrocephaly is detected in approximately 45% of cases of NF1.[28] OPGs are the most common cerebral tumor in patients affected by NF1 and usually arise within the first decade.[29] If NF1 is suspected in the macrocephalic child, serial MRI studies may be required to monitor for the development of intracranial neoplasms.

PTEN Hamartoma Tumor Syndrome

The term *PTEN* Hamartoma tumor syndrome (PHTS) encompasses a range of genetic syndromes all attributed to aberrant expression of the *PTEN* tumor suppressor gene (namely, Cowden Syndrome, autism with macrocephaly, Bannayan-Riley Ruvalcaba syndrome). These mutations have reported associations in macrocephalic children with developmental delay or autism spectrum disorders.[30] The presence of macrocephaly in children with PHTS is one of the major diagnostic criteria. Neuroimaging findings of children with these syndromes include Chiari I malformations, cerebrovascular malformations, and maldevelopment of the cerebral cortex.

Clinics Care Points

- Although rare, genetic or syndromic causes of macrocephaly should be suspected when signs of more common causes (ie, family history or hydrocephalus) are not present.
- Pediatricians should closely monitor OFC in children with a family history of genetic disorders that can cause macrocephaly.
- Pediatricians should consistently use achondroplasia head circumference charts for children with achondroplasia.

OSSEOUS ABNORMALITIES

Thalassemia Major

Although a very rare diagnosis, children with Thalassemia major can present with macrocephaly secondary to extramedullary hematopoiesis with extensive calvarial thickening and a "hairy" appearance of the cranium on radiographic images.

MEGALENCEPHALY

Megalencephaly is a condition in which the size or weight of the brain is greater than 2 SD above the age-related mean.[16] It is organized into 3 main categories on the basis of its underlying etiology: idiopathic/benign, anatomic, and metabolic.[31] The benign entity is characterized by a large head and an absence of neurologic impairment. Children with benign megalencephaly demonstrate a gradual increase in OFC until 18 months of age when growth becomes stable. Otherwise, these patients will exhibit normal cerebral development.

Anatomic megalencephaly describes a group of disorders characterized by developmental megalencephaly due to an underlying genetic mutation that ultimately affects early neurocellular growth, replication, or apoptosis.[31] This developmental error results in an excess of neurons and therefore more brain tissue than physiologically normal (**Fig. 6**). These disorders typically involve other abnormalities depending on the syndromic characteristics associated with the underlying mutation.

Metabolic megalencephaly occurs secondary to an inborn error of metabolism that causes an excess buildup of metabolic products within the brain (**Fig. 7**). These disorders are broadly categorized into defects of organic acids, metabolic encephalopathies, and lysosomal storage disorders.[31] In addition to macrocephaly, children with defects of organic acids are often neurologically impaired, and in severe variants, may present with debilitating epilepsy.[32–34] Metabolic encephalopathies may result in severe neurologic deficits in addition to megalencephaly, such as hypertonia, seizures, and poor growth. In the setting of Canavan disease, children die within the first decade of life.[35] Alexander disease is a primary genetic astrocyte disorder that results

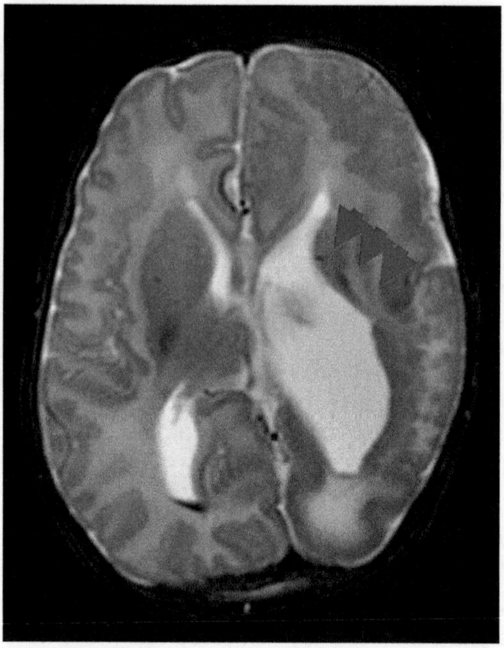

Fig. 6. MRI of a child with macrocephaly demonstrating a classic appearance of hemimegalencephaly. Ventricular enlargement seen in the involved hemisphere (*arrows*).

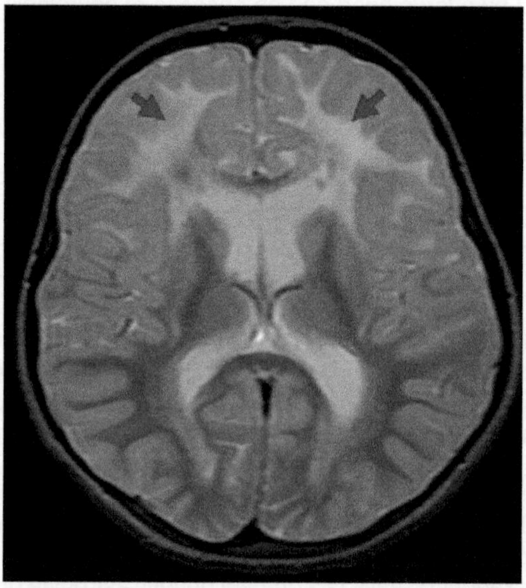

Fig. 7. Image of a child with Alexander disease with the classic abnormality in the periventricular white matter (*arrows*) with associated ventriculomegaly and macrocephaly.

in progressive neurologic impairment, megalencephaly, and characteristic periventricular white matter on neuroimaging (see **Fig. 7**).

Lysosomal storage disorders are often associated with macrocephaly.[31] The severity of the associated neurologic impairment is directly related to the underlying genetic abnormality. For example, Tay-Sachs disease is associated with severe neurologic consequences in which affected children exhibit hypotonia, seizures, and developmental delay due to the toxic accumulation of glycosphingolipids (GM2 ganglioside) in the brain.

SUMMARY

Macrocephaly is a common entity that has a broad spectrum of etiologies. Although some causes of macrocephaly are benign, such as BFM and BESSI, others require thorough evaluation with neurologic examination and neuroimaging. In rare instances, macrocephaly may reflect a genetic or syndromic cause that necessitates referral to a specialist for the long-term care of the patient. If acute pathology is expected, immediate referral is essential to the preservation of the child's neurologic function. Using an algorithmic approach to managing macrocephaly can provide the clinician with a useful decision-making tool and ensure the safest care for their patient.

DISCLOSURE

The authors have nothing to disclose.

REFERENCES

1. Winden KD, Yuskaitis CJ, Poduri A. Megalencephaly and macrocephaly. Semin Neurol 2015;35:277–87.
2. Nellhaus G. Head circumference from birth to 18 years. Practical composite international and interracial graphs. Pediatrics 1968;41:106–14.
3. Weaver D, Christian J. Familial variation of head size and adjustment for parental head circumference. J Pediatr 1980;96:990–4.
4. Jones S, Samanta D. Macrocephaly. In: StatPearls. Treasure Island, FL: StatPearls Publishing Copyright © 2020, StatPearls Publishing LLC; 2020.
5. Ounsted M, Moar V, Scott A. Head circumference charts updated. Arch Dis Child 1985;60:936–9.
6. Rollins J, Collins J, Holden K. United States head circumference growth reference charts: birth to 21 years. J Pediatr 2010;156:907–13.e2.
7. James HE, Perszyk AA, MacGregor TL, et al. The value of head circumference measurements after 36 months of age: a clinical report and review of practice patterns. J Neurosurg Pediatr 2015;16:186.
8. Sampson MA, Berg AD, Huber JN, et al. Necessity of intracranial imaging in infants and children with macrocephaly. Pediatr Neurol 2019;93:21–6.
9. Orrù E, Calloni SF, Tekes A, et al. The child with macrocephaly: differential diagnosis and neuroimaging findings. AJR Am J Roentgenol 2018;210:848–59.
10. Haws ME, Linscott L, Thomas C, et al. A retrospective analysis of the utility of head computed tomography and/or magnetic resonance imaging in the management of benign macrocrania. J Pediatr 2017;182:283–9.e1.

11. Tucker J, Choudhary AK, Piatt J. Macrocephaly in infancy: benign enlargement of the subarachnoid spaces and subdural collections. J Neurosurg Pediatr 2016;18: 16–20.
12. van Wezel-Meijler G, Steggerda SJ, Leijser LM. Cranial ultrasonography in neonates: role and limitations. Semin Perinatol 2010;34:28–38.
13. Missios S, Quebada PB, Forero JA, et al. Quick-brain magnetic resonance imaging for nonhydrocephalus indications. J Neurosurg Pediatr 2008;2:438–44.
14. Williams CA, Dagli A, Battaglia A. Genetic disorders associated with macrocephaly. Am J Med Genet A 2008;146a:2023–37.
15. Alvarez LA, Maytal J, Shinnar S. Idiopathic external hydrocephalus: natural history and relationship to benign familial macrocephaly. Pediatrics 1986;77:901–7.
16. DeMyer W. Megalencephaly: types, clinical syndromes, and management. Pediatr Neurol 1986;2:321–8.
17. Schreier H, Rapin I, Davis J. Familial megalencephaly or hydrocephalus? Neurology 1974;24:232–6.
18. Asch AJ, Myers GJ. Benign familial macrocephaly: report of a family and review of the literature. Pediatrics 1976;57:535–9.
19. Kuruvilla LC. Benign enlargement of sub-arachnoid spaces in infancy. J Pediatr Neurosci 2014;9:129–31.
20. Kendall B, Holland I. Benign communicating hydrocephalus in children. Neuroradiology 1981;21:93–6.
21. Acres MJ, Morris JA. The pathogenesis of retinal and subdural haemorrhage in non-accidental head injury in infancy: assessment using Bradford Hill criteria. Med Hypotheses 2014;82:1–5.
22. Recinos PF, Rahmathulla G, Pearl M, et al. Vein of Galen malformations: epidemiology, clinical presentations, management. Neurosurg Clin N Am 2012;23: 165–77.
23. Starke RM, McCarthy D, Sheinberg D, et al. Genetic drivers of vein of galen malformations. Neurosurgery 2019;85:E205–6.
24. Hoang S, Choudhri O, Edwards M, et al. Vein of Galen malformation. Neurosurg Focus 2009;27:E8.
25. Alvarez H, Garcia Monaco R, Rodesch G, et al. Vein of Galen aneurysmal malformations. Neuroimaging Clin N Am 2007;17:189–206.
26. Chiu S, Wegelin JA, Blank J, et al. Early acceleration of head circumference in children with fragile x syndrome and autism. J Dev Behav Pediatr 2007;28:31–5.
27. Anderson JL, Gutmann DH. Neurofibromatosis type 1. Handb Clin Neurol 2015; 132:75–86.
28. Riccardi VM. Type 1 neurofibromatosis and the pediatric patient. Curr Probl Pediatr 1992;22:66–106 [discussion 7].
29. Tan AP, Mankad K, Gonçalves FG, et al. Macrocephaly: solving the diagnostic dilemma. Top Magn Reson Imaging 2018;27:197–217.
30. Butler MG, Dasouki MJ, Zhou XP, et al. Subset of individuals with autism spectrum disorders and extreme macrocephaly associated with germline PTEN tumour suppressor gene mutations. J Med Genet 2005;42:318–21.
31. Pavone P, Praticò AD, Rizzo R, et al. A clinical review on megalencephaly: a large brain as a possible sign of cerebral impairment. Medicine (Baltimore) 2017;96: e6814.

32. Steenweg ME, Jakobs C, Errami A, et al. An overview of L-2-hydroxyglutarate dehydrogenase gene (L2HGDH) variants: a genotype-phenotype study. Hum Mutat 2010;31:380–90.
33. Jafari P, Braissant O, Bonafé L, et al. The unsolved puzzle of neuropathogenesis in glutaric aciduria type I. Mol Genet Metab 2011;104:425–37.
34. Nyhan WL, Shelton GD, Jakobs C, et al. D-2-hydroxyglutaric aciduria. J Child Neurol 1995;10:137–42.
35. Matalon R, Michals-Matalon K. Canavan disease. In: GeneReviews®[Internet]. Seattle, WA: University of Washington; 2015.

Incidental Intracranial Cysts in Children

Whitney E. Muhlestein, MD, Cormac O. Maher, MD*

KEYWORDS

• Benign • Intracranial • Cyst • Pediatrics

KEY POINTS

- Benign intracranial cysts are usually incidental findings and rarely require treatment or even imaging follow-up in the absence of symptoms.
- These lesions may rarely cause symptoms, usually caused by mass effect on nearby structures.

INTRODUCTION

Neurologic complaints, including headache, developmental delay, seizures, failure to thrive, macrocrania, and nocturnal incontinence, are common in the pediatric practice. For example, 20% of adolescents in the United States report headache one or more times per week, whereas 6% report headaches several times a week or every day.[1,2] Advanced brain imaging is also increasingly available and used for evaluation of these common symptoms. Between 1996 and 2010, MRI examinations increased from 17 per 1000 patients to 65 per 1000 patients, a four-fold increase in MRI use over that period.[3] Ten percent to 20% of children who undergo imaging have radiographic abnormalities, including vascular abnormalities (eg, developmental venous anomalies, telangiectasia), Chiari malformations, lipomas, intracranial cysts, abnormal ventricle size, benign macrocrania, and syrinx, which may or may not explain patient complaints.[4]

In a retrospective review of 225 MRIs obtained on neurologically normal children, four subjects (1.8%) were found to have benign intracranial cyst.[5]

Benign intracranial cysts in the pediatric population are almost universally incidentally discovered in the context of work-up for an unrelated neurologic symptom. Although nearly all of these lesions are asymptomatic, these imaging findings are of great concern to patients and their families. The intersection of common neurologic

The authors report no commercial or financial conflicts of interest.
Department of Neurosurgery, University of Michigan, 1500 East Medical Center Drive, SPC 5337, Ann Arbor, MI 48109, USA
* Corresponding author.
E-mail address: cmaher@med.umich.edu

Pediatr Clin N Am 68 (2021) 775–782
https://doi.org/10.1016/j.pcl.2021.04.005
0031-3955/21/

symptoms with common radiologic findings can trigger a cascade of additional testing and evaluation, often driven by parental anxiety, which may ultimately result, in rare circumstances, in inappropriate surgical intervention.[6]

Here, we describe three common benign intracranial cysts found in the pediatric population: (1) arachnoid cysts, (2) choroid cysts, and (3) pineal cysts. A good understanding of the natural history and clinical course of these lesions can help clinicians to provide reassurance to families and also assist clinicians in determining when a referral for neurosurgical evaluation is appropriate.

ARACHNOID CYSTS

Arachnoid cysts are cerebrospinal fluid–filled collections that form within the arachnoid membrane. With increasing use of intracranial imaging, identification of these lesions, which is almost always incidental, is becoming more frequent.[5,7,8] On MRI, arachnoid cysts tend to be well-circumscribed, can exert mass effect on local structures, and have characteristics consistent with cerebrospinal fluid (hyperintense on T2-weighted sequences and without FLAIR signal) (**Fig. 1**). Arachnoid cysts are common intracranial lesions, with prevalence estimates in the general population range from 1.1% to 2.6% depending on study population and imaging modality.[7,9,10] There are up to 1.95 million children in the United States with arachnoid cysts on imaging. Arachnoid cysts are most commonly located in the anterior aspect of the middle fossa, the cerebellopontine angle, the retrocerebellar space, or the suprasellar space, but can present adjacent to any arachnoid membrane (see **Fig. 1**A–D).[5]

The natural history of arachnoid cysts is variable, with reports of spontaneous enlargement, shrinking, and even complete resolution, but the clinical course is almost universally benign, requiring no surgical intervention in most cases.[7,11–17] Most cysts do not grow over time, especially in patients older than 5 years of age at the time of diagnosis.[7] Although most do not require treatment, the exception to this rule is arachnoid cysts that cause clear neurologic symptoms that are localized specifically to the cyst.[18–20] This most frequently occurs with arachnoid cysts in the suprasellar space, which can manifest with clinically meaningful symptoms caused by mass effect on

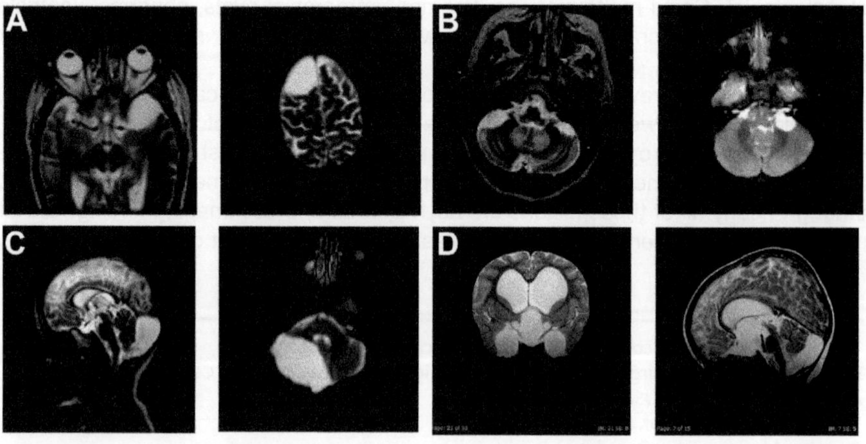

Fig. 1. Typical radiographic appearance of arachnoid cysts. T2-weighted MRIs demonstrating typical (*A*) temporal and convexity arachnoid cysts, (*B*) cerebellopontine angle arachnoid cyst, (*C*) retrocerebellar arachnoid cyst, and (*D*) coronal and sagittal views of the same suprasellar arachnoid cyst with hydrocephalus.

local structures.[21] These rare lesions account for approximately 1.6% of all arachnoid cysts, and can occasionally lead to loss of vision caused by compression of the optic nerves, endocrine abnormalities caused by compression of the pituitary stalk, or hydrocephalus caused by obstruction of the ventricular system.[7,22,23] Pediatricians caring for children with suprasellar cysts should be vigilant in monitoring patients for vision changes, headaches with associated lethargy and nausea/vomiting, and precocious or delayed puberty, which may suggest that a lesion is symptomatic. Symptomatic suprasellar arachnoid cysts are often managed using endoscopic surgical approaches for cyst fenestration.[24]

Arachnoid cysts can rarely undergo intracyst hemorrhage or rupture, leading to the development of acute subdural hygromas. In retrospective studies, risk of cyst rupture was associated with cyst size greater than 5 cm and with head trauma.[25–27] Because of these findings, some have advised that children with arachnoid cysts are not allowed to play contact sports or have even recommended prophylactic surgery to avoid perceived complications of cyst rupture.[28] Subsequent studies have demonstrated, however, no substantially increased risk of long-term neurologic sequelae after head injury for most children with arachnoid cysts compared with those without cysts.[25–30] Furthermore, acute subdural hygromas associated with arachnoid cysts, although often symptomatic, can often be managed expectantly, avoiding surgical intervention.[27] Finally, prophylactic surgery can in and of itself lead to the development of iatrogenic subdural hygromas.[18,31,32] For all of these reasons, it is our practice not to recommend prophylactic fenestration of arachnoid cysts in children who play contact sports nor to bar children with arachnoid cysts from participating in contact sports.

Because greater than 98% of arachnoid cysts follow a benign course, follow-up imaging is not generally indicated. Referral for neurosurgical evaluation is warranted in the rare case of arachnoid cysts causing clear neurologic symptoms that are localized to the cyst location.

Clinics Care Points

- Arachnoid cysts are almost always incidentally discovered and have a benign course.
- When symptomatic, symptoms arise from compression of surrounding structures, particularly in the suprasellar space. This can result in hydrocephalus, vision changes, and endocrine abnormalities.
- There is no evidence to suggest that children with arachnoid cysts are at substantially higher risk from head trauma than their peers without arachnoid cysts and therefore should not be barred from participating in sports.

CHOROID PLEXUS CYSTS

Choroid plexus cysts are fluid-filled collections found associated with the choroid plexus of the ventricular system. Choroid plexus cysts are most commonly encountered as incidental findings on prenatal or neonatal ultrasound. Prevalence estimates for choroid plexus cysts range from 0.6% to 2.3%.[33–35] These cysts are usually isolated findings; however, in the presence of other anomalies, choroid plexus cysts may serve as a marker of underlying fetal aneuploidy, particularly trisomy 18.[35–37]

Isolated choroid plexus cysts almost always have a benign course and regress during the third trimester or shortly after birth. Although choroid plexus cysts can exert mass effect and cause hydrocephalus, it is unusual for a choroid plexus cyst to become clinically important and require treatment.[36] Choroid plexus cysts resulting in hydrocephalus certainly warrant neurosurgical referral, but there is no clear evidence to support neurosurgical referral or surveillance imaging for smaller, incidentally discovered choroidal cysts.[4,38,39]

Clinics Care Points

- Only choroid plexus cysts resulting in hydrocephalus require neurosurgical referral or surveillance imaging.

PINEAL CYSTS

Pineal cysts are fluid-filled spaces within the pineal gland, an endocrine organ found behind the third ventricle. The prevalence of pineal cysts increases with age during childhood but decreases again during adulthood, with prevalence estimates of 1.9% of children and 1.1% to 4.3% of adults depending on the age of the population studied.[40–48] The natural history of pineal cysts is generally benign. Most pineal cysts grow during childhood and then involute in adulthood (**Fig. 2**).[49,50] Regardless of stage of natural history, pineal cysts are rarely symptomatic and almost never require surgical intervention.

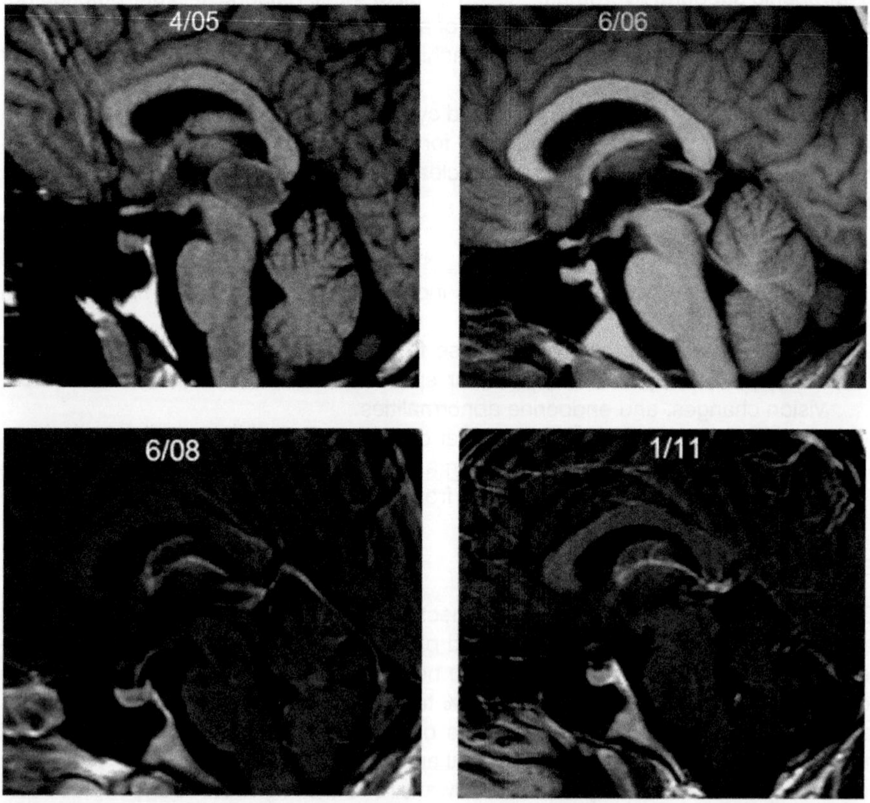

Fig. 2. Natural history of pineal cysts. Sagittal, T1-weighted MRIs demonstrating the natural course on surveillance imaging of a pineal cyst in the same patient, with interval involution and regression over the course of 6 years. Dates are indicated at the top of each image.

Rarely, large pineal cysts (typically >2 cm) may present with hydrocephalus through obstruction of the cerebral aqueduct, a channel that connects the third and fourth ventricles.[50–53] Hydrocephalus in children may present with headaches, nausea/vomiting, lethargy, and upgaze palsy. Additionally, large pineal cysts have also been reported to cause gaze palsies and Parinaud syndrome caused by brainstem compression.[50,53–57] The development of clinically significant symptoms remains rare, however, and even very large, asymptomatic pineal cysts can be managed expectantly.[41,43,47–49,58]

Pineal cysts are not infrequently diagnosed in the work-up for headache in children. Although there are reports of surgical management of pineal cysts for chronic headache, most surgeons would not consider headache without associated radiographic hydrocephalus as an indication for surgical resection.[52,53,59,60]

For the pediatrician, small pineal cysts likely do not require referral to a neurosurgeon or surveillance imaging. Patients with very large and potentially symptomatic cysts (eg, clinical and/or radiographic concerns for hydrocephalus or brainstem compression) warrant neurosurgical evaluation, but are unlikely to require surgical intervention.

Clinical Care Point

- Typically, only large pineal cysts (>2 cm) are symptomatic, potentially causing hydrocephalus or brainstem compression. However, even most large pineal cysts are asymptomatic and require no surgical intervention.

SUMMARY

As the use of intracranial imaging rises, clinicians are increasingly likely to diagnose pediatric patients with benign intracranial cysts. In general, benign intracranial cysts are asymptomatic and incidentally discovered and do not typically require follow-up imaging in the absence of symptoms. When benign intracranial cysts cause symptoms, it is typically through direct compression of nearby structures, including the ventricular system and the brainstem. Symptomatic lesions are rare, however, and even symptomatic lesions do not necessarily require surgical intervention.

REFERENCES

1. Kernick D, Reinhold D, Campbell JL. Impact of headache on young people in a school population. Br J Gen Prct 2009;59(566):678–81.
2. Kernick D, Campbell J. Measuring the impact of headache in children: a critical review of the literature. Cephalgia 2009;29(1):3–16.
3. Smith-Bindman R, Miglioretti DL, Johnson E, et al. Use of diagnostic imaging studies and associated radiation exposure for patients enrolled in large integrated health care systems, 1996-2010. JAMA 2012;307(22):2400–9.
4. Maher CO, Piatt JH. Incidental findings on brain and spine imaging in children. Pediatrics 2015;135(4):e1084–96.
5. Kim BS, Illes J, Kaplan RT, et al. Incidental findings on pediatric MR images of the brain. AJNR Am J Neuroradiol 2002;23:1674–7.
6. Mold JW, Stein HF. The cascade effect in the clinical care of patients. N Engl J Med 1986;314(8):512–4.
7. Al-Holou WN, Yew AY, Boomsaad ZE, et al. Prevalence and natural history of arachnoid cysts in children. J Neurosurg Pediatr 2010;5:578–85.
8. Weber F, Knopf H. Incidental findings in magnetic resonance imaging of the brains of healthy young men. J Neurol Sci 2006;240:81–4.

9. Rogers AJ, Maher CO, Schunk JE, et al. Incidental findings in children with blunt head trauma evaluated with cranial CT scans. Pedatrics 2013;132:e356–63.
10. Vernooij MW, Ikram MA, Tanghe HL, et al. Incidental findings on brain MRI in the general population. N Engl J Med 2007;357:1821–8.
11. Go KG, Houthoff HJm Hartsuiker J, Blaauw EH, et al. Fluid secretion in arachnoid cysts as a clue to cerebrospinal fluid absorption at the arachnoid granulation. J Neurosurg 1986;65:642–8.
12. Golash A, Mitchell G, Mallucci C, et al. Prenatal diagnosis of suprasellar arachnoid cyst and postnatal endoscopic treatment. Childs Nerv Syst 2001;17:739–42.
13. Rao G, Anderson RC, Feldstein NA, et al. Expansion of arachnoid cysts in children: report of two cases with review of the literature. J Neurosurg 2005;102(3 Suppl):314–7.
14. Russo N, Domeniccucci M, Beccaglia MR, et al. Spontaneous reduction of intracranial arachnoid cysts: a complete review. Br J Neurosurgy 2008;22:626–9.
15. Seizeur R, Forlodou P, Coustans M, et al. Spontaneous resolution of arachnoid cysts: review and features of an unusual case. Acta Neurochir (Wien) 2007; 149:75–8.
16. Thomas BP, Pearson MM, Wushensky CA. Active spontaneous decompression of a suprasellar-prepontine arachnoid cyst detected with routine magnetic resonance imaging. Case report. J Neurosurgy Pediatr 2009;3:70–2.
17. Wbere R, Voit T, Lumenta C, et al. Spontaneous regression of a temporal arachnoid cyst. Childs Nerv Syst 1991;7:414–5.
18. Fewel ME, Levy ML, McComb JG. Surgical treatment of 95 children with 102 intracranial arachnoid cysts. Pediatr Neurosurg 1996;25(4):165–73.
19. Gangemi M, Seneca V, Colella G, et al. Endoscopy versus microsurgical cyst excision and shunting for treating intracranial arachnoid cysts. J Neurosurg Pediatr 2011;8(2):158–64.
20. Kan JK, Lee Ks, Lee IW, et al. Shunt-independent surgical treatment of middle cranial fossa arachnoid cysts in children. Chils Nerv Syst 2000;16(2):111–6.
21. Ciricillo SF, Cogen PH, Harsh GR, et al. Intracranial arachnoid cysts in children. A comparison of the effects of fenestration and shunting. J Neurosurg 1991;74: 230–5.
22. Faris AA, Bale GF, Cannon B. Arachnoidal cyst of the third ventricle with precocious puberty. South Med J 1971;64:1139–42.
23. Hoffman HJ, Hendrick EB, Humphreys RP, et al. Investigation and management of suprasellar arachnoid cysts. J Neurosurg 1982;57:597–602.
24. Maher CO, Goumnerova L. The effectiveness of ventriculocystocisternostomy for suprasellar arachnoid cysts. J Neurosurg Pediatr 2011;7:64–72.
25. Rogers AJ, Kuppermann N, Thelen AE, et al. Children with arachnoid cysts who sustain blunt head trauma: injury mechanisms and outcomes. Acad Emerg Med 2016;23:358–61.
26. Albuquerque FC, Giannotta SL. Arachnoid cyst rupture producing subdural hygroma and intracranial hypertension: case reports. Neurosurgery 1997;41: 951–5 [discussion 5-6].
27. Maher CO, Garton HJ, Al-Holou WN, et al. Management of subdural hygromas associated with arachnoid cysts. J Neurosurg Pediatr 2013;12:434–43.
28. Cress M, Kestle JR, Holubkov R, et al. Risk factors for pediatric arachnoid cyst rupture/hemorrhage: a case-control study. Neurosurgery 2013;72:716–22.
29. Tamburrini G, Dal Gabbro M, Di Rocco C. Sylvian fissure arachnoid cysts: a survey on their diagnostic workout and practical management. Childs Nerv Syst 2008;24:593–604.

30. Strahle J, Selzer B, Geh N, et al. Sports participation with arachnoid cysts. J Neurosurg Pediatr 2016;17:410–7.
31. Di Rocco C. Sylvian fissure arachnoid cysts: we do operate on them but should it be done? Childs Nerv Syst 2008;24(5):593–604.
32. Tamburrini G, Caldarelli M, Massimi L, et al. Subdural hygroma: an unwanted result of Sylvian arachnoid cyst marsupialization. Childs Nerv Syst 2003;19(3): 159–65.
33. Geary M, Patel S, Lamon R. Isolated choroid plexus cysts and association with fetal aneuploidy in an unselected population. Ultrasound Obstet Gynecol 1997; 10(3):171–3.
34. Digiovanni Lm, Guinlan MP, Verp MS. Choroid plexus cysts: infant and early childhood developmental outcome. Obstet Gynecol 1997;90(2):191–4.
35. Reinsch RC. Choroid plexus cysts – association with trisomy: prospective review of 16,059 patients. Am J Obstet Gynecol 1997;176(6):1381–3.
36. Naeini RM, Yoo JH, Hunter JV. Spectrum of choroid plexus lesions in children. AJR Am J Roentgenol 2009;192:32–40.
37. Becker S, Niemann G, Schoning M, et al. Clinically significant persistence and enlargement of an antenatally diagnosed isolated choroid plexus cyst. Ultrasound Obstet Gynecol 2002;20(6):620–2.
38. Spennato P, Chiaramonte C, Cicala D, et al. Acute triventricular hydrocephalus caused by choroid plexus cysts: a diagnostic and neurosurgical challenge. Neurosurg Focus 2016;41(5):E9.
39. Filardi T, Finn L, Gabikan P, et al. Treatment of intermittent obstructive hydrocephalus secondary to a choroid plexus cyst. J Neurosurg Pediatr 2009;4(6):571–4.
40. Di Vaostanzo A, Tedeschi G, Di Salle F, et al. Pineal cysts: an incidental MRI finding? J Neurol Neurosurg Psychiatry 1993;56:207–8.
41. Golzarian J, Baleriaux D, Bank WO, et al. Pineal cyst: normal or pathological? Neuroradiology 1993;35:251–3.
42. Lee DH, Norman D, Newton TH. MR imaging of pineal cysts. J Comput Assist Tomogr 1987;11:586–90.
43. Mamourian AC, Towfighi J. Pineal cysts: MR imaging. AJNR Am J Neuroradiol 1986;7:1081–6.
44. Petitcolin V, Garcier JM, Mohammedi R, et al. [Prevalence and morphology of pineal cysts discovered at pituitary MRI: review of 1844 examinations]. J Radiol 2002;83:141–5 (Fr).
45. Sawamura Y, Ikeda J, Ozawa M, et al. Magnetic resonance images reveal a high incidence of asymptomatic pineal cysts in young women. Neurosurgery 1995; 37:11–6.
46. Sener RN. The pineal gland: a comparative MR imaging study in children and adults with respect to normal anatomical variations and pineal cysts. Pediatr Radiol 1995;25:245–8.
47. Al-Holou WN, Garton HJL, Muraszko KM, et al. Prevalence of pineal cysts in children and young adults. J Neurosurg Pediatr 2009;4:230–6.
48. Al-Holou WN, Maher CO, Muraszko KM, et al. The natural history of pineal cysts in children and young adults. J Neurosurg Pedaitr 2010;5(2):162–6.
49. Al-Holou WN, Terman SW, Kiburg C, et al. Prevalence and natural history of pineal cysts in adults. J Neurosurg 2011;115(6):1106–14.
50. Wisoff JH, Epstein F. Surgical management of symptomatic pineal cysts. J Neurosurg 1992;77(6):896–900.
51. Tapp E, Huxley M. The histological appearance of the human pineal gland from puberty to old age. J Pathol 1972;108(2):137–44.

52. Fleege MA, Miller GM, Fletcher GP, et al. Benign glial cysts of the pineal gland: unusual imaging characteristics with histologic correlation. AJNR Am J Neuroradiol 1994;15(1):161–6.
53. Klein P, Rubinstein LJ. Benign symptomatic glial cysts of the pinal gland: a report of seven cases and review of the literature. J Neurol Neurosurg Psychiatry 1989; 52(8):991–5.
54. Mandera M, Marcol W, Bierzynaska-Macyszyn G, et al. Pineal cysts in childhood. Childs Nerv Syst 2003;19(10–11):750–5.
55. Fain JS, Tomlinson FH, Scheithauer BW, et al. Symptomatic glial cysts of the pineal gland. J Neurosurg 1994;80(3):454–60.
56. Mena H, Armonda RA, Ribas JL, et al. Nonneoplastic pineal cysts: a clinicopathologic study of twenty-one cases. Ann Daign Pathol 1997;1(1):11–8.
57. Michielsen G, Benoit Y, Baert E, et al. Symptomatic pineal cysts: clinical manifestations and management. Acta Neurochir (Wien) 2002;144(3):233–42 [discussion 242].
58. Barboriak DP, Leel L, Provenzale JM. Serial MR imaging of pineal cysts: implications for natural history and follow-up. AJR Am J Roentgenol 2001;176(3):737–43.
59. Gore PA, Gonzalez LF, Rekate HL, et al. Endoscopic supracerebellar infratentorial approach for pineal cyst resection: technical case report. Neurosurgery 2008; 62(3 suppl 1):108–9 [discussion 109].
60. Stevens QE, Colen CB, Ham SD, et al. Delayed lateral rectus palsy following resection of a pineal cyst in sitting position: direct or indirect compressive phenomenon? J Child Nuerol 2007;22(12):1411–4.

Chiari Malformation in Children

Gregory W. Albert, MD, MPH

KEYWORDS

• Chiari malformation • Syringomyelia • Scoliosis

KEY POINTS

- Chiari malformation type 1 (CM1) is often found incidentally.
- Most patients with CM1 will not require surgical intervention.
- Patients with CM1 who have symptoms or signs referable to CM1 or who have a syrinx are candidates for surgical intervention.
- Pediatric patients with CM1 should be referred to a pediatric neurosurgeon for evaluation.

DESCRIPTION/CLASSIFICATION

Hans Chiari, an Austrian pathologist, was the first to describe the conditions that now bear his name. His initial manuscript, published in 1891, described Chiari malformations 1, 2, and 3. In an 1896 publication, Dr Chiari postulated on the pathogenesis of Chiari malformations and described Chiari 4 malformation. In reality, Chiari 2 malformation, which is associated with myelomeningocele, had been previously described in the seventeenth century by Nicholas Tulp, a Dutch anatomist. In 1894, Dr Julius Arnold also described a case of Chiari 2 malformation associated with myelomeningocele. Two of his students later used the term "Arnold-Chiari malformation" in 1907 to describe 4 patients with myelomeningocele and hindbrain herniation. Now, when used at all, Arnold-Chiari malformation only refers to Chiari 2 malformation associated with myelomeningocele.[1]

Classically, the Chiari malformations are classified into 4 types: Chiari types 1, 2, 3, and 4. Chiari malformation type 1 (CM1) is by far the most common type of Chiari malformation. CM1 is characterized by extension of the cerebellar tonsils by at least 5 mm below the foramen magnum. Chiari malformation type 2 (CM2) is found in patients with myelomeningocele and involves a greater degree of hindbrain displacement, which may include the cerebellar vermis, brainstem, and fourth ventricle. Chiari malformation types 3 (CM3) and 4 (CM4) are extremely rare. CM3 is an encephalocele of the

The author has no commercial or financial conflicts of interest nor funding source for this article.
Arkansas Children's Hospital, 1 Children's Way, Slot 838, Little Rock, AR 72202, USA
E-mail address: galbert2@uams.edu

Pediatr Clin N Am 68 (2021) 783–792
https://doi.org/10.1016/j.pcl.2021.04.015
pediatric.theclinics.com

posterior fossa with herniation of portions of the cerebellum and brainstem into the encephalocele sac. CM4 is aplasia or hypoplasia of the cerebellum.[2]

Over the years, largely thanks to the work of Dr Jerry Oakes and his colleagues, 2 additional types of Chiari malformation have been described and are now widely accepted in the pediatric neurosurgical community. Chiari malformation 0 (CM0) is rare. Patients with CM0 have syringomyelia but no displacement of the cerebellar tonsils. They may have caudal displacement of the cervicomedullary junction and often have intradural obstruction of cerebrospinal fluid (CSF) flow. In patients with CM0, the syrinx resolves with posterior fossa decompression and restoration of CSF flow at the cervicomedullary junction.[3,4] Chiari malformation 1.5 is a severe variant of CM1 in which there is caudal displacement of the brainstem in addition to the cerebellar tonsils below the foramen magnum.[5]

The types of Chiari malformation are summarized in **Table 1**. Each type of Chiari malformation is really a different condition, not stages of a single pathologic process. The remainder of this monograph focuses on CM1, as this is the most commonly encountered type. The same principles of diagnosis and management apply to CM1.5.

EPIDEMIOLOGY

Most of the patients diagnosed with CM1 are found to have this condition as an incidental finding on imaging performed for other reasons. Because most of the patients with CM1 are asymptomatic, determining the true prevalence of this condition has proved difficult. Attempts at estimating the population prevalence have used large databases of brain and spine imaging performed for a variety of conditions. These studies suggest that 1% to 3.6% of children have CM1.[6,7]

Deciding how many patients are truly symptomatic from CM1 is challenging, for reasons that will become clear in the later discussion of symptoms and signs. Although patients presenting for neurosurgical consultation are a selected group, these data can provide some insight into the prevalence of symptomatic versus asymptomatic CM1. In our experience, only 15% of patients seen in the pediatric neurosurgery clinic with CM1 are deemed symptomatic from CM1 and undergo surgery.[8]

There is no gender predilection for CM1.[7] Age at initial neurosurgical evaluation is roughly 8 years on average across multiple studies. However, the range of ages is very large.[9–11] Therefore, no strong conclusion can be made regarding age and CM1 diagnosis.

Table 1
Summary of types of Chiari malformations

Chiari Malformation Type	Description
0	Syrinx without caudal descent of cerebellar tonsils. Syrinx resolves with posterior fossa decompression
1	Caudal displacement of the cerebellar tonsils at least 5 mm below the foramen magnum
1.5	Caudal displacement of the brainstem and cerebellar tonsils below the foramen magnum
2	Caudal displacement of hindbrain structures below the foramen magnum in a patient with myelomeningocele
3	Posterior fossa encephalocele containing brainstem and cerebellar tissue
4	Aplasia or hypoplasia of the cerebellum

REVIEW OF SYMPTOMS AND PHYSICAL EXAMINATION FINDINGS

The most common symptom of CM1 is headache, found roughly in 80% of patients.[12] However, headache is a very common diagnosis in general, and therefore care must be taken in distinguishing "Chiari headache" from "non-Chiari headache." CM1 causes headache by preventing changes in CSF flow at the foramen magnum. Normally, the transient elevation in intracranial pressure (ICP) that occurs with Valsalva maneuvers is relieved by displacement of the CSF from the cranium to the spine. Although patients with CM1 do not typically have hydrocephalus or elevated ICP, the dynamic change in CSF flow during Valsalva can be impaired by the displaced cerebellar tonsils at the foramen magnum. In 1980, Williams reported on 2 patients with CM1 and headaches whose ventricular and spinal CSF pressures were measured invasively before and after CM1 decompression. Preoperatively, both patients had "craniospinal pressure dissociation," which resolved after Chiari decompression.[13] More recently, MRI has been used to demonstrate correlation with obstructed CSF flow and occipital headache as well as correlation between obstructed CSF flow preoperatively and resolution of headache following surgery.[14] Headaches that are reliably attributable to CM1 occur at the back of the head, are precipitated by Valsalva maneuvers, and are short in duration.[12] It has been demonstrated with regard to headaches that brevity, severity, precipitation by Valsalva maneuvers, and posterior location are all positive predictors of headache resolution following Chiari decompression.[15] Other headache types (migraine, tension headaches, cluster headaches, sinus headaches, etc) are often seen in children with CM1 because they are common in the general population. These headaches are not attributable to CM1 and are not expected to improve with surgery for CM1.

Other signs and symptoms of CM1 are much less common than headache and can be broadly classified into 3 categories: brainstem dysfunction, cerebellar dysfunction, and spinal cord dysfunction.[12] Each of these categories will be considered in turn.

Brainstem Dysfunction

Sleep apnea and dysphagia both have well-known associations with CM1. Oropharyngeal dysfunction, presenting as sleep-disordered breathing and/or dysphagia, is a common presentation in children younger than 3 years.[16] Studies looking at cohorts of children with CM1 have found rates of sleep-disordered breathing of 24% to 60%. The sleep apnea may be obstructive, central, or mixed. The mechanisms by which CM1 leads to central sleep apnea (CSA) or obstructive sleep apnea (OSA) are not fully understood but likely relate to dysfunction of the medullary respiratory center (CSA) and cranial nerves IX and X (OSA), both of which are in the anatomic vicinity of the ectopic cerebellar tonsils that are the hallmark of CM1.[17,18]

CM1 malformation also causes dysphagia. Patients with neurogenic dysphagia may present with coughing and choking while eating, longer feeding times, regurgitation into the nasal cavity, recurrent aspiration pneumonia, weight loss, failure to thrive, and absent gag reflex.[19] In a large study of 500 children who all had Chiari decompression performed, 20 (4%) had reported dysphagia.[20] A study of 11 surgical adult patients evaluated swallowing function prospectively in a comprehensive fashion. Four patients (36%) had dysphagia, 2 of which were mild cases.[21] The pathophysiology of neurogenic dysphagia secondary to CM1 is likely multifactorial, potentially involving all phases of swallowing. The medullary swallowing center may be dysfunctional. In addition, function of the afferent and efferent nerves of the oropharynx and esophagus may be impaired leading to difficulty with initiating swallowing, protecting the airway during swallowing, and peristalsis of the esophagus.[19]

Cerebellar Dysfunction

Ataxia has been reported in 9.5% of pediatric patients with nonoperative CM1.[22] Cerebellar signs or ataxia have been reported in up to 40% of patients in a surgical series of CM1.[23] Signs of cerebellar dysfunction may include ataxic gait, clumsiness with hands, and nystagmus.[12] Although cerebellar dysfunction is widely consider to be associated with CM1, it has not been systematically studied. Whether the cerebellar dysfunction is truly caused by the CM1 is less clear, and only 38% of patients with ataxia as a presenting symptom improved with surgery.[23]

Spinal Cord Dysfunction and Scoliosis

CM1 is a well-known cause of syrinx (syringomyelia, hydromyelia, syringohydromyelia) formation (**Fig. 1**). In their series of 500 pediatric patients treated surgical for CM1, Tubbs and colleagues reported a 57% prevalence of syrinx. The plurality of these were holocord syringes (39.3%). The remaining regions of the spinal cord involved, in decreasing order of involvement, were cervicothoracic junction (24.9%), cervical (15.4%), thoracic (14.7%), and lumbar (3.5%).[20] In a large study of 14,116 pediatric patients undergoing MRI for a variety of indications, 3.6% had CM1. Of the patients with CM1, 23% also had a syrinx, and 86% of the syringes were located in the cervical spinal cord.[7] The pathophysiology of CM1-related syrinx is an area of debate and beyond the scope of this review.

Although a syrinx may be asymptomatic, larger syringes do cause myelopathy. One classic, but infrequently seen, finding is dissociated sensory loss with loss of pain and temperature sensation in a "cape-like" distribution (affecting arms and upper trunk but not lower trunk or legs) but preservation of sensation to light touch and proprioception,

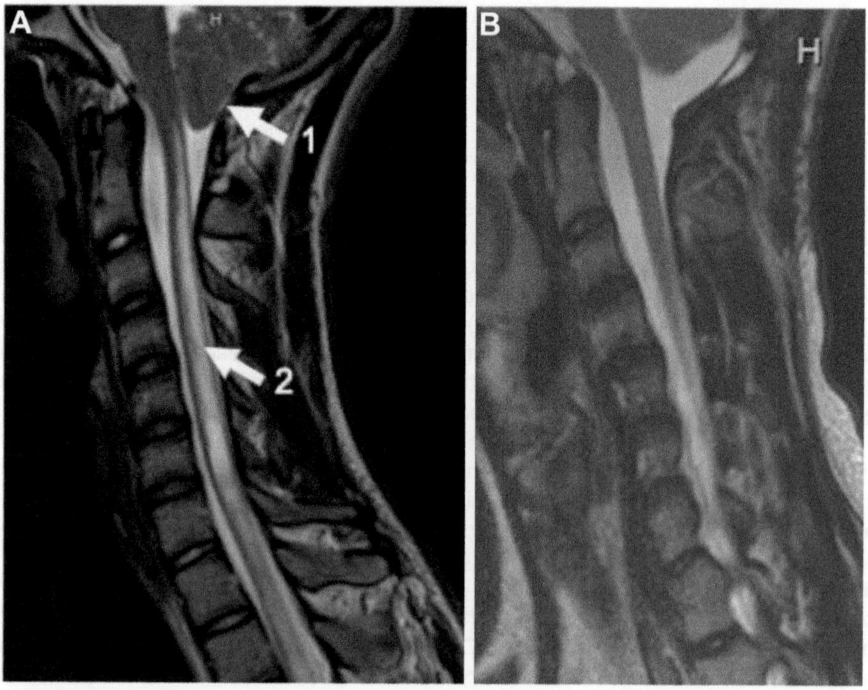

Fig. 1. (*A*) A 16-year-old boy with Chiari malformation type 1 (*arrow 1*) and syringomyelia (*arrow 2*). (*B*) Postoperative MRI reveals decompression of the Chiari malformation and resolution of the syrinx.

which occurs due to interruption of the crossing spinothalamic fibers in the spinal cord. Other findings include weakness of the extremities, hyperreflexia, and presence of a Babinski response.[2] Rarely, the syrinx will extend into the brainstem (syringobulbia), leading to cranial nerve dysfunction (facial numbness, facial weakness, impaired ocular motility, dysphagia, tongue weakness, tongue atrophy).

Patients with CM1 and a syrinx are at increased risk of scoliosis.[24] The prevalence of scoliosis in patients with CM1 without a syrinx is the same as the general population, suggesting that CM1 alone is not a cause of scoliosis. However, the prevalence of scoliosis in patients with CM1 and a syrinx is markedly elevated, suggesting that the syrinx is the cause of scoliosis, not CM1 directly.[25] The prevalence of scoliosis in pediatric patients with CM1 and syrinx is approximately 30%.[24] This finding favors the theory that asymmetric effects of the syrinx on the anterior horn cells of the spinal cord leads to asymmetric paraspinal muscle weakness and subsequent scoliosis.[26] Patients may also have a syrinx without obvious CM1. In these cases, the syrinx may be idiopathic, caused by a spinal cord tumor, posttraumatic, or represent CM0 (discussed earlier). Regardless of the cause, patients with a syrinx should be evaluated by a neurosurgeon.

Associated Conditions

Most patients with CM1 do not have an underlying genetic condition. However, several conditions have been associated with CM1 including, but not limited to, neurofibromatosis type 1, growth hormone deficiency, hydrocephalus, basilar invagination, Klippel-Feil syndrome, and multisuture or syndromic craniosynostosis.[2,20] Ehlers-Danlos syndrome and other hypermobility disorders have also been associated with CM1.[27] A detailed discussion of these associations is beyond the scope of this review.

Clinics Care Points

Symptoms of Chiari I malformation that pediatricians should be aware of include

- Headache precipitated by Valsalva maneuvers (most common)
- Obstructive, central, or mixed sleep apnea
- Dysphagia
- Scoliosis

DIAGNOSIS AND TREATMENT

The 2 primary questions that a neurosurgeon considers when evaluating a patient with CM1 are

1. Is surgery indicated for this patient?
2. If surgery is indicated, what operation should be performed?

Indications for Chiari Decompression

As indicated earlier, most of the patients with CM1 are diagnosed incidentally and do not require surgical intervention. The actual rate of symptomatic versus asymptomatic CM1 is difficult to assess due to heterogeneity in the literature. However, in our own experience, only 15% of patients with CM1 evaluated by a pediatric neurosurgeon were thought to be symptomatic from CM1 and had surgery performed.[8] However, surveys of pediatric neurosurgeons have indicated varying indications for surgical intervention. Most of the pediatric neurosurgeons agree that asymptomatic patients with CM1, but without syrinx, should be followed conservatively and not offered surgical decompression. There is also general consensus that presence of a syrinx in a patient with CM1 is an indication for surgery. Most neurosurgeons also recommend decompression for patients with neurologic deficits referable to the CM1 (brainstem/cranial nerve dysfunction, sensory loss, weakness, etc). Suboccipital headache as an indication for surgery is more controversial, but over time there has been greater acceptance of surgery for this indication.[28]

The International Headache Society (IHS) has presented criteria to define CM1-related headache, referencing occipital/suboccipital location, causation by Valsalva maneuvers, and brevity in a patient with radiographic findings of CM1. Studies have shown that the IHS criteria are predictive of resolution of headache following Chiari decompression. Approximately 80% of patients meeting IHS criteria for CM1-related headache will have headache resolution after Chiari decompression. Only half of patients with other headache types had improved after Chiari decompression.[15,29] Care should be taken when recommending surgery for CM1 when headache is the only symptom. Patients with headaches that are tolerable and/or well managed medically may not need surgery even if the headache is believed to be due to the CM1. The neurosurgeon must have a discussion with the patient and family, as observation in this case is a perfectly reasonable alternative to surgery.

Surgical Technique

The underlying goal of surgery for CM1 is to relieve the compression at the cervicomedullary junction; this typically involves a posterior fossa craniectomy (removal of occipital bone including the posterior rim of the foramen magnum) and a C1 laminectomy (removal of the posterior portion of the C1 ring) (**Fig. 2**). In addition, further cervical laminectomies, duraplasty, shrinkage or resection of the cerebellar tonsils, etc. may be performed. Rarely patients will require ventral decompression (removal of the odontoid process of C2) and/or occipitocervical fusion. The literature does not demonstrate the superiority of any one surgical approach for all patients. The surgery must be tailored to each individual patient.

Depending on the approach used, surgery time, including anesthesia, is typically 2 to 3 hours. Patients are admitted to the hospital postoperatively for 2 to 5 days, shorter for patients in whom the dura is left intact and longer for patients in whom a duraplasty is performed. Pain control is the primary issue postoperatively. Muscle spasms develop in the neck due to retraction during surgery. Although narcotics can be used for breakthrough pain, muscle relaxants (diazepam in particular) and acetaminophen (intravenous initially then enteral) are most effective. Usually, the patients are asked to avoid strenuous activities and heavy lifting for 1 month after surgery. The complication rate of the procedure is very low. Infection and CSF leak are the most common complications. The risk of neurologic deficit from injury to the cerebellum, brainstem, or spinal cord is extremely low.

Alternatives to surgery for symptomatic patients depend on the presentation. For patients with syringomyelia, surgery is almost always recommended, as this condition is expected to worsen without surgery. Headaches may be treated with medications. Sleep apnea may be managed with continuous positive airway pressure. Dysphagia can be addressed with adjustments in feeding such as thickening of liquids.

Occasionally, patients or their families will ask to see a "Chiari expert." Evaluation and management of Chiari malformation is a standard part of any pediatric neurosurgical practice, and all pediatric neurosurgeons are familiar with this condition.

APPROACH TO INCIDENTAL CHIARI I MALFORMATION

Patients with CM1 but without symptoms referable to the imaging findings and without syrinx are typically not offered surgery. Those patients who are initially selected for

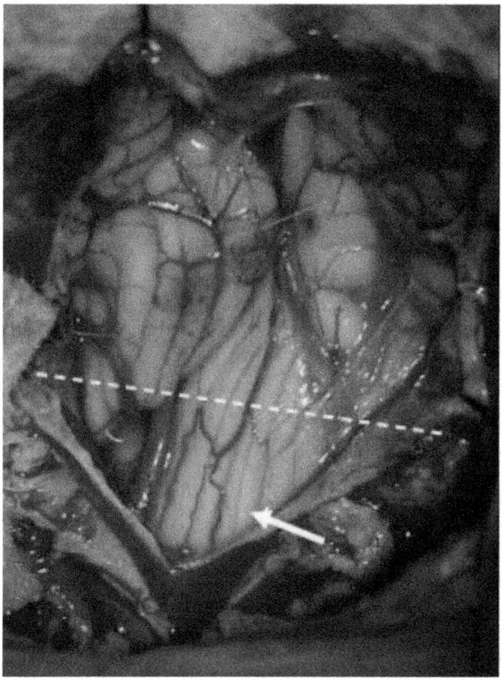

Fig. 2. Intraoperative view after the posterior fossa craniectomy, C1 laminectomy, and opening of the dura. The level of the foramen magnum is indicated by the dashed line. The left cerebellar tonsil (*arrow*) extends substantially below the foramen magnum.

conservative management will rarely require surgical intervention in the future. In a study of 427 patients who did not undergo surgery for CM1 initially, Leon and colleagues[9] found that 3.5% ultimately underwent surgery at a median of 21 months after initial evaluation. Our own experience with 197 patients with CM1 who were asymptomatic at initial presentation showed that 2.6% of the patients developed new symptoms leading to surgery during the follow-up period. No patient needed surgery more than 2 years after initial presentation.[8] Indications for delayed surgery included development of a syrinx, new or worsening headache, onset of sleep apnea, and worsening of dysphagia.[8,9]

Although it is well accepted that most patients with CM1 who are asymptomatic at initial presentation will not require surgery in the future, the need for follow-up clinical or radiologic evaluation and/or imaging is not standardized across centers. In general, a pediatric patient who has been diagnosed with CM1 should be evaluated by a pediatric neurosurgeon. The treating neurosurgeon will then use his or her own experience and the specific features of the patient (signs, symptoms, radiographic findings) to guide decisions regarding follow-up evaluation. Development of new symptoms referable to CM1 (as discussed earlier) or findings that suggest syrinx formation (back pain, myelopathy, etc) should prompt rereferral to a pediatric neurosurgeon. Long-term follow-up studies on the natural history of CM1 have not been done; however, our experience following-up children into adolescence has demonstrated that no patient needed surgery more than 2 years after initial diagnosis.[8]

Participation in contact sports is a frequent concern of patients with CM1, their families, and their medical providers. Two large retrospective studies have suggested that the risk of significant neurologic injury from contact sports in patients with asymptomatic CM1 is very low.[30,31] However, there are case reports of cardiorespiratory arrest in patients with CM1 following head injury, possibly due to compression of the cervicomedullary junction. Therefore, it has been recommended that patients with CM1 and associated symptoms, syrinx, significant impaction of the cerebellar tonsils at the foramen magnum, and/or anterior compression of the medulla oblongata should be restricted from contact sports.[32] Ultimately, the decision of whether or not a particular patient can participate in contact sports should be made between the patient, family, and neurosurgeon after review of the patient's clinical condition and imaging.

Clinics Care Points

- Most children with Chiari I malformation are not symptomatic at presentation, will not develop symptoms, and will not require surgery for CM1.
- Participation in contact sports is likely safe for most patients with CM1. However, each patient should be considered individually and the ultimate decision be made by the patient and family in conjunction with the neurosurgeon.

SUMMARY

CM1 is a relative common incidental finding on neuroimaging. Surgical intervention is reserved for patients who have signs or symptoms referable to the CM1 or who have a syrinx. However, most patients with CM1 do not require surgical intervention at presentation and will not require surgery in the future. Decisions regarding follow-up depend on several patient-specific factors and should be left to the discretion of the treating neurosurgeon. Children who develop new signs of symptoms that could be referrable to CM1 should be rereferred to a pediatric neurosurgeon.

REFERENCES

1. Massimi L, Peppucci E, Peraio S, et al. History of Chiari type I malformation. Neurol Sci 2011;32(S3):263–5.
2. Tubbs RS, Griessenauer CJ, Oakes WJ. Chiari malformations. In: Albright AL, Pollack IF, Adelson PD, editors. Principles and practice of pediatric neurosurgery. 3rd edition. New York: Thieme Publishers; 2015. p. 192–204.
3. Iskandar BJ, Hedlund GL, Grabb PA, et al. The resolution of syringohydromyelia without hindbrain herniation after posterior fossa decompression. J Neurosurg 1998;89(2):212–6.
4. Chern JJ, Gordon AJ, Mortazavi MM, et al. Pediatric Chiari malformation Type 0: a 12-year institutional experience. J Neurosurg Pediatr 2011;8(1):1–5.
5. Tubbs RS, Iskandar BJ, Bartolucci AA, et al. A critical analysis of the Chiari 1.5 malformation. J Neurosurg 2004;101(2 Suppl):179–83.
6. Aitken LA, Lindan CE, Sidney S, et al. Chiari type I malformation in a pediatric population. Pediatr Neurol 2009;40(6):449–54.
7. Strahle J, Muraszko KM, Kapurch J, et al. Chiari malformation Type I and syrinx in children undergoing magnetic resonance imaging. J Neurosurg Pediatr 2011; 8(2):205–13.
8. Carey M, Fuell W, Harkey T, et al. Natural history of Chiari I malformation in children: a retrospective analysis. Child's Nerv Syst 2020;37(4):1185–90.
9. Leon TJ, Kuhn EN, Arynchyna AA, et al. Patients with "benign" Chiari I malformations require surgical decompression at a low rate. J Neurosurg Pediatr 2019; 23(4):498–506.

10. Novegno F, Caldarelli M, Massa A, et al. The natural history of the Chiari Type I anomaly. J Neurosurg Pediatr 2008;2(3):179–87.
11. Pomeraniec IJ, Ksendzovsky A, Awad AJ, et al. JAJ. Natural and surgical history of Chiari malformation Type I in the pediatric population. J Neurosurg Pediatr 2016;17(3):343–52.
12. Ciaramitaro P, Ferraris M, Massaro F, et al. Clinical diagnosis—part I: what is really caused by Chiari I. Child's Nerv Syst 2019;35(10):1–7.
13. Williams B. Cough headache due to craniospinal pressure dissociation. Arch Neurol 1980;37(4):226–30.
14. Mcgirt MJ, Nimjee SM, Floyd J, et al. Correlation of cerebrospinal fluid flow dynamics and headache in Chiari I malformation. Neurosurgery 2005;56(4): 716–21 [discussion 716-21].
15. Grangeon L, Puy L, Gilard V, et al. Predictive Factors of Headache Resolution After Chiari Type 1 Malformation Surgery. World Neurosurg 2018;110:e60–6. Pediatr Neurol 40 2009.
16. Albert GW, Menezes AH, Hansen DR, et al. Chiari malformation Type I in children younger than age 6 years: presentation and surgical outcome. J Neurosurg Pediatr 2010;5(6):554–61.
17. Losurdo A, Dittoni S, Testani E, et al. Sleep disordered breathing in children and adolescents with Chiari malformation type I. J Clin Sleep Med 2013;9(4):371–7.
18. Dauvilliers Y, Stal V, Abril B, et al. Chiari malformation and sleep related breathing disorders. J Neurol Neurosurg Psychiatry 2007;78(12):1344.
19. Pollack IF, Pang D, Kocoshis S, et al. Neurogenic dysphagia resulting from chiari malformations. Neurosurgery 1992;30(5):709–19.
20. Tubbs RS, Beckman J, Naftel RP, et al. Institutional experience with 500 cases of surgically treated pediatric Chiari malformation Type I. J Neurosurg Pediatr 2011; 7(3):248–56.
21. Almotairi F, Andersson M, Andersson O, et al. Swallowing dysfunction in adult patients with chiari I malformation. J Neurol Surg B Skull Base 2018;79(06):606–13.
22. Killeen A, Roguski M, Chavez A, et al. Non-operative outcomes in Chiari I malformation patients. J Clin Neurosci 2015;22(1):133–8.
23. Furtado SV, Thakar S, Hegde AS. Correlation of functional outcome and natural history with clinicoradiological factors in surgically managed pediatric Chiari I malformation. Neurosurgery 2011;68(2):319–28.
24. Strahle JM, Taiwo R, Averill C, et al. Radiological and clinical associations with scoliosis outcomes after posterior fossa decompression in patients with Chiari malformation and syrinx from the Park-Reeves Syringomyelia Research Consortium. J Neurosurg Pediatr 2020;1–7.
25. Strahle J, Smith BW, Martinez M, et al. The association between Chiari malformation Type I, spinal syrinx, and scoliosis. J Neurosurg Pediatr 2015;15(6):607–11.
26. Noureldine MHA, Shimony N, Jallo GI, et al. Scoliosis in patients with Chiari malformation type I. Child's Nerv Syst 2019;35(10):1853–62.
27. Milhorat TH, Bolognese PA, Nishikawa M, et al. Syndrome of occipitoatlantoaxial hypermobility, cranial settling, and Chiari malformation Type I in patients with hereditary disorders of connective tissue. J Neurosurg Spine 2007;7(6):601–9.
28. Hersh DS, Groves ML, Boop FA. Management of Chiari malformations: opinions from different centers—a review. Child's Nerv Syst 2019;35(10):1869–73.
29. Raza-Knight S, Mankad K, Prabhakar P, et al. Headache outcomes in children undergoing foramen magnum decompression for Chiari I malformation. Arch Dis Child 2017;102(3):238–43.

30. Meehan WP, Jordaan M, Prabhu SP, et al. Risk of athletes with chiari malformations suffering catastrophic injuries during sports participation is low. Clin J Sport Med 2015;25(2):133–7.
31. Strahle J, Geh N, Selzer BJ, et al. Sports participation with Chiari I malformation. J Neurosurg Pediatr 2016;17(4):403–9.
32. Miele VJ, Bailes JE, Martin NA. Participation in contact or collision sports in athletes with epilepsy, genetic risk factors, structural brain lesions, or history of craniotomy. Neurosurg Focus 2006;21(4):E9.

Pediatric Hydrocephalus and the Primary Care Provider

Smruti K. Patel, MD[a], Rabia Tari, MD[a], Francesco T. Mangano, DO[b,*]

KEYWORDS

- hydrocephalus (HCP) • Ventriculomegaly • Primary care
- CSF (Cerebrospinal fluid) shunting • Pediatric neurosurgery

KEY POINTS

- Hydrocephalus is a complex disorder that often presents in infancy or childhood and may require lifelong monitoring and repeated assessments by a clinician.
- Understanding the etiology of hydrocephalus in individual patients is critical in treatment decision making, patient and family counseling, prognosis, and long-term outcome.
- Signs and symptoms of hydrocephalus may vary with patient age, and surgical treatment may differ based on multiple factors but may include temporary cerebrospinal fluid (CSF) diversion procedures, CSF shunting, or endoscopic third ventriculostomy.
- Patients with suspected shunt malfunction or infection should be referred urgently to the nearest emergency room for evaluation.
- This article will assist the primary care provider with fielding common questions posed by patients and families with shunted hydrocephalus to include activity restrictions, need for prophylactic antibiotics, and exposure to magnetic fields in the patient with a programmable shunt valve.

INTRODUCTION

With a global prevalence of 88 per 100,000, hydrocephalus (HCP) is the most common disease process treated by pediatric neurosurgeons and results in nearly $2 billion of health expenditures in the United States each year.[1,2] Given the significant morbidity and mortality related to HCP within the pediatric population and its significant societal impact, vigilance must be maintained by all health care professionals caring for these patients. In particular, the pediatrician or primary care physician plays a significant role in recognizing the early signs and symptoms of HCP and initiating the appropriate workup.

[a] Pediatric Neurosurgery, Cincinnati Children's Hospital Medical Center, 3333 Burnet Avenue, MLC 2016, Cincinnati, OH 45229-3026, USA; [b] Department of Neurological Surgery, Pediatric Neurosurgery, Cincinnati Children's Hospital Medical Center, University of Cincinnati College of Medicine, 3333 Burnet Avenue, MLC 2016, Cincinnati, OH 45229-3026, USA
* Corresponding author.
E-mail address: francesco.mangano@cchmc.org

Pediatr Clin N Am 68 (2021) 793–809
https://doi.org/10.1016/j.pcl.2021.04.006
0031-3955/21/

ANATOMY AND PHYSIOLOGY OF CEREBROSPINAL FLUID PATHWAYS

Cerebrospinal fluid (CSF) is a clear, colorless fluid contained within the brain that functions in waste removal, nutrition, cushioning of the brain, and regulation of brain function through soluable neuortransmitters and hormones. In a healthy individual, most of the circulating volume of CSF is secreted by the choroid plexus within the lateral ventricles (**Fig. 1**).[3] In general, the rate of production of CSF (0.35 mL/min or approximately 400–500 mL/d) is equal to the rate of absorption. The total volume of CSF within the ventricles and the intracranial and spinal subarachnoid space is primarily age-dependent (65–140 mL in children) and reaches the adult volume of 150 mL at approximately 5 years of age.[4] Traditionally, 2 patterns of normal CSF circulation have been described. These are known as the major and minor pathways.[5] In the major pathway, CSF flows from the lateral ventricles to the third ventricle and through the aqueduct of Sylvius into the fourth ventricle (**Fig. 2**). From the fourth ventricle, CSF circulates through the foramina of Luschka and Magendie into the basilar cisterns and subarachnoid spaces and ultimately is reabsorbed by the arachnoid villi and granulations. The minor pathway involves absorption through alternative sites, such as along nerve root sleeves, venous capillaries, and glymphatic channels. This pathway is particularly significant in neonates and infants in whom arachnoid granulations have not yet formed.[6]

CLASSIFICATION OF HYDROCEPHALUS

Classification by Type

Although there is no universally accepted classification system, HCP has been divided into 2 broad radiographic and functional subsets: communicating and noncommunicating (or obstructive) hydrocephalus.[7] Despite the terminology, HCP occurs due to restricted flow, except for the rare instances in which it is caused by an overproduction of CSF. For the purposes of this article, we simply define obstructive HCP (OH) as that which occurs when there is a physical obstruction of CSF flow within the ventricular system (**Fig. 3**A). Communicating HCP (CH) is defined as restriction of CSF flow or absorption within the subarachnoid spaces (**Fig. 3**B).[8,9]

Classification by Etiology

The most practical classification may be one based on etiology. HCP can occur at any age, but it is more commonly seen in neonates or infants.[10,11] The 2 primary subdivisions are congenital versus acquired. More than half of all cases of HCP are

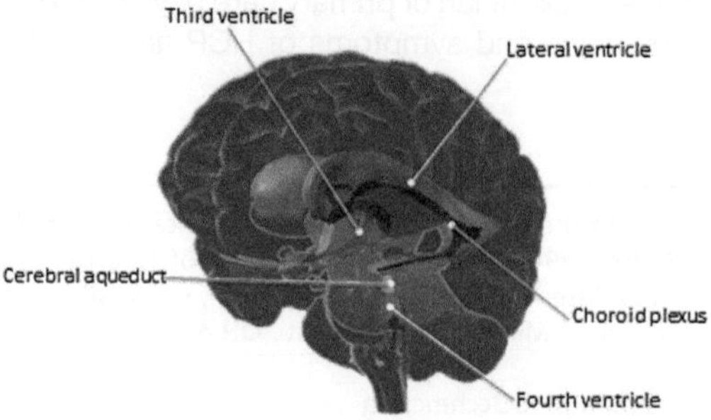

Fig. 1. Illustration of the ventricular system to include the lateral, third, and 4th ventricles. The cerebral aqueduct is the narrowest point of the ventricular system, connecting the 3rd and 4th ventricles.

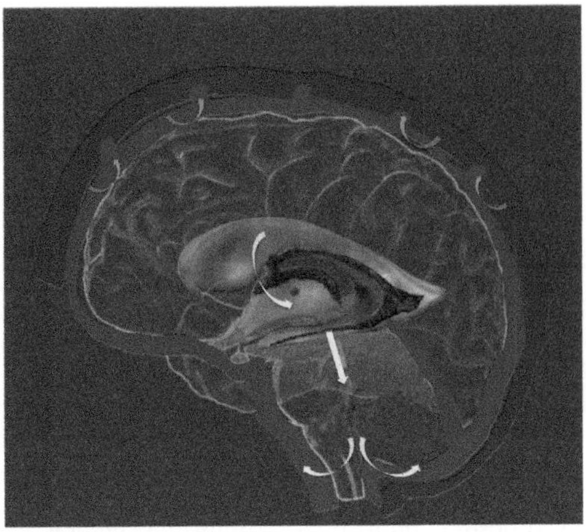

Fig. 2. Diagram illustrating the normal flow of CSF through the major pathway. Spinal fluid flows through the ventricular system to the outlet foramen of the 4th ventricle (yellow arrows). Once in the subarachnoid space, spinal fluid proceeds to arachnoid villi (orange arrows) where it passively flows into the low-pressure venous sinuses.

congenital; that is, they are present at birth and usually become clinically symptomatic in the neonatal period or during infancy.[4,12] Primary aqueductal stenosis accounts for approximately 5% of cases with congenital HCP. It is a form of OH that occurs due to partial or complete obstruction of CSF flow through the cerebral aqueduct (**Fig. 4**A, B). Approximately 75% of these patients are prenatally diagnosed on routine obstetric ultrasound due to ventriculomegaly and can be followed up with fetal MRI.[13] The most common inheritable form of congenital HCP is X-linked HCP.[14] This is a single gene disorder caused by mutations in the neural cell adhesion molecule, L1CAM.[4,14]

Clinics Care Points

Risk factors associated with congenital hydrocephalus[15]

- Birth weight less than 1500 g
- Prematurity
- Male gender
- Maternal diabetes
- Maternal hypertension
- Preeclampsia
- Lack of prenatal care
- Maternal obesity
- Alcohol use during pregnancy

Another subpopulation of patients at risk for developing CH are those with a diagnosis of myelomeningocele or spina bifida (MMC) (**Figure 4**C,D). HCP can occur in up to 80% of patients who undergo postnatal MMC repair with approximately one-half requiring treatment for HCP within 1 month of age.[16] Myelomeningocele can cause HCP secondary to third and fourth ventricular outlet obstruction, altered venous compliance, and arachnoid or ependymal scarring. With the advent of fetal repair or prenatal closure of myelomeningocele defects, the rates of shunted HCP have decreased to approximately 40%; however, this population is considered an at-risk group for HCP-related complications.[17]

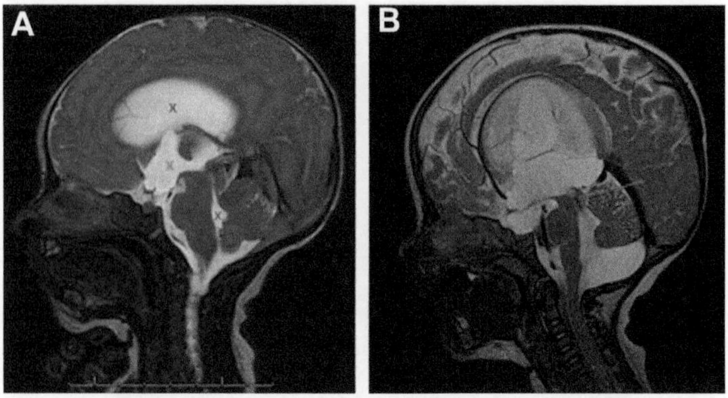

Fig. 3. Classification of hydrocephalus by type. A. Obstructive hydrocephalus. Note enlargement of the lateral (red X) and third ventricles (green X) without enlargement of the 4th ventricle (blue X) due to obstruction of flow through the cerebral aqueduct (red arrow). B. Communicating hydrocephalus. Note all ventricles are enlarged with fluid movement (blue arrow) indicating spinal fluid passing through the cerebral aqueduct.

In acquired HCP (AH), an extrinsic cause is often apparent based on history or imaging findings.[12] A detailed discussion regarding each of these etiologies is outside the scope of this article; however, it is prudent to note that a post-hemorrhagic etiology is the most common form of AH in infants, primarily due to intraventricular hemorrhage (IVH) of prematurity (**Fig. 4**E, F). Secondary, or acquired, aqueductal stenosis can occur due to arachnoid scarring related to IVH. The development of HCP can be slow and progress over the course of 2 to 6 weeks. Rates of hydrocephalus in patients with intraventricular hemorrhage range from 8-10%.[18] Other forms of acquired hydrocephalus include intracranial neoplasms. Tumors can cause HCP

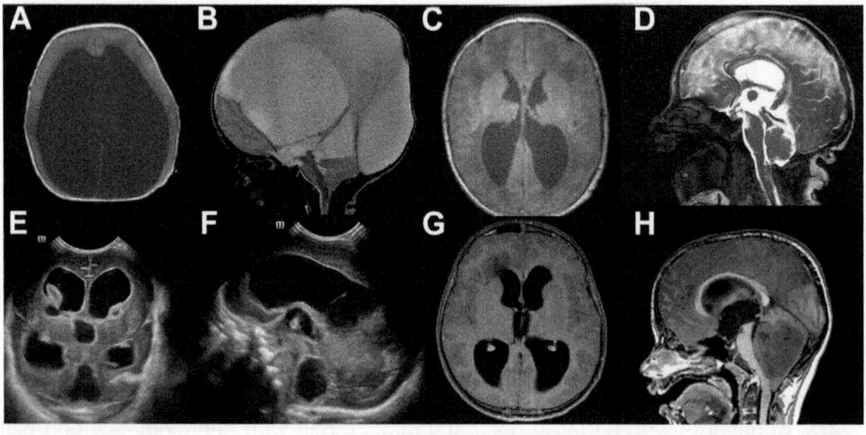

Fig. 4. Axial and sagittal MRI of a newborn boy with OH (*A* and *B*) secondary to congenital aqueductal stenosis. Axial and sagittal MRI of a patient with OH (*C*) and Chiari II malformation (*D*) in a patient with myelomeningocele, who underwent postnatal repair. Coronal and sagittal views (*E, F*) of head ultrasound in a premature neonate born at 23 weeks' gestational age that shows communicating HCP in the setting of grade IV intraventricular hemorrhage of prematurity. Axial and sagittal MRI demonstrating OH (*G*) secondaryto posterior fossa mass (*H*).

through the obstruction of the CSF pathway through blockage in the ventricular system or overproduction of CSF.[4] HCP is present in up to 80% of all cases with posterior fossa tumors (**Fig. 4**G, H).[19] Resolution of HCP has been reported in 60% to 90% of pediatric patients after posterior fossa tumor resection. Other etiologies of acquired hydrocephalus include post-traumatic and post-infectious, typically due to impairment of spinal fluid absorption at the level of arachnoid granulations.[20]

Clinics Care Points

Etiologies of acquired HCP include the following:

- Post-hemorrhagic
- Neoplastic
  - Posterior fossa tumors, third ventricle tumors, tectal glioma (OH)
  - Choroid plexus tumors (CSF overproduction)
- Other
  - Post-infectious
  - Posttraumatic

Clinical Presentation

The clinical presentation of HCP is challenging for the primary care provider due to similarity of signs and symptoms of common childhood disease to include otitis media, gastroenteritis, and urinary tract infection. In the neonatal period, prolonged or frequent apneic or bradycardic events (not related to cardiopulmonary etiology) increasing head circumference (HC) (especially crossing percentiles on growth curves), presence of sunsetting eyes or upward gaze palsy, evidence of full or tense anterior/posterior fontanelle(s), and splayed cranial sutures are signs of increased intracranial pressure (**Table 1**).

Infants with HCP commonly present with progressive macrocephaly or increasing HC crossing percentiles, nausea/vomiting, poor appetite, irritability, and regression of developmental milestones. Physical examination findings may include prominent scalp veins, full or tense anterior fontanelle, lethargy, eye deviation, or new esotropia. It is important to note isolated changes in the patient's head growth curve in relationship to the body growth curves for height and weight. Conversely, it is also important to consider familial macrocephaly in which a large head size is a familial trait (see the article by Bryant and colleagues' article, "Macrocephaly in the Primary Care Provider's Office," in this issue).

Younger children (>2 years of age) generally present with signs and symptoms of intracranial hypertension such as early morning headaches and worsening symptoms with increased effort, lethargy, somnolence, gait changes, visual disturbances, cognitive deficits, and/or regression of developmental milestones. In older children (>10 years of age), depending on the acuity of development of HCP, the presentation may be striking or subtle. Symptoms may vary from decline in academic studies, memory loss, and behavioral disturbances to severe headache, lethargy, vomiting, nausea, blurry vision, and gait abnormalities.

Clinics Care Points

Ophthalmologic examination can be helpful in both younger and older children:

- Assessment of intraocular pressure
- Presence or absence of papilledema
- Papilledema may not be seen before closure of the anterior fontanelle.

Table 1
Signs and symptoms of hydrocephalus, stratified by age

Infants	Toddlers	Children and adolescents
• Macrocephaly • Full fontanelle • Prominent scalp veins • Vomiting • Irritability • Lethargy • Sundowning	• Macrocephaly • Vomiting • Headache • Irritability • Lethargy • New strabismus • Loss of developmental milestones	• Vomiting • Headache • Visual complaints • Irritability and personality changes • Lethargy • Loss of coordination or balance • Decline in academic performance

DIAGNOSTIC TESTING

Diagnostic imaging plays a key role in the evaluation of the patient with suspected or established hydrocephalus. We provide a brief overview of imaging below; for more detailed discussion, please see the article by Wood and colleagues "Neuroimaging for the Primary Care Provider: A Review of Modalities, Indications, and Pitfalls," in this issue.

Head Ultrasound

Ultrasonography is often used as a bedside screening test for evaluation of IVH and ventriculomegaly in neonates. Ultrasound provides excellent images of supratentorial structures to include the lateral and third ventricles. However, imaging of posterior fossa structures is limited. It is highly operator-dependent and rarely used as a singular diagnostic test for evaluation of HCP. Thus, ultrasound is best used as a cursory screening test and follow-up before or after treatment when the anterior fontanelle is open.[21]

Computed Tomography

Computed tomography (CT) of the head is one of the most used studies in diagnostic radiology and serves as a fast, reliable, and rapidly available means of obtaining images. It is the study of choice during an emergency. Because many children with HCP require long-term follow-up over the course of their lifetime, the primary concern with the repeated use of CT for surveillance is the effect of ionizing radiation on the developing brain. Thus, CT investigation should be used sparingly.[21] Low-dose protocol CTs should be used when available and appropriate to minimize radiation exposure.[22]

MRI

MRI is the study of choice to assess ventricular size and morphology, and the identification of the underlying etiology of HCP. The MRI of the brain can also be used to assess for cerebral edema or transependymal flow (CSF around the ventricle in the surrounding white matter) as well as signs of brain herniation in severe cases.[21]

There are additional imaging modalities (plain radiographs, nuclear medicine studies[23,24]) that may be utilized for the evaluation of the patient with shunted hydrocephalus. It is acceptable to let the neurosurgery specialist decide on the proper imaging modality after referral.

SURGICAL MANAGEMENT OF HYDROCEPHALUS

Clinics Care Points

Temporary management of HCP

- Though temporary measures are unlikely to be encountered in primary care, understanding of their use and utility is helpful to primary care providers in their communication with families. An external ventricular drain can be placed for rapid CSF drainage as well as monitoring of intracranial pressure (**Fig. 5**A).
  - Although temporary, this is the preferred route of management in an emergent scenario.
- In special cases or patients who are critically ill, such as those with HCP secondary to IVH of prematurity, a temporary ventricular access device (VAD) can be considered for treatment.
  - In this case, a small catheter is placed into the ventricular system attached to a reservoir that can be accessed to remove CSF from the ventricular system as needed (**Fig. 5**B).
- VADs are typically indicated for underweight infants (typically <2 kg) or those who may not be ready for definitive CSF shunting due to other comorbidities.

Cerebrospinal fluid shunting

- Most common form of surgical treatment for HCP and globally available in the neurosurgeon's armamentarium.
- Involves diverting CSF from the intracranial ventricular system into a distal cavity, most commonly the peritoneum.

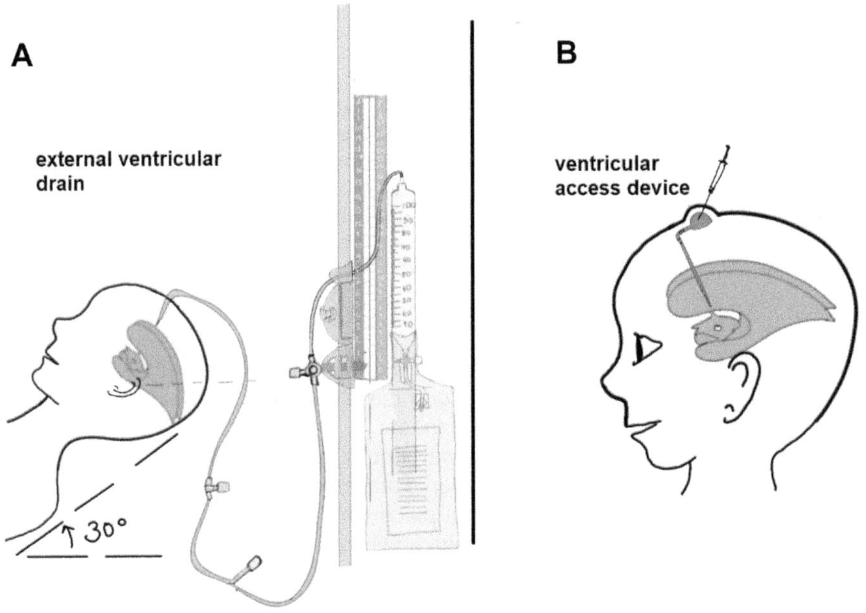

Fig. 5. Illustration demonstrating (*A*) an external ventricular drain system that is typically set to drain at a certain opening pressure and can easily be adjusted or clamped; and a VAD (*B*), which can be accessed using a needle and syringe through the scalp to aspirate CSF.

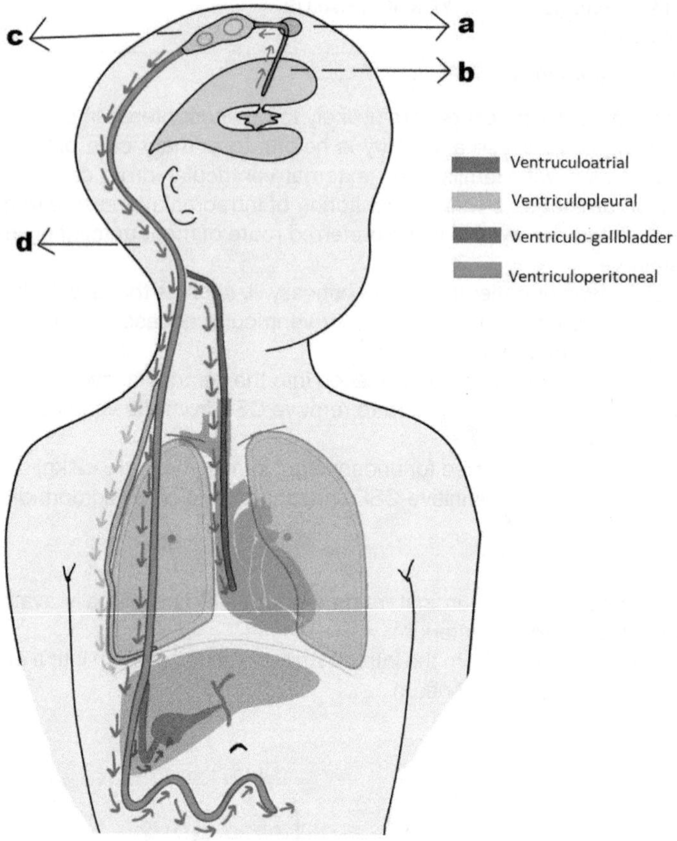

Fig. 6. Types of CSF shunt systems. Each shunt system includes a proximal ventricular catheter (a), proximal reservoir placed at the burr hole site that can be placed in the frontal (b) or occipital region (not shown here), and the valve (c). The different cavities in which the distal catheter (d) may terminate include the peritoneum (*blue arrows*), pleura (*yellow arrows*), atria of the heart (*red arrows*), and gall bladder (*green arrows*). The different colored arrows and color legend within the figure show the direction of flow through the corresponding catheters (D: distal system; E: to the atria; F: to the pleural cavity; G: to the gall bladder, and H: to the peritoneal cavity).

- If the peritoneal cavity is not found to be amenable for this procedure, other distal areas for shunt placement may include the pleural space, the right atria of the heart, and less commonly, the gall bladder.
- Three standard components: proximal ventricular catheter, a valve, and a distal catheter that terminates in the chosen distal cavity (**Fig. 6**).
- Overall complication rates for shunt placement can reach 40%, with the most common complications being hardware failure and infection[25].
- Intervening valves come in different shapes, sizes, and models (none has been proven more effective than the others).
  - Flow-regulated valves and differential pressure fixed-type valves (these will not be altered by MRI).
  - Programmable valves

  - Valve settings can be altered if exposed to a large magnet, such as an MRI.
  - Must be interrogated and reprogrammed after such exposures (see Magnetic Field Exposures section).

Endoscopic third ventriculostomy

- Alternative to CSF shunting
- Procedure in which a fenestration is made in the floor of the third ventricle to re-establish CSF circulation (**Figs. 7** and **8**).
- ETV avoids the need for foreign body implantation and restoration of more physiologic CSF circulation.
- Success rates range from 50-90%, with success equating to life-long freedom of potential shunt complications.
- ○ Although the risk of injury to critical brain structures is small (less than 1%), parents must be aware of these heightened short term risks with ETV in comparison to shunt placement/revision.

Clinics Care Points: The success[26] of the ETV procedure is dependent on:

- Patient age
- Etiology of HCP
- Prior need for shunt

MONITORING A CHILD WITH HYDROCEPHALUS: THE PRIMARY CARE PERSPECTIVE

Monitoring a child with HCP who has been surgically treated can be difficult given the heterogeneity of the etiologies related to the condition. It is paramount to note a

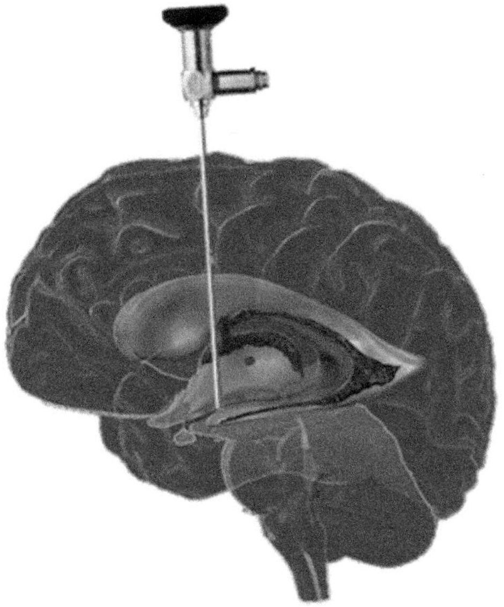

Fig. 7. Endoscopic third ventriculostomy. Using an endoscope, the neurosurgeon bypasses obstructed anatomy by fashioning a hole in the floor of the third ventricle, allowing spinal fluid to escape the ventricular system into the subarachnoid space, re-establishing access to the major pathway for spinal fluid resorption.

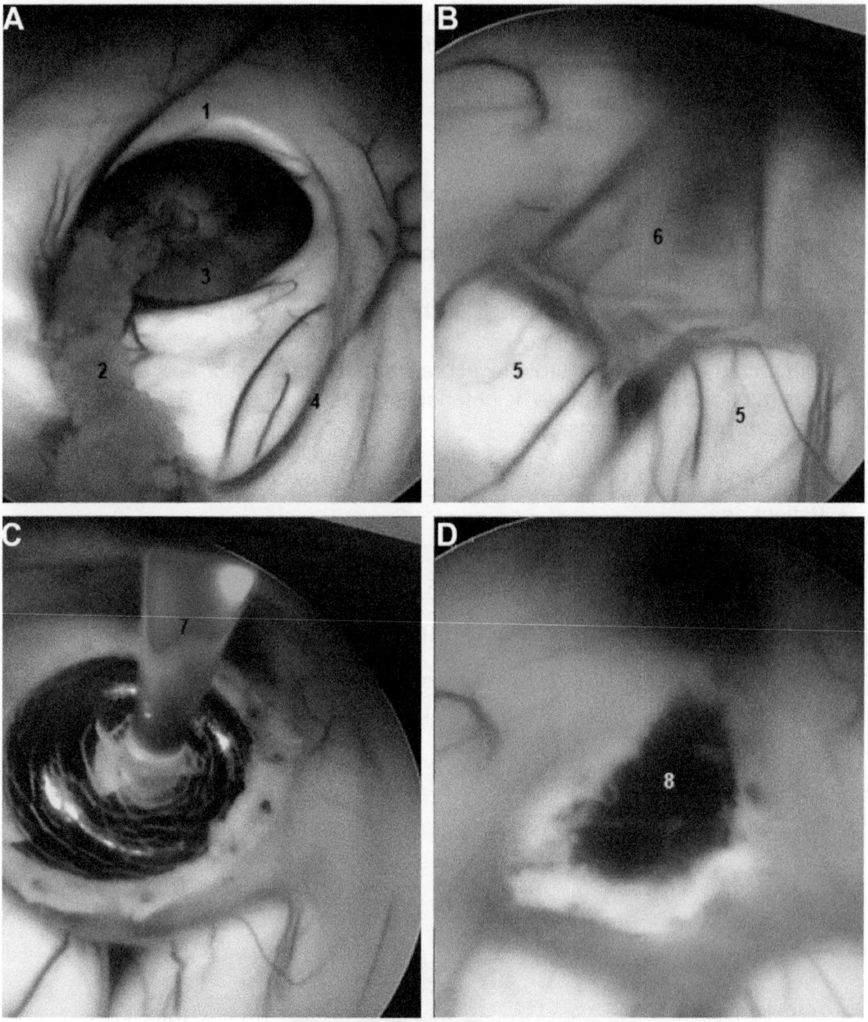

Fig. 8. Intraoperative photographs from an ETV procedure. The endoscope is placed into the right ventricle (*A*) and the ipsilateral fornix (1), choroid plexus (2), foramen of Monro (3), and thalamostriate veins are visualized. It is then advanced into the third ventricle, where the mammillary bodies (6) and floor of the third ventricle (6) are seen. An opening is made in this thin, nearly transparent membrane anterior to the mammillary bodies and expanded using a small Fogarty catheter (7). This creates an opening or ostomy through which CSF can now flow obviating the need for a shunt, in some cases.

patient's initial symptomatology before surgical intervention and have a thorough understanding of medical history. In general, most patients are at highest risk of ventriculoperitoneal shunt (VPS)-related complications within the first year of insertion. Overall, complication rates are high after VPS, and have been reported to be between 17% and 33%.[25] Close surveillance during the first year after VPS insertion is critical to decrease or prevent related complications. At many centers, follow-up is done with a limited brain MRI, which involves a rapid survey of the ventricular system with the benefit of not requiring sedation in most cases. Shunt complications can be subdivided into 3 basic categories: shunt malfunction, shunt infection, or an imbalance in drainage causing either overdrainage or underdrainage of CSF.

Shunt Malfunction

Shunt malfunction is the most common shunt complication and usually presents with similar signs and symptoms present before shunting. It is important to listen to parents and caregivers when symptomatology is not clear cut. If there is a high suspicion for shunt malfunction, the child should be referred to the nearest emergency room for evaluation.

Shunt Infection

Shunt infections are a serious and unfortunate complication of shunt surgery, with an estimated risk of 7% in high volume centers. The number of past shunt revisions is a significant risk factor for developing a shunt infection.[27] This risk is also higher in patients born with prematurity, younger age, and a history of prior shunt infection.[28] The risk is highest in the first 90 days following shunt surgery. In the setting of shunt infection, it is possible that the intracranial imaging remains stable and may not reveal any changes of the ventricular system. An inflammatory response to infected spinal fluid may result in 'walling off' of the distal end of the shunt producing a pseudocyst that may be palpable on physical exam, or detected on abdominal imaging such as ultrasound[29] A "shunt tap" or diagnostic test in which the reservoir is accessed with a small-gauge butterfly needle to assess for spontaneous proximal flow and obtain CSF sampling, can also be done by a trained neurosurgical provider. Urgent referral to the emergency room is recommended if a possible shunt infection is suspected.

Clinics Care Points: Signs and Symptoms of Shunt Infection

- Pain and erythema along the shunt tract
- Development of swelling around the shunt
- Fever
- Hypothermia
- Irritability/fussiness
- Abdominal pain
- Meningitic signs
- Peritoneal signs
- Tenderness along shunt catheter or valve

Overdrainage Syndromes

While shunt systems are lifesaving, they can not replicate the normal physiology of spinal fluid production and absorption. Overdrainage is thought to occur due to intracranial hypotension with ventricular collapse and can result in the development of subdural fluid collections or slit-ventricle syndrome (SVS). The management of the extra-axial collections often involves decreasing the overdrainage by making adjustments to the shunt valve, if programmable. Alternatively, the subdural fluid can be drained if symptomatic and persistent.[30]

Spinal fluid plays an important physiologic role in buffering changes in brain volume that occur with varying activities. Shunt placement in early childhood can interfere with the development of normal intracranial spinal fluid volume that allows for changes in brain volume related to activity-driven changes in cerebral blood flow. The result is a patient with small slit-like ventricles and frequent intermittent symptoms that are similar to shunt failure. SVS occurs secondary to symptomatic ventricular collapse. SVS typically develops in a delayed fashion after shunt insertion. The reported incidence of this syndrome ranges from 1% to 2% in some series, and more than 50% in others.[31] The classic triad of this syndrome has been defined as intermittent headache that interferes with activities of daily living, small or slitlike ventricles on imaging, and slow filling of the valve reservoir on palpation. Patients often state that they feel an improvement in headache when in a recumbent position.[31,32]

Clinics care point
Management of slit-ventricle syndrome[33,34]

- Conservative measures including the following:
  - Intravenous fluids and antimigraine therapy
  - Placement of an ICP monitor has been described in some situations to help distinguish high or low intracranial pressure and guide further treatment.
  - Surgical treatments include shunt revision, cranial vault expansion procedures, lumboperitoneal shunt placement, and ETV with possible shunt removal.

COMMON QUESTIONS RELATED TO SHUNTS AND HYDROCEPHALUS

Clinics Care Pearls

Activity restrictions after surgery

- Avoidance of strenuous activity should be followed in the early postoperative period.
- Avoidance of swimming until the wound heals or stitches are removed (usually 2–3 weeks after surgery).
- Avoidance of any activity that places constant pressure on the valve or shunt tract under the skin, causing irritation, abrasion, or ulceration.
- Physical activity level can typically commence after appropriate surgical wound healing.
- Alternate head positioning to prevent plagiocephaly in an infant.

General activity restrictions and recommendations[35–38]

- No consensus exists among neurosurgeons regarding sports-related activity, driving, air travel, pregnancy, SCUBA diving, and sexual intercourse in patients with shunted hydrocephalus.
  - Activity-related restrictions will largely be clinician dependent and related advice should ideally be the result of a mutual agreement among the pat ient, primary care provider, and neurosurgeon.
- Antibiotic prophylaxis[39,40]
  - Antibiotic prophylaxis is NOT required for patients with ventriculoperitoneal shunts prior to dental care.
  - Antibiotic prophylaxis IS recommended for patients with ventriculoatrial shunts prior to dental care.
- Gastrointestinal or abdominal surgery in the setting of an indwelling VPS.[41–43]
  - Minimal risk for VPS malfunction or infection exists in patients who undergo clean or clean-contaminated abdominal surgeries.
- A child with a shunt has a fever. Is this concerning?
  - Children with shunts have coughs and colds like any other kids. In most cases, a fever with accompanying symptoms can be managed conservatively by the family and/or pediatrician. Fever in a child who had their shunt placed within 30 days should be discussed with the neurosurgeon. Fever in a child who had

their shunt placed within 6 months may be discussed with the neurosurgeon following evaluation and exclusion of other potential sources.

- Are all headaches in shunted patients concerning?
  - No, but shunt patients require an extra level of attention when they develop headaches. Headaches that are more concerning for shunt failure include one or more of these features: Severe (>7/10), Persistent (> 1 hour), Increasing over time, or associated with emesis. When in doubt about a patient with a shunt and headaches, discussion and/or evaluation by a neurosurgeon is always a good idea.
- Can a child become 'shunt independent' after a shunt is placed?
  - Resolution of hydrocephalus after shunt placement is exceedingly rare. Children with a history of shunted hydrocephalus require serial monitoring, even if they have not had symptoms for an extended period of time.

MAGNETIC FIELD EXPOSURES

Unknown external magnetic forces (if strong enough) can have an influence over programmable valve mechanisms and modify the opening pressure setting.[44,45] Magnetic fields emitted by many devices including handheld portable tablets, mobile devices, headphones, and other wearable technology can often be a concern for patients and parents of children with shunted HCP who carry programmable valves. if a patient undergoes an MRI study, the conservative recommendation is for valve interrogation by a neurosurgery provider afterward to ensure the valve is at the correct setting.

Clinics Care Points

Based on the reported literature and guidelines available, it is recommended that commonly used magnetic devices such as those mentioned as follows should be kept at a distance of at least 2 inches from the programmable valve.[46]

- Implanted hearing devices
- Mobile devices
- Tablet devices
- Metal detectors
- Earbuds and headphones
- Common household magnets
- Magnetic toys
- Smart badges used in health care facilities

HYDROCEPHALUS EDUCATION

It is critical that parents and caregivers are aware of the symptoms of a possible shunt malfunction or infection. Parental recognition of shunt failure has been shown to be accurate about 57% of the time.[47] We advocate for structured shunt education with distribution of appropriate resources and verbal feedback of understanding. Useful resources that all families should be provided before discharge from the hospital after shunt insertion or revision include the shunt manufacturers' pamphlets, online resources such as the Hydrocephalus Association booklet for families (http://www.hydroassoc.org/docs/AboutHydrocephalus-A_Book_for_Families_Dec08.pdf), and mobile applications like HydroAssist (http://www.hydroassoc.org/hydroassist-mobile-application/). Wallet cards containing implant-related information should also be provided to the patient and/or caregivers.[48]

SUMMARY

Hydrocephalus is a complex disorder that often requires lifelong treatment and monitoring. The role of the primary care provider or pediatrician in these patients' care is key to early recognition of subtle changes or neurologic decline related to HCP or shunt malfunction. An understanding of the basic pathophysiology and clinical signs and symptoms of HCP facilitates prompt initiation of workup or referral to the emergency department or neurosurgery provider when appropriate. In addition, a thorough understanding of risks and restrictions related to implanted shunt systems can further help avoid related complications.

DISCLOSURE

The authors have nothing to disclose.

REFERENCES

1. Isaacs AM, Riva-Cambrin J, Yavin D, et al. Age-specific global epidemiology of hydrocephalus: systematic review, metanalysis and global birth surveillance. PLoS One 2018;13(10):e0204926.
2. Simon TD, Riva-Cambrin J, Srivastava R, et al. Hospital care for children with hydrocephalus in the United States: utilization, charges, comorbidities, and deaths. J Neurosurg Pediatr 2008;1(2):131–7.
3. Wright Z, Larrew TW, Eskandari R. Pediatric hydrocephalus: current state of diagnosis and treatment. Pediatr Rev 2016;37(11):478–90.
4. Abou-Hamden A, Drake JM. Hydrocephalus. In: Albright AL, Pollack IF, Adelson PD, editors. Principles and practice of pediatric neurosurgery. 3rd edition. New York: Thieme Medical Publishers, Inc.; 2015. p. 89–99.
5. Symss NP, Oi S. Theories of cerebrospinal fluid dynamics and hydrocephalus: historical trend. J Neurosurg Pediatr 2013;11(2):170–7.
6. Drake JM. The surgical management of pediatric hydrocephalus. Neurosurgery 2008;62(Suppl 2):633–40 [discussion: 640–2].
7. Dandy W, Blackfan K. An experimental and clinical study of internal hydrocephalus. JAMA 1913;61:2216–7.
8. Zahl SM, Egge A, Helseth E, et al. Benign external hydrocephalus: a review, with emphasis on management. Neurosurg Rev 2011;34(4):417–32.
9. Sun M, Yuan W, Hertzler DA, et al. Diffusion tensor imaging findings in young children with benign external hydrocephalus differ from the normal population. Childs Nerv Syst 2012;28(2):199–208.
10. Oi S. Hydrocephalus research update–controversies in definition and classification of hydrocephalus. Neurol Med Chir (Tokyo) 2010;50(9):859–69.
11. Oi S. Classification of hydrocephalus: critical analysis of classification categories and advantages of "Multi-categorical Hydrocephalus Classification" (Mc HC). Childs Nerv Syst 2011;27(10):1523–33.
12. Tully HM, Dobyns WB. Infantile hydrocephalus: a review of epidemiology, classification and causes. Eur J Med Genet 2014;57(8):359–68.
13. Rodis I, Mahr CV, Fehrenbach MK, et al. Hydrocephalus in aqueductal stenosis–a retrospective outcome analysis and proposal of subtype classification. Child's Nerv Syst 2016;32(4):617–27.
14. Adle-Biassette H, Saugier-Veber P, Fallet-Bianco C, et al. Neuropathological review of 138 cases genetically tested for X-linked hydrocephalus: evidence for

closely related clinical entities of unknown molecular bases. Acta Neuropathol 2013;126(3):427–42.
15. Kalyvas AV, Kalamatianos T, Pantazi M, et al. Maternal environmental risk factors for congenital hydrocephalus: a systematic review. Neurosurg Focus 2016; 41(5):E3.
16. Tuli S, Drake J, Lamberti-Pasculli M. Long-term outcome of hydrocephalus management in myelomeningoceles. Childs Nerv Syst 2003;19(5–6):286–91.
17. Tulipan N, Wellons JC 3rd, Thom EA, et al. Prenatal surgery for myelomeningocele and the need for cerebrospinal fluid shunt placement. J Neurosurg Pediatr 2015;16(6):613–20.
18. Raybaud C. MR assessment of pediatric hydrocephalus: a road map. Childs Nerv Syst 2016;32(1):19–41.
19. Anania P, Battaglini D, Balestrino A, et al. The role of external ventricular drainage for the management of posterior cranial fossa tumours: a systematic review. Neurosurg Rev 2020. https://doi.org/10.1007/s10143-020-01325-z.
20. Dewan MC, Lim J, Shannon CN, et al. The durability of endoscopic third ventriculostomy and ventriculoperitoneal shunts in children with hydrocephalus following posterior fossa tumor resection: a systematic review and time-to-failure analysis. J Neurosurg Pediatr 2017;19(5):578–84.
21. Dinçer A, Özek MM. Radiologic evaluation of pediatric hydrocephalus. Childs Nerv Syst 2011;27(10):1543–62.
22. Jończyk-Potoczna K, Frankiewicz M, Warzywoda M, et al. Low-dose protocol for head CT in evaluation of hydrocephalus in children. Pol J Radiol 2012; 77(1):7–11.
23. Ouellette D, Lynch T, Bruder E, et al. Additive value of nuclear medicine shuntograms to computed tomography for suspected cerebrospinal fluid shunt obstruction in the pediatric emergency department. Pediatr Emerg Care 2009;25(12): 827–30.
24. May CH, Aurisch R, Kornrumpf D, et al. Evaluation of shunt function in hydrocephalic patients with the radionuclide 99mTc-pertechnetate. Childs Nerv Syst 1999;15(5):239–44 [discussion: 245].
25. Merkler AE, Ch'ang J, Parker WE, et al. The rate of complications after ventriculoperitoneal shunt surgery. World Neurosurg 2017;98:654–8.
26. Kulkarni AV, Riva-Cambrin J, Rozzelle CJ, et al. Endoscopic third ventriculostomy and choroid plexus cauterization in infant hydrocephalus: a prospective study by the Hydrocephalus Clinical Research Network. J Neurosurg Pediatr 2018;21(3): 214–23.
27. Simon TD, Schaffzin JK, Stevenson CB, et al. Cerebrospinal fluid shunt infection: emerging paradigms in pathogenesis that affect prevention and treatment. J Pediatr 2019;206:13–9.
28. McGirt MJ, Zaas A, Fuchs HE, et al. Risk factors for pediatric ventriculoperitoneal shunt infection and predictors of infectious pathogens. Clin Infect Dis 2003;36(7): 858–62.
29. Yuh SJ, Vassilyadi M. Management of abdominal pseudocyst in shunt-dependent hydrocephalus. Surg Neurol Int 2012;3:146.
30. Kalra R, Kestle J. Treatment of hydrocephalus with shunts. In: Albright AL, Pollack IF, Adelson PD, editors. Principles and practice of pediatric neurosurgery. 3rd edition. New York: Thieme Medical Publishers, Inc.; 2015. p. 100–18.
31. Ros B, Iglesias S, Martín Á, et al. Shunt overdrainage syndrome: review of the literature. Neurosurg Rev 2018;41(4):969–81.

32. Rekate HL. Shunt-related headaches: the slit ventricle syndromes. Childs Nerv Syst 2008;24(4):423–30.
33. Baskin JJ, Manwaring KH, Rekate HL. Ventricular shunt removal: the ultimate treatment of the slit ventricle syndrome. J Neurosurg 1998;88(3):478–84.
34. Reddy K, Fewer HD, West M, et al. Slit ventricle syndrome with aqueduct stenosis: third ventriculostomy as definitive treatment. Neurosurgery 1988;23(6):756–9.
35. Blount JP, Severson M, Atkins V, et al. Sports and pediatric cerebrospinal fluid shunts: who can play? Neurosurgery 2004;54(5):1190–6 [discussion: 1196–8].
36. Shastin D, Zaben M, Leach P. Can patients with a CSF shunt SCUBA dive? Acta Neurochir (Wien) 2016;158(7):1269–72.
37. Shastin D, Zaben M, Leach P. Life with a cerebrospinal fluid (CSF) shunt. BMJ 2016;355:i5209.
38. Zaben M, Manivannan S, Petralia C, et al. Patient advice regarding participation in sport in children with disorders of cerebrospinal fluid (CSF) circulation: a national survey of British paediatric neurosurgeons. Childs Nerv Syst 2020;36(11):2783–7.
39. Helpin ML, Rosenberg HM, Sayany Z, et al. Antibiotic prophylaxis in dental patients with ventriculo-peritoneal shunts: a pilot study. ASDC J Dent Child 1998;65(4):244–7.
40. Acs G, Cozzi E. Antibiotic prophylaxis for patients with hydrocephalus shunts: a survey of pediatric dentistry and neurosurgery program directors. Pediatr Dent 1992;14(4):246–50.
41. Li G, Dutta S. Perioperative management of ventriculoperitoneal shunts during abdominal surgery. Surg Neurol 2008;70(5):492–5 [discussion: 495–7].
42. Bui CJ, Tubbs RS, Pate G, et al. Infections of pediatric cerebrospinal fluid shunts related to fundoplication and gastrostomy. J Neurosurg 2007;107(5 Suppl):365–7.
43. Mortellaro VE, Chen MK, Pincus D, et al. Infectious risk to ventriculo-peritoneal shunts from gastrointestinal surgery in the pediatric population. J Pediatr Surg 2009;44(6):1201–4 [discussion: 1204–5].
44. Medtronic. Strata Valves and Magnetic Fields; 2012.
45. Strata Valves and Magnetic Fields. 2012. Available at: https://nam03.safelinks.protection.outlook.com/?url=http%3A%2F%2Fwww.hydrocephaluskids.org%2Ffiles%2FMagnetInfoStrataMedtronic.pdf&data=04%7C01%7Cr.mayakrishnan%40elsevier.com%7C7adffdb339f242708c8608d91166b0a3%7C9274ee3f94254109a27f9fb15c10675d%7C0%7C0%7C637559956937448770%7CUnknown%7CTWFpbGZsb3d8eyJWIjoiMC4wLjAwMDAiLCJQIjoiV2luMzIiLCJBTiI6Ik1haWwiLCJXVCI6Mn0%3D%7C1000&sdata=PT4kF7aQaSFfCryifRc8LYEW9d%2Bwv8ccwBBpOzyspq0%3D&reserved=0. Accessed September 16, 2020.
46. Magnetic Field Influences and Your Strata TM Valve. Medtronic EN UC201504957A; 2017. Available at: https://nam03.safelinks.protection.outlook.com/?url=https%3A%2F%2Fwww.medtronic.com%2Fus-en%2Fhealthcare-professionals%2Fproducts%2Fneurological%2Fshunts%2Fstrata-nsc-adjustable-pressure-valve%2Fmagnetic-field-influences.html&data=04%7C01%7Cr.mayakrishnan%40elsevier.com%7C7adffdb339f242708c8608d91166b0a3%7C9274ee3f94254109a27f9fb15c10675d%7C0%7C0%7C637559956937448770%7CUnknown%7CTWFpbGZsb3d8eyJWIjoiMC4wLjAwMDAiLCJQIjoiV2luMzIiLCJBTiI6Ik1haWwiLCJXVCI6Mn0%3D%7C1000&sdata=2FjTqqTp8cztFwzaLJqCg%2FmgkQBteuDBx0auZO%2Ff1dk%3D&reserved=0. Accessed December 7, 2020.

47. Naftel R, Tubergen E, Shannon C, et al. Parental recognition of shunt failure: a prospective single-institution study. J Neurosurg Pediatr 2012;9:363–71.
48. Ackerman LL, Fulkerson DH, Jea A, et al. Parent/guardian knowledge regarding implanted shunt type, setting, and symptoms of malfunction/infection. J Neurosurg Pediatr 2018;21(4):359–66.

Brain and Spinal Cord Tumors in Children

Jignesh Tailor, MD, PhD, Eric M. Jackson, MD*

KEYWORDS

• Brain tumor • Spinal cord tumors • Neuro-oncology

KEY POINTS

- Brain tumors can present with signs and symptoms of raised intracranial pressure, epilepsy, or neurologic deficit.
- The clinical presentation depends on age of patient, location, and invasiveness of the tumor.
- Nocturnal or early morning headaches in children or back pain that wakes a child up at night are red flags that should be taken seriously.
- The first line in treatment of brain tumors usually is surgery, which may be gross total resection, debulking surgery, or biopsy. The surgical option depends on the likely pathology, surgical accessibility, and proximity to eloquent areas.
- Most malignant tumors require radiation therapy and chemotherapy; however, radiation usually is spared in children less than 3 years of age due to significant risks of cognitive impairment.

INTRODUCTION

Primary tumors of the central nervous system (CNS) constitute the largest group of solid tumors in children.[1] Approximately 3000 to 3500 children develop brain tumors in the United States each year (5.26 per 100,000 population).[2–4] The incidence has increased over the past 2 decades. Despite advances in surgical therapy, radiation, and chemotherapy, the outlook for children with malignant tumors generally is poor, and brain cancer has overtaken leukemia as the leading cause of cancer mortality in children.[5] Many children, however, are found with benign brain tumors that may be treated successfully, especially when in a favorable location. The management of brain tumors requires accurate diagnosis and careful estimation of the risks of treatment. Discussion between neurosurgeons and neuro-oncologists within a multidisciplinary team often is needed at initial diagnosis as well as at follow-up visits.

Division of Pediatric Neurosurgery, Department of Neurosurgery, Johns Hopkins University School of Medicine, 600 North Wolfe Street, Phipps 5, Baltimore, MD 21287, USA
* Corresponding author.
E-mail address: ejackson@jhmi.edu

Pediatr Clin N Am 68 (2021) 811–824
https://doi.org/10.1016/j.pcl.2021.04.007

This article reviews the general principles involved in the diagnosis and treatment of childhood brain and spinal cord tumors and discusses special circumstances that may be encountered by pediatricians in the community.

DISTRIBUTION OF PEDIATRIC CENTRAL NERVOUS SYSTEM TUMORS

The distribution of tumors differs markedly in children from the pattern seen in adults[1] (**Fig. 1**). Adult brain tumors usually occur in and around the cerebral hemispheres, whereas the most common site of brain tumors in children of all ages is the posterior fossa.[4] Supratentorial tumors predominate, however, in infants less than 1 year of age and in children 10 to 14 years of age.

The most common histologic subtype overall in children is glioma (52.9%), which consists predominantly of glial cells. A majority of these glioma are benign tumors, such as pilocytic astrocytoma (33.2%), or low-grade gliomas (27.1%).[4] High-grade gliomas are relatively uncommon in children. Meningiomas, pituitary tumors, and metastatic tumors, which are common in adults, rarely are seen in children.

In infants less than 1 year of age, low-grade glioma, embryonal tumors, and choroid plexus tumors predominate (**Fig. 2**). The most common embryonal tumor in infants is atypical teratoid/rhabdoid tumor. In older children, glioma and embryonal tumors are most common, with the most common embryonal tumor being medulloblastoma (MB) (**Fig. 3**). The primary differential diagnosis of a posterior fossa mass in a child includes

- MB
- Ependymoma
- Cerebellar astrocytoma (**Fig. 4**)

Intramedullary spinal cord tumors in the pediatric population usually are astrocytoma or ependymoma. Astrocytoma is more common in infants and young children and usually present as infiltrative/diffuse lesions in the upper spinal cord (**Fig. 5**). Spinal cord ependymoma are more common in older children and adults.

CLINICAL PRESENTATION OF BRAIN TUMORS

In general, brain tumors can present with

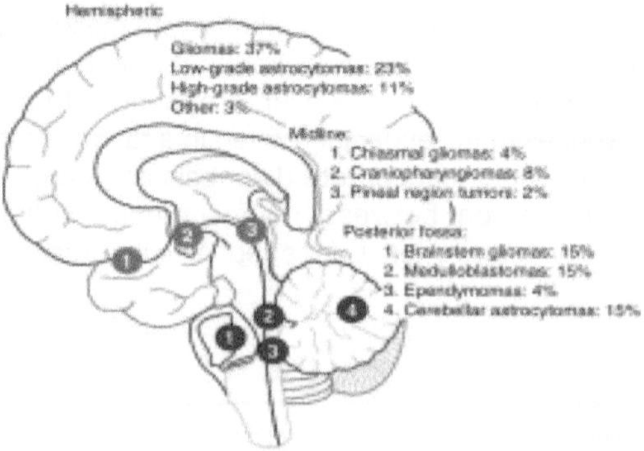

Fig. 1. Brain tumors in childhood. Childhood brain tumors occur at any location within CNS. The relative frequency of brain tumor histologic types and the anatomic distribution are shown. The numbers in green circles refer to the location of midline tumors, and the numbers in purple refer to the location of the posterior fossa tumors. (*From* Nelson Textbook of Pediatrics. Zaky, Wafik; Ater, Joann L.; Khatua, Soumen. Published January 1, 2020. Pages 2666-2678. Elsevier © 2020.)

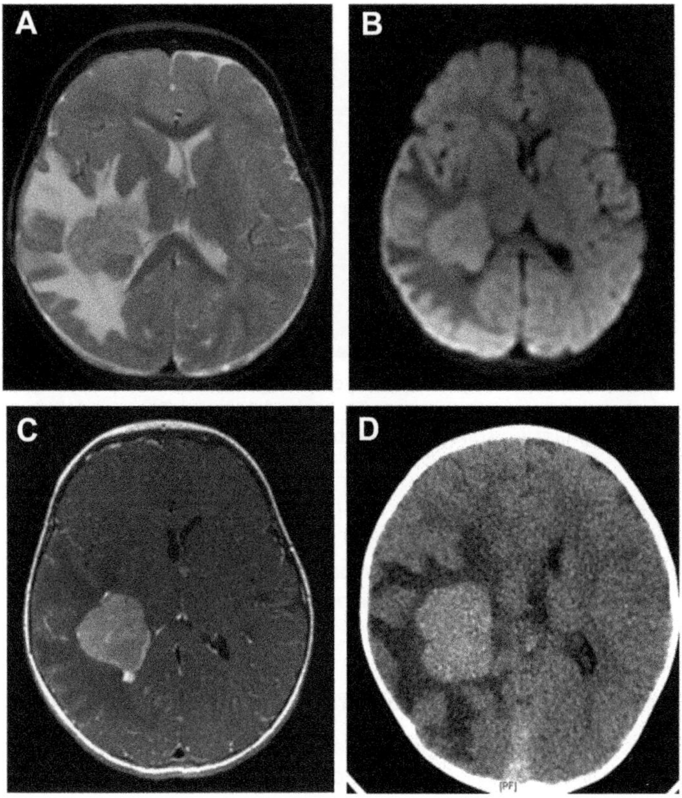

Fig. 2. Choroid plexus carcinoma. A 16-month-old girl who presented with intractable vomiting for 2 weeks. The T2 axial MRI scan (*A*), diffusion-weighted imaging (DWI) (*B*), and T1 axial (*C*) postcontrast MRI (*C*) show an enhancing intraventricular tumor with surrounding edema. The lesion was hyperdense on CT imaging (*D*).

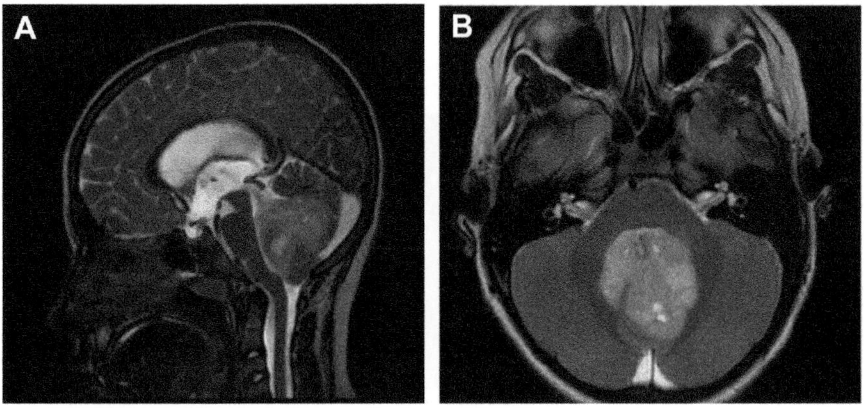

Fig. 3. MB. An 11-year-old boy who presented with headaches associated with nausea/vomiting. T2 sagittal MRI (*A*) and T2 axial MRI (*B*) show a heterogeneous cerebellar mass at the roof of the fourth ventricle. The mass is obstructing CSF flow and causing obstructive hydrocephalus.

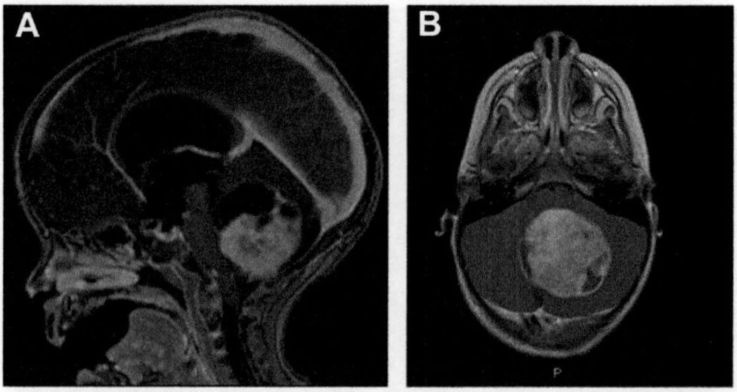

Fig. 4. Cerebellar pilocytic astrocytoma. A 2-year-old girl presented with 6-week history of nausea/vomiting and more recent ataxia. T1 sagittal (*A*) and T1 axial MRI with contrast (*B*) show an avidly enhancing solid/cystic cerebellar mass with associated hydrocephalus.

- Raised intracranial pressure (ICP) (due to an expanding tumor mass or hydrocephalus)
- Epilepsy (usually simple or complex partial seizures)
- Neurologic deficit (usually progressive but occasionally can be abrupt if hemorrhage occurs into the tumor)
- Incidental finding on imaging done for other reasons (eg, trauma)

Three important factors determine the presentation of a brain tumor:

- Age of the child (infants present differently to older children because of their stage of development and nonfusion of sutures)
- Location (proximity to eloquent areas and/or ventricular system)
- Histologic grade (rate of growth and local invasiveness)

The brain is classically divided into eloquent and silent areas. Eloquent areas are regions in which a tumor produces significant neurologic signs and symptoms before the tumor has grown sufficiently large to raise ICP. Eloquent areas include

- Speech pathway (left temporal and frontal lobe)
- Motor pathway (primary motor cortex and corticospinal tracts)

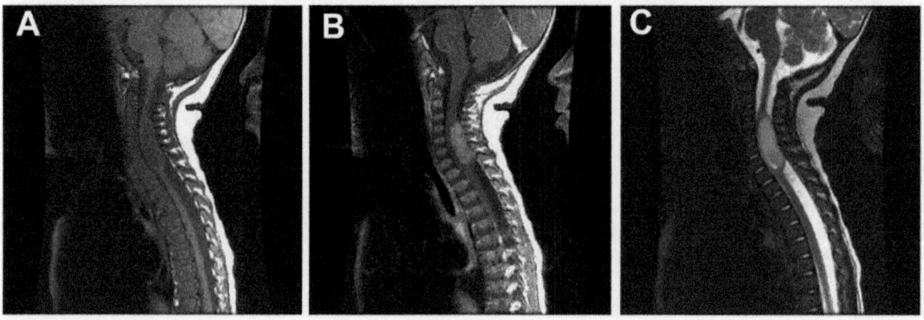

Fig. 5. Spinal astrocytoma. A 9-month-old girl who presented with subtle weakness of left arm. T1 sagittal MRI of cervical spine without contrast (*A*), T1 sagittal MRI postcontrast (*B*), and T2 sagittal MRI (*C*) show a homogeneously contrast enhancing expansile mass in the cervical cord.

- Visual pathway (occipital lobe, optic nerve, and radiations)

The silent areas are regions where tumors can grow to a remarkably large size without causing obvious neurologic impairment. They instead eventually produce symptomatic raised ICP. Silent areas can include the right temporal and frontal lobe.

Raised Intracranial Pressure

The symptoms of raised ICP in infants are notoriously inconsistent and may include irritability, lethargy, vomiting, failure to thrive, or developmental regression. Because the cranial sutures are not fused, an expanding mass or hydrocephalus can lead to a rapidly increasing head circumference (crossing percentiles) and a bulging fontanelle. In severe cases, infants may develop apneic or bradycardic episodes from pressure on the brainstem.

Older children usually complain of headache. The classic description is a headache that

- Is worse in the morning
- Can occur at night
- Is worse with straining
- Can be associated with nausea and vomiting

Nocturnal headache is a red flag and should be taken seriously in any child because it is highly suggestive of raised ICP. Papilledema (optic disc swelling) can occur in patients with raised ICP. This important clinical sign is considered a medical emergency because of the risk to vision and underlying raised ICP.[6] In severe cases, children with raised ICP may develop deteriorating consciousness. The decline in consciousness can occur rapidly, so children with concerns of raised ICP should be transferred to an emergency department immediately for evaluation. The initial signs of life-threatening deterioration are increasing drowsiness and confusion. These often are recorded in the hospital setting using the Glasgow Coma Scale,[7] which provides an accurate and reproducible way of describing the level of consciousness (www.glasgowcomascale.org).

Hydrocephalus

Children with brain tumors that are located close to the ventricular system can develop hydrocephalus due to obstruction to cerebrospinal fluid (CSF) flow (see **Figs. 3** and **4**). For example, a posterior fossa tumor can obstruct the fourth ventricular outflow and lead to a buildup of CSF in the ventricles upstream (third and lateral ventricles). Hydrocephalus causes elevated ICP and can present with the signs and symptoms, discussed previously, such as headaches, nausea/vomiting, and lethargy.

Epilepsy

Epilepsy is a variable phenomenon with brain tumors; many patients with brain tumors do not develop epilepsy. Epilepsy can be common, however, with some pathologic types of tumors for example, slow-growing tumors, such as subtypes of low-grade glioma.[8] Tumors in certain locations, such as the temporal lobe, also are more likely to present with seizures.

Neurologic Deficit

A neurologic deficit (speech difficulty, limb weakness, or loss of visual fields) can develop if the tumor is near an eloquent area. It is more likely to develop if the tumor is intrinsic (ie, in the brain substance) and if it is growing rapidly and invasively (eg, high-grade glioma). Malignant intrinsic tumors grow quickly over weeks to months and usually are associated with rapidly progressive neurologic deficit. Slow-growing benign extrinsic tumors (eg, craniopharyngioma) can take years to produce a slowly progressive deficit. Occasionally, hemorrhage can occur into a previously asymptomatic tumor and this can present acutely with neurologic deficit, similar to a stroke. Most cases of hemorrhage occur in malignant tumors, such as high-grade glioma.

CLINICAL PRESENTATION OF SPINAL CORD TUMORS

In general, spinal cord tumors can present with

- Neurologic deficit
  - Weakness, numbness, bowel, or bladder function changes
- Back pain
  - Back pain that regularly wakes a child up at night from sleep is a tumor until proved otherwise
- Spinal deformity

DIAGNOSTIC WORK-UP

Red flags for elevated ICP and a suspected brain tumor are highlighted in **Fig. 6**. Infants and children with a suspected brain tumor should be transferred immediately to an emergency room for an urgent brain scan. Initially, either a CT scan or,

Red flags for raised intracranial pressure and brain tumors in both		
	Symptoms	**Signs**
Infants	Persistent irritability Lethargy Poor feeding Neurological deficit • Weakness • Sensory loss Seizures	Head circumference crossing percentiles Bulging fontanelle Distended scalp veins Suture splay Papilledema Lateral gaze palsy (false localizing sign) Deteriorating GCS
Children	Headache • Nocturnal • Worse in morning • Associated with nausea/vomiting Vision loss Neurological deficit • Weakness • Sensory loss Seizures	Papilledema Lateral gaze palsy (false localizing sign) Confusion/disorientation Deteriorating GCS

Fig. 6. Red flag signs and symptoms of raised ICP and brain tumors in infants and children.

preferably, fast spin-echo, T2-sequence magnetic resonance imaging (MRI) scan can be used to rule out a mass lesion. If a tumor is found, however, most children require more detailed MRI with and without contrast.

Children with brain tumors subsequently have preoperative blood work, including complete blood cell count, metabolic panel, coagulation screen, and type and screen. For children with suspected germ cell tumors (**Fig. 7**), blood and/or CSF can be obtained for the measurement of tumor markers, including α-fetoprotein and ß-subunit of human chorionic gonadotrophin. A diagnosis of these tumors can be made on these laboratory tests and may obviate surgery for the tumor itself.

For malignant tumors with a high incidence of dissemination within the CSF and leptomeningeal disease (LMD), such as MB or posterior fossa ependymoma, a whole-spine MRI is performed prior to surgical intervention. In addition, a sample of CSF usually is taken for cytology, usually 2 weeks postoperatively and prior to the commencement of oncological treatment. The presence of LMD significantly affects the prognosis and treatment of pediatric patients with malignant tumors, such as MB. Both CSF cytology and spinal MRI are used routinely to diagnose LMD. With the use of either CSF cytology or spinal MRI alone, LMD is missed in up to 14% to 18% of patients with malignant embryonal tumors.[9] Primary brain tumors, such as glial neoplasms, rarely spread beyond the CNS at the time of diagnosis; therefore, a systematic staging work-up usually is not necessary.

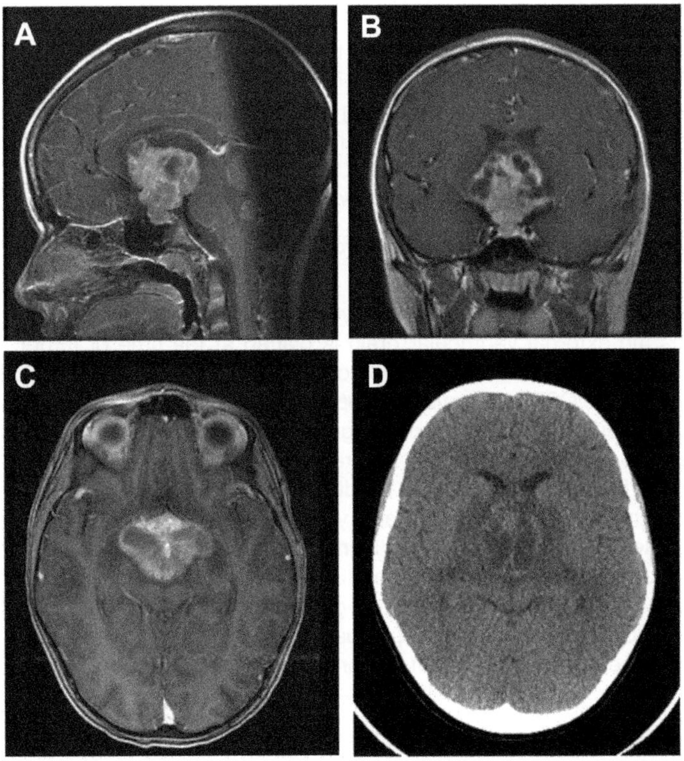

Fig. 7. Suprasellar germ cell tumor. A 10-year-old girl who presented with headaches, visual changes, lethargy, and elevated sodium. T1-weighted MRIs postcontrast in sagittal (*A*), coronal (*B*), and axial (*C*) views show vivid enhancement of a large suprasellar mass extending into the hypothalamic region and third ventricle. CT scan shows no calcification (*D*).

SURGICAL TREATMENT

The initial step in treatment of brain tumors usually is surgery. In general, the surgical options for brain tumors depend on the location of the tumor and suspected pathology. They include

1. GTR—the goal is to establish histopathologic diagnosis as well as to macroscopically remove the entire tumor. For a majority of tumors, GTR often provides the best outcomes. Benign tumors, such as pilocytic astrocytoma, can be cured by GTR. Some others, such as ependymoma, do not respond well to adjuvant therapies; thus, GTR, if it can be done safely, is the best treatment.[10] Therefore, GTR is recommended for most pediatric brain tumors, unless they are in surgically inaccessible locations.
2. Surgical debulking—the goal is to establish histopathologic diagnosis and to reduce tumor burden while preserving neurologic function. Tumor in eloquent locations may be left in order to prevent significant neurologic deficit.
3. Biopsy—a small sample of the tumor is taken only for histopathologic diagnosis. This option usually is performed for unresectable tumors, such as diffuse gliomas and deep-seated tumors, where the risk of surgical resection outweighs the potential benefits of cytoreduction. The biopsy typically is performed using stereotactic navigation.[11] Surgical biopsy has become particularly valuable in the current molecular era because the genetic phenotype of the tumor may influence the subsequent oncological course or establish candidates for targeted drug therapy.

Neurosurgeons may use several adjuncts to improve the extent of resection, including neuronavigation, intraoperative ultrasound, and intraoperative MRI. Image-guided surgery or neuronavigation involves registering the MRI scan of the patient to the head in real space, thereby allowed the surgeon to navigate regions of the brain using the MRI as a map.[11] This allows accurate planning of surgical trajectories, localization of the margins of the tumor following resection, and avoidance of eloquent structures.

Management of Common Perioperative Problems

Obstructive hydrocephalus

Patients with raised ICP from obstructive hydrocephalus may require CSF diversion. In many cases, an external ventricular drain is placed at the time of tumor resection. Alternatively, endoscopic third ventriculostomy (ETV) may be performed. Following tumor resection, if the CSF pathways open up, the external ventricular drain can be discontinued. Patients who develop progressive ventriculomegaly or significant pseudomeningocele post–resection of brain tumors may require permanent CSF diversion in the form of a shunt or ETV. Predictors of CSF shunting in patients with posterior fossa tumors include age less than 2 years (score of 3), papilledema (score of 1), moderate to severe hydrocephalus at diagnosis (score of 2), presence of CSF metastases (score of 3), and specific estimated tumor pathologies, such as MB or ependymoma (score of 1).[12] Patients with score of greater than 5 are thought to be at high risk of developing postresection hydrocephalus. Although shunt-related extraneural metastases from peritoneal seeding of tumors have been described in literature, they are extremely rare.

Peritumoral edema

Vasogenic edema associated with tumors may cause mass effect on eloquent brain areas. In that context, consideration is given to perioperative dexamethasone (0.05–0.1 mg per kg/4 times daily). Steroids usually are tapered within several days of surgery, especially if there has been extensive resection of the tumor.

Seizures
An antiepileptic agent, such as levetiracetam (Keppra) or phenytoin (Dilantin) can be started preoperatively and continued during surgery for cortical lesions that present with seizures, or if a substantial amount of cortical retraction is expected during surgery. The antiepileptics often are continued for a week after surgery in the absence of seizures. Children with a history of seizures usually are assessed by neurologists, and the decision to continue antiepileptics depends on their postoperative electroencephalographic activity and clinical seizure freedom.

Hypothalamic-pituitary hormonal insufficiency
Endocrine abnormalities typically occur with tumors in and around the sellar region, such as craniopharyngioma. Preoperatively, a full endocrine profile usually is performed as part of the initial blood work and stress-dose steroids often are given for patients with tumors in this region. Surgery near the hypothalamus/pituitary region can result in central diabetes insipidus due to insufficient vasopressin release from posterior pituitary gland, which can lead to the production of copious amount of dilute urine (> 4cc/kg/hour) and hypernatremia. A vasopressin analog (desmopressin) can be administered to patients for treatment of diabetes insipidus if necessary. Postoperatively, steroid treatment usually can be decreased to physiologic levels under the guidance of endocrinologists. Fluid balance and electrolytes are monitored closely and follow-up with endocrinology is important to determine the need for long-term hormone replacement.

RADIATION THERAPY

Ionizing radiation can be delivered to tumors by 2 sources:

- High-energy photons (x-rays or gamma rays)
- Accelerated charged particles (protons or helium)

Conventional radiation therapy involves the delivery of hypofractionated photons to tissue. Hypofractionated radiation therapy is based on the premise that normal tissues are better able than tumor cells to repair sublethal damage between doses. The delivery of multiple daily fractions also increases the likelihood of irradiating proliferating tumor cells in a radiosensitive portion of the cell cycle.

Hypofractionated craniospinal radiation therapy remains appropriate for tumors that are prone to disseminate throughout the neuroaxis, such as MB. Children with MB typically receive craniospinal irradiation (CSI) to the entire neuroaxis, followed by a radiation boost to the posterior fossa.[13] For locally invasive tumors, such as malignant glioma, radiation usually is administered to the tumor bed and margins of the surrounding brain. Despite being efficacious, radiation can lead to long-term cognitive impairment and should be avoided in children under 3 years of age if possible.

Stereotactic radiosurgery (SRS) involves the stereotactic delivery of a highly focused photon dose to the tumor. The ideal objective is the destruction of the targeted area (mainly through vascular necrosis) without damaging any surrounding normal tissue. SRS differs from conventional radiotherapy in several ways. The efficacy of radiotherapy depends primarily on the greater sensitivity of tumor cells to radiation relative to normal brain tissue. In standard radiotherapy, the spatial accuracy of the treatment is a secondary concern as normal tissues are protected by administering the radiation dose over multiple sessions (fractions) daily for a period of several weeks. Radiosurgery requires much greater targeting accuracy. SRS protects normal tissues by both selectively targeting only the abnormal lesion and using cross-firing techniques to minimize the exposure of the adjacent normal tissue. There are 2 main types of SRS:

- Gamma Knife uses cobalt-60 gamma rays and focuses multiple channels onto a single target
- LINAC uses high-energy x-rays and has an arm that projects a single beam from multiple angles.

The main use in children is in skull base tumors, arteriovenous malformations, and brain metastases.

Proton beam radiotherapy uses accelerated charged particles or protons instead of photons. The main difference with proton therapy is that that the proton beam stops at the tumor and does not exit the body. This principle limits the impact of ionizing radiation on the surrounding brain. Proton therapy is particularly useful in children, because it lowers the risk to developing brain by reducing the exposed areas.[14] There is reduced risk of cognitive impairment and less risk of secondary tumors in children receiving CSI.[15] In addition, it can be useful in pregnant women who need CSI, because it reduces the dose to the fetus. With conventional radiation therapy, the fetus is irradiated by photons. The disadvantage of proton therapy is that it is costly to set up a center; thus, it is available at more limited centers throughout the country.

CHEMOTHERAPY

For most malignant tumors, chemotherapy is offered. There is limited role for chemotherapy in some CNS tumors, however, such as ependymoma due to lack of efficacy.[10] Occasionally, chemotherapy may be given to infants and young children under the age of 3 years with malignant tumors as a therapeutic strategy to delay radiation therapy.

The first major role of chemotherapy in treating MB was based on the discovery that adjuvant chemotherapy after GTR and radiation resulted in improved survival rates[16] and allowed for the delivery of a lower dose of CSI in those without metastatic disease.[17] This discovery contributed to the stratification of these tumors into 2 risk groups:

- Standard-risk MBs have less than a 1.5-cm^2 measurable residual after surgical resection, no metastases on staging MRI of the spine, and no tumor cells seen in CSF obtained via lumbar puncture
- High-risk MBs have greater than a 1.5-cm^2 residual tumor at the primary site after surgical resection or metastases on staging as seen either on MRI or in the CSF. More recently, anaplastic or large-cell pathology has been considered to identify a high-risk tumor.

The specific chemotherapy regimen for MB may vary between oncology centers. For standard-risk MB, children typically receive CSI with boost to the posterior fossa, followed chemotherapy. For high-risk MB, children typically receive chemotherapy during radiation (higher-dose CSI with posterior fossa boost), followed by maintenance chemotherapy. Complications of these chemotherapy regimens include

- Bone marrow suppression—low platelets, neutropenia
- Gastrointestinal distress—nausea, vomiting
- Hearing loss—cisplatin and carboplatin are ototoxic.
- Nephrotoxicity—cisplatin is nephrotoxic; monitoring renal function and avoiding about nephrotoxic agents, such as aminoglycosides, is recommended.
- Neuropathy—vincristine-induced motor and sensory polyneuropathy is common, and children may require splints or ankle/foot orthotics to ambulate. Autonomic neuropathy also is common and can lead to ileus, bowel obstruction, or bladder retention.

In recent years, the genetic profiling of brain tumors has opened up the opportunity for targeted drug therapy. For example, BRAF mutations and MAPK pathway activation in pediatric low-grade gliomas have been the driving factor for research and novel therapeutic approaches in these patients, especially for recurrent or refractory tumors.[18–20]

Novel agents and modifications to chemotherapy regimens usually go through several treatment trial phases before they become mainstream practice. The trial phases are outlined in **Fig. 8**. Briefly, a phase I trial is safety driven and aims to find the best dose of a new drug with the fewest side effects. The drug usually is tested in a small group of 15 to 30 patients. A phase II trial further assess the safety of a drug. It is often tested among patients with a specific cancer and in larger groups compared with phase I. If the drug is found to work, it is tested in a phase III trial. This phase compares the new drug to a standard of care drug in the setting of a randomized controlled trial. The aim is to assess the efficacy and side effects of the new drug.

New cancer drug trials usually are studied collaboratively in consortiums, such as the Pediatric Brain Tumor Consortium (www.pbtc.org) and the Pacific Pediatric Neuro-Oncology Consortium (PNOC) (www.pnoc.us). PNOC is a network of children's hospitals across the United States and world that perform clinical trials of therapies that are specific to the molecular profiles of a patient's tumor (targeted therapy). PNOC trials aim to provide patients with therapies optimized for their tumor type. The Children's Oncology Group is another cooperative group that combines the efforts of pediatric clinical trials groups based in North America to accelerate the search for a cure and prevention of cancer in children and adolescents (www.childrensoncologygroup.org).

SPECIAL CIRCUMSTANCES

Screening

Currently, there are no widely recommended screening tests for brain and spinal cord tumors in children or adults. In general, patients only require further evaluation if they are found to have symptoms or signs of a suspected brain tumor. Patients with a strong family history of brain cancer may be monitored clinically on a regular basis or referred to genetics for testing and counseling.

Inherited syndromes, such as neurofibromatosis, tuberous sclerosis or Li-Fraumeni syndrome, may predispose a child to a brain tumor. These children may benefit from frequent physical examinations and surveillance from a young age. This monitoring could be performed in the community or in specialist clinics, if available, for example, a neurofibromatosis clinic. Not all tumors related to these syndromes may need to be treated right away. Finding them early, however, could help them to be monitored and treated quickly if they begin to grow or cause symptoms.

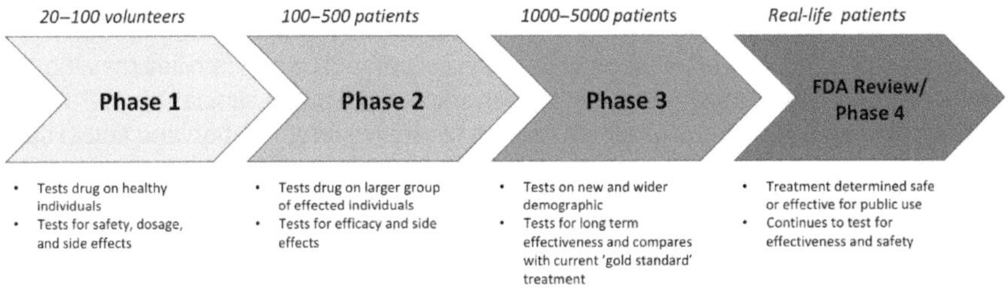

Fig. 8. Phases of clinical trials. Phases 1 to 3 are necessary prior to Food and Drug Administration (FDA) approval. Brain tumor clinical trials usually are conducted within a large consortium.

Incidental Tumors

Some brain tumors are found incidentally on MRI scans performed for other reasons. These cases should be brought to the attention of a neurosurgeon and discussed in a neuro-oncology multidisciplinary conference. Tumors that show worrying radiological features (eg, restricted diffusion, enhancement, local invasion, and tumor growth) may require surgery to determine pathology. A majority of incidentally found lesions on MRI scans, however, are benign and do not end up requiring intervention. They require surveillance MRI, initially at short intervals (eg, 3 months) and subsequently at longer intervals if the appearances are stable (eg, 1 year). Radiological changes in the lesion or clinical symptoms may prompt surgical intervention.

FUTURE DIRECTIONS

The past decade has witnessed an explosion of information on the genetic landscape of pediatric CNS tumors.[21–23] Next-generation sequencing has provided deep insight into the broad molecular blueprints of childhood cancer and has identified important genes and signaling pathways that serve to drive tumor growth.[18] This insight has greatly impacted the field by providing potential therapeutic targets for these diseases, and the opportunity for targeted drug therapy. Moreover, it is changing the way CNS tumors are classified and the way children with disease are risk-stratified. For example, MB now can be subdivided into 4 molecular subgroups: WNT, SHH, group 3, group 4. Each of these MB subgroups behaves as a separate entity, with different clinical and risk profiles. An exciting era of personalized medicine is being entered that aims to tailor oncological treatment to the unique molecular and genetic profile of the individual with cancer.

SUMMARY

Brain tumors come in different varieties with significant variation in aggressiveness. The most important steps in the initial management of brain tumor and spinal cord tumors are recognizing that a tumor may be present and initiating the appropriate investigations. The early warning signs of brain tumors may include persistent headache (which may be severe and worsen with activity or in the early morning), especially when associated with nausea/vomiting, developmental regression, or lethargy. Patients also can present with intermittent neurologic symptoms or signs representing focal seizures. Any child with a suspected CNS tumor should be referred for immediate evaluation. The mainstay of treatment in most cases is surgical; however, factors, such as surgical accessibility and radiological appearance, are taken into consideration. Some tumors can be observed due to their benign growth pattern; however, the risk of malignant progression or effects on neighboring structures must be monitored carefully. Diagnosis and further oncological management of brain tumors now are highly influenced by the genetics of the tumor. Although many families may inquire about targeted drug therapy, most of these therapies still are in clinical trials. Patients with brain and spinal cord tumors often require extensive rehabilitation and social support after treatment, including both physical and neurocognitive therapy.

Clinics Care Points

- A critical step in the diagnosis of brain tumors is recognition of the signs and symptoms of raised ICP in an infant (irritability, enlarging head, and bulging fontanelle) or a child (headache worse in morning or nocturnal, associated with nausea/vomiting and papilledema)

- Brain tumors also may present with epilepsy or neurologic deficit or may be found incidentally on a brain scan performed for other reasons (eg, trauma). The presentation of a brain tumor depends on the age of patient, location of tumor, and aggressiveness of the tumor, that is, the histologic grade.
- A child with a suspected symptomatic CNS tumor should be referred immediately for imaging and neurologic evaluation.
- The surgical treatment options for CNS tumors include GTR, surgical debulking, and biopsy. Depending on the pathology, surgery may be followed by radiation therapy and/or chemotherapy. Conventional radiation therapy (photons) is avoided in children less than 3 years old to prevent cognitive impairment. Proton beam radiotherapy may reduce these risks, but it does not eliminate the risks and not always is available.
- Children may require coordinated and multidisciplinary care for many years, including visits with neurosurgery (for surgical follow-up), medical and radiation oncology (for chemotherapy and radiation and surveillance imaging), neurology (for seizure management), endocrinology (especially for sellar/suprasellar tumors), ophthalmology (for tumors that affect the brainstem cranial nerves or visual fields), neuropsychology, physical therapy, and social care services (for their physical, emotional, and social well-being).

DISCLOSURE

The authors have nothing to disclose.

REFERENCES

1. Pollack IF. Brain tumors in children. N Engl J Med 1994;331(22):1500–7.
2. Johnson KJ, Cullen J, Barnholtz-Sloan JS, et al. Childhood brain tumor epidemiology: a brain tumor epidemiology consortium review. Cancer Epidemiol Biomarkers Prev 2014;23(12):2716–36.
3. Ostrom QT, Gittleman H, Farah P, et al. CBTRUS statistical report: primary brain and central nervous system tumors diagnosed in the United States in 2006-2010. Neuro Oncol 2013;15(suppl 2):ii1–56.
4. Ostrom QT, de Blank PM, Kruchko C, et al. Alex's Lemonade Stand Foundation Infant and childhood primary brain and central nervous system tumors diagnosed in the United States in 2007–2011. Neuro Oncol 2015;16(Suppl 10):x1.
5. Curtin SC, Miniño AM, Anderson RN. Declines in cancer death rates among children and adolescents in the United States. 1999. Available at: http://www.cdc.gov/nchs/. Accessed May 12, 2020.
6. Peragallo JH. Visual function in children with primary brain tumors. Curr Opin Neurol 2019;32(1). https://doi.org/10.1097/WCO.0000000000000644.
7. Teasdale G, Jennett B. Assessment of coma and impaired consciousness. Lancet 1974;304(7872):81–4.
8. Wells EM, Gaillard WD, Packer RJ. Pediatric brain tumors and epilepsy. Semin Pediatr Neurol 2012;19(1):3–8.
9. Fouladi M, Gajjar A, Boyett JM, et al. Comparison of CSF cytology and spinal magnetic resonance imaging in the detection of leptomeningeal disease in pediatric medulloblastoma or primitive neuroectodermal tumor. J Clin Oncol 1999;17(10). https://doi.org/10.1200/JCO.1999.17.10.3234.
10. Pajtler KW, Mack SC, Ramaswamy V, et al. The current consensus on the clinical management of intracranial ependymoma and its distinct molecular variants. Acta Neuropathol 2017;3:5–12.

11. Orringer DA, Golby A, Jolesz F. Neuronavigation in the surgical management of brain tumors: current and future trends. Expert Rev Med Devices 2012;9(5):491.
12. Riva-Cambrin J, Detsky AS, Lamberti-Pasculli M, et al. Predicting postresection hydrocephalus in pediatric patients with posterior fossa tumors. J Neurosurg Pediatr 2009;3(5). https://doi.org/10.3171/2009.1.PEDS08298.
13. Northcott PA, Robinson GW, Kratz CP, et al. Medulloblastoma. Nat Rev Dis Primers 2019;5(1):11.
14. Kirsch DG, Tarbell NJ. New technologies in radiation therapy for pediatric brain tumors: the rationale for proton radiation therapy. Pediatr Blood Cancer 2004; 42(5):461–4.
15. Clair WHS, Adams JA, Bues M, et al. Advantage of protons compared to conventional X-ray or IMRT in the treatment of a pediatric patient with medulloblastoma. Int J Radiat Oncol Biol Phys 2004. https://doi.org/10.1016/S0360-3016(03)01574-8.
16. Evans AE, Jenkin RDT, Sposto R, et al. The treatment of medulloblastoma. Results of a prospective randomized trial of radiation therapy with and without CCNU, vincristine, and prednisone. J Neurosurg 1990;72(4):572–82.
17. Deutsch M, Thomas PRM, Krischer J, et al. Results of a prospective randomized trial comparing standard dose neuraxis irradiation (3,600 cGy/20) with reduced neuraxis irradiation (2,340 cGy/13) in patients with low-stage medulloblastoma. Pediatr Neurosurg 1996;24(4):167–77.
18. Cacciotti C, Fleming A, Ramaswamy V. Advances in the molecular classification of pediatric brain tumors: a guide to the galaxy Division of Pediatric Hematology/ Oncology , McMaster Children ' s Hospital , Hamilton , ON Hospital for Sick Children , Toronto , ON Programme in Developmental an. J Pathol 2020. https://doi.org/10.1002/path.5457.
19. Fangusaro J, Onar-Thomas A, Poussaint TY, et al. Selumetinib in paediatric patients with BRAF-aberrant or neurofibromatosis type 1-associated recurrent, refractory, or progressive low-grade glioma: a multicentre, phase 2 trial. Lancet Oncol 2019;20. https://doi.org/10.1016/S1470-2045(19)30277-3.
20. Banerjee A, Jakacki RI, Onar-Thomas A, et al. A phase I trial of the MEK inhibitor selumetinib (AZD6244) in pediatric patients with recurrent or refractory low-grade glioma: a Pediatric Brain Tumor Consortium (PBTC) study. Neuro Oncol 2017; 19(8):1135–44.
21. Parsons DW, Li M, Zhang X, et al. The genetic landscape of the childhood cancer medulloblastoma. Science 2011. https://doi.org/10.1126/science.1198056.
22. Dubuc AM, Northcott PA, Mack S, et al. The genetics of pediatric brain tumors. Curr Neurol Neurosci Rep 2010. https://doi.org/10.1007/s11910-010-0103-9.
23. Northcott PA, Buchhalter I, Morrissy AS, et al. The whole-genome landscape of medulloblastoma subtypes. Nature 2017. https://doi.org/10.1038/nature22973.

Intracranial Vascular Abnormalities in Children

Alaa Montaser, MD, PhD, Edward R. Smith, MD*

KEYWORDS

• Moyamoya • Arteriovenous malformations • Cavernous malformations
• Intracranial vascular abnormalities • Arteriopathy • Stroke • Pediatric

KEY POINTS

- Intracranial vascular abnormalities in children can be categorized as vascular malformations (arteriovenous malformations/arteriovenous fistulae and cavernous malformations), structural arteriopathies (aneurysms and moyamoya), and incidental developmental anomalies of the vasculature.
- These entities are unique in typically being occult, with few (if any) indications of their presence in history or physical examination for long periods of time.
- Acute hemorrhagic or ischemic stroke is the most common presentation in a majority of symptomatic cases, often incurring significant morbidity and mortality.
- The primary care provider has an essential role in recognizing relevant diagnostic cues and key associations to genetic and syndromic risk factors and comanaging the critical efforts of screening for disease and ensuring appropriate follow-up after diagnosis and treatment.

INTRODUCTION

Although encountered rarely in routine pediatric practice, the potential severe morbidity of pathologic intracranial vascular malformations, coupled with the typical acuity of their presentation, merits ongoing awareness of current relevant diagnostic and therapeutic strategies (**Fig. 1**). The major clinical concern is stroke, including ischemic infarction, hemorrhagic infarction, intracerebral hemorrhage (ICH), and subarachnoid hemorrhage (SAH).

Knowing how to identify at-risk populations, perform the proper evaluation, and refer a patient to surgical treatment puts primary care providers (PCPs) in a leading position to protect children from the sequelae of stroke.[1] This review defines key intracranial vascular abnormalities, discusses indications for screening, provides a general overview of key history and examination features of suspected vascular lesions in the primary care setting, and concludes with an overview of frequently asked questions encountered in practice.

Department of Neurosurgery, Boston Children's Hospital, Harvard Medical School, 300 Longwood Avenue, Boston, MA 02115, USA
* Corresponding author.
E-mail address: edward.smith@childrens.harvard.edu

Pediatr Clin N Am 68 (2021) 825–843
https://doi.org/10.1016/j.pcl.2021.04.010
pediatric.theclinics.com

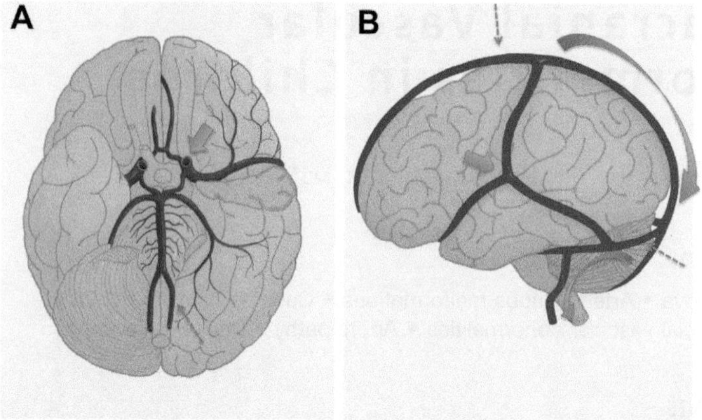

Fig. 1. Normal vascular anatomy of the brain. (*A*) Inferior view of the brain illustrating the arterial supply to the brain, with contributions from the vertebral artery (*dashed arrow*) and ICA (*solid arrow*). (*B*) Lateral view of the brain demonstrating centrifugal venous drainage of the brain to include cortical surface veins (*solid arrow*) leading to dural venous sinuses (*dashed arrows*), ultimately draining to the jugular veins in the neck. Direction of flow is indicated by curved arrows.

VASCULAR MALFORMATIONS (ARTERIOVENOUS MALFORMATIONS/ ARTERIOVENOUS FISTULAE AND CAVERNOUS MALFORMATIONS)

Arteriovenous Malformations and Arteriovenous Fistulae

Pathophysiology

Arteriovenous malformations (AVMs) and arteriovenous fistulae (AVF) lesions encompass a spectrum from simple single-point connections between 1 artery and 2 veins (AVF) to large concatenations of tangled, dysplastic vessels with multiple feeding and draining channels (AVM) (**Fig. 2**). An AVM is a tangle of dysplastic vessels (nidus) consisting of direct arterial-to-venous connections without intervening capillaries, forming a high-flow low-resistance shunt between the arterial and venous systems.[2] Central nervous system (CNS) AVMs lack functional neural tissue within the lesions. The AVM nidus can change over time and is prone to rupture with progressive weakening.

Intracerebral AVM usually is an isolated lesion.[3] Multiple AVMs are rare but exist in 2 conditions.[4] First is Wyburn-Mason syndrome, characterized by ipsilateral retinal and optic pathway cerebral AVMs with cutaneous capillary malformations.[4] Second is hereditary hemorrhagic telangiectasia (HHT), an autosomal dominant disorder with telangiectasias of the skin in association with AVMs of deep structures, including the lungs and CNS, making up approximately 3.4% of all AVMs.[5]

Epidemiology and risk

ICH comprises approximately 50% of pediatric stroke, with an incidence of approximately 1/100,000/year, caused by either structural lesions or hematological disorders.[6] Nontraumatic, spontaneous ICH are caused by structural lesions in up to approximately 75% of cases, with AVM found most commonly, and approximately 10% of hemorrhage remaining idiopathic.[7–12] Vein of Galen malformation (VOGM) is far more rare, comprising less than 1% of all pediatric vascular cases in the United States, with 1 case to 2 cases on average per high-volume center annually.[13] The prevalence of AVFs ranges between 0.1/100,000 and 1/100,000, with no clear sex

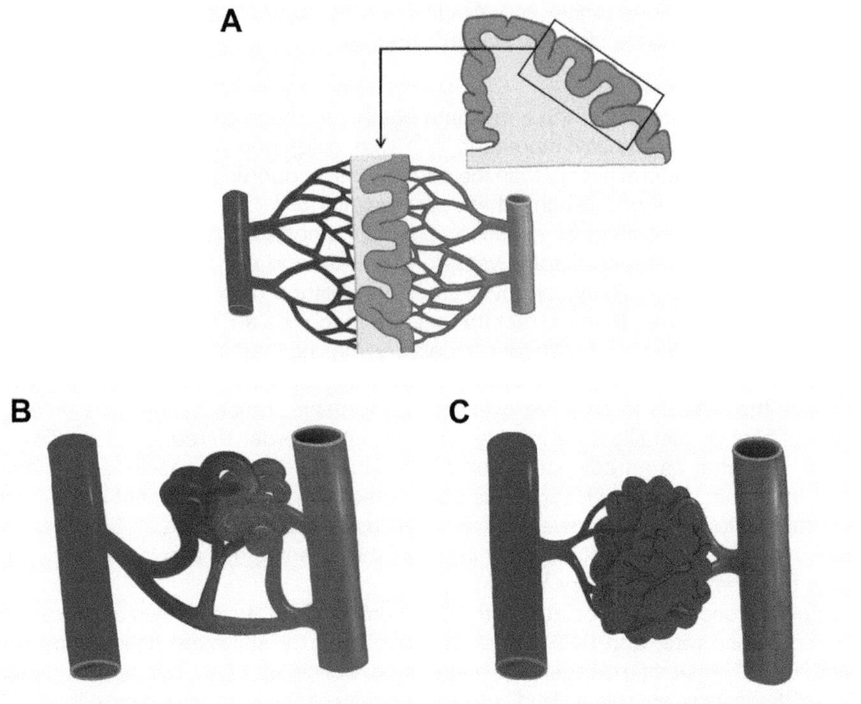

Fig. 2. Vascular malformations of the CNS. (*A*) Conceptualization of normal blood flow from artery to vein. Note intervening cortex/tissue bed that prevents direct conveyance of arterial pressure to draining veins. Cortex of brain (inset). (*B*) AVM, illustrating dysplastic vessels of the AVM nidus and high-flow connection between arteries and veins without intervening capillaries and tissue. This leads to pressurization of vessels unaccustomed to high transmural pressure gradients and potential hemorrhage. (*C*) CMs are mulberry-like vascular lesions consisting of compact clusters of sponge-like vascular spaces. Unlike AVMs, they are low-pressure, low-flow lesions with hemorrhage occurring less commonly and with lower consequence than AVMs.

predilection, and AVFs comprise approximately 4% of pediatric cerebral vascular malformations.[14,15]

AVMs may exist in up to 1.4% of the general population but are symptomatic in approximately 1/100,000 individuals. Pediatric AVMs have equal male and female distribution, with an average presentation at 11 years old.[5,16] AVMs typically are silent, with symptomatic AVMs presenting most commonly with hemorrhage (52%), headache without bleeding (20%), seizures without bleeding (12%), and incidental discovery (16%).[5] Mortality from the initial rupture is approximately 12% to 25%.[17]

Diagnostic evaluation

It can be challenging for PCPs to detect asymptomatic AVMs in children, because the physical examination typically is normal in AVM patients without hemorrhage. For symptomatic children, computed tomography (CT) is the most common initial study. Unexplained ICH on CT should be considered for evaluation with CT arteriogram (CTA) emergently, followed by magnetic resonance imaging (MRI)/magnetic resonance angiography (MRA) and a digital subtraction angiogram (DSA) if AVM is suspected (if the child is clinically stable)[18] (**Fig. 3**).

Treatment and follow-up

Rebleeding rates are low in the immediate posthemorrhage period (3%–6%/y), then approximately 2% annually thereafter.[16,19] That said, pediatric AVMs have a far more aggressive natural history than the adult AVMs, supporting the stance of aggressive treatment in this population, whenever possible.[19,20]

Treatment includes surgical resection, radiation, embolization, or observation. Surgery entails cauterizing or clipping vessels that enter and exit the AVM, followed by cutting out the nidus. Radiation involves using photons or protons (essentially the same in efficacy, other than the fact that photon machines are more widely available, whereas protons have a sharper edge in delivery, making them better for select lesions abutting critical structures) in either single doses or multiple treatments (fractionated) to cause the vessels to sclerose over months to years. Embolization uses different forms of glue or metallic coils to plug AVM vessels in order to reduce blood flow in the lesion, either as an adjunct to surgery/radiation or—in rare cases—as a standalone treatment. In general, surgery is considered the primary treatment in anatomically favorable lesions, followed by radiation as a second choice.[1,5] Embolization alone in complex cases actually may increase the bleeding risk and make outcomes worse than the natural history.[19]

Surgical resection is associated with 0.3% hemorrhage rate in 5 years and less than 1% recurrence rate, and 94% of patients are stable or improved neurologically at follow-up.[5,16] Risk of perioperative neurologic deficit is 17%, but approximately 80% of these were only visual field cuts, the majority of which improved or recovered.[5] Following operation, radiographic obliteration of the AVM is reported in 86% to 100% of cases.[5,21,22]

If surgery is not feasible (inaccessible AVMs or children unable to tolerate general anesthesia due to severe medical conditions), radiation therapy is an excellent treatment, particularly in smaller lesions (<3 cm).[23] Radiographic obliteration of the AVM at 5 years is approximately 50% to 80%, with bleeding rates of 1.3% annually.[23–26] New neurologic deficits occurred in approximately 16% of cases and re-radiation was performed in up to approximately 35% of cases.[23,25,27]

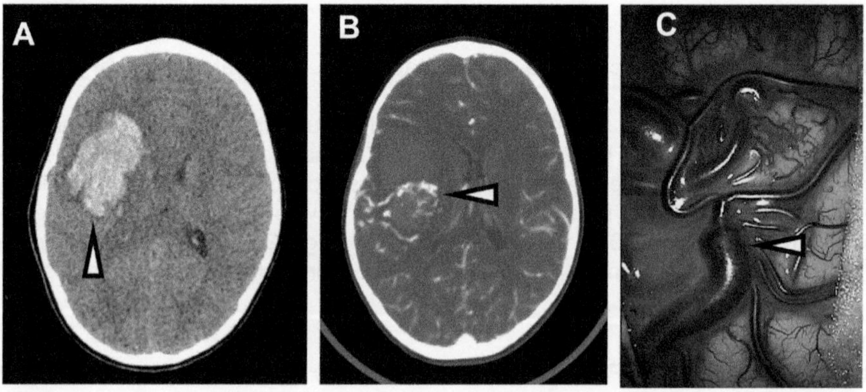

Fig. 3. (*A*) Noncontrast axial CT of the brain showing a large hemorrhage in the right frontal lobe (*arrowhead*). (*B*) CTA of the same patient, showing serpiginous vessels in the posterior part of the clot, indicative of an AVM (*arrowhead*). (*C*) Intraoperative image of an AVM with markedly dilated cortical vein (a common site of rupture) (*arrowhead*).

Ultimately, many AVMs may require multimodality treatment, combining embolization with surgery or other interventions. In some cases, the risk of any treatment may be unacceptable, making observation the safest option. Whether or not treated, pediatric AVMs mandate careful follow-up. In many series, a DSA is obtained 1 year after treatment, followed by annual MRI/MRA for at least 3 to 5 years.

Screening

In patients with AVF, approximately 9% have germline mutations.[28–30] RASA-1 and HHT-related mutations (ENG and ACVRL1) are most common, with clinical findings including multiple cranial lesions, spinal AVF/AVM, hypercoagulable states, and capillary hemangioma (in RASA-1).[28–31] In VOGM, there are few indications for familial screening.[32]

Although most AVMs are thought to be isolated developmental lesions, there are known genetic conditions predisposing individuals to multiple AVMs. Mutations in RASA-1 are associated with abnormal vessel development, including familial high-flow arteriovenous lesions.[31] For individuals with HHT, guidelines recommend AVM screening with MRI in the first 6 months of life or at the time of diagnosis.[33,34]

Cavernous Malformations

Pathophysiology

Cavernous malformations (CMs), also known as cavernous hemangiomas, cavernous angiomas, and cavernomas, are low-flow capillary lesions consisting of compact clusters of sponge-like vascular spaces without intervening neural parenchyma.[35,36] They can be familial with several associated germline mutations, but a majority are sporadic. Developmental venous anomalies (DVAs)—essentially, normal veins in an abnormal configuration)—commonly are seen (approximately 20%–40%) in association with CMs.[37–39]

Three genes have been strongly associated with the formation of CMs: CCM1 (also known as *KRIT1*), CCM2 (also known as, malcaverin), and CCM3 (also known as, programmed cell death 10). De novo CMs can develop over the life of a given patient. The CCM1 genotype is associated with a higher number of lesions with increased age than the CCM2 or CCM3 genotypes.[40] In contrast, although CCM3 mutation carriers generally have fewer lesions, they have a higher risk of hemorrhage. Other systems may be affected (skin, eyes, and visceral organs), most commonly with CCM1 mutations.[41,42]

Epidemiology and risk

CMs are found in approximately 0.5% to 1% in autopsy studies.[36,40–42] An incidence of 0.43/100,000 people per year has been reported.[43] There is no difference in incidence based on sex. Most cases are sporadic (50%–80%), although familial variants exist, with nearly all familial (genetic) cases demonstrating multiple lesions on imaging.[40] If multiple CMs are seen on imaging, a familial or postradiation etiology should be considered. Few (<10%) sporadic cases have multiple lesions.[36,39]

CMs can cause symptoms from hemorrhage or progressive enlargement with mass effect.[39] Seizure is the presenting symptom in 25% to 30% of cases.[34,39] The overall annual bleeding rate is 0.5% to 1% for incidental lesions but increases to greater than 18% for lesions that have previously bled, with clustering of rebleeding within 3 years of the initial presentation.[39] These data support observation for many asymptomatic, small lesions (especially if multiple in familial cases), but promote treatment in hemorrhagic or larger lesions.

Diagnostic evaluation

Patients with known family histories of CCM should be considered for screening with MRI (discussed later). DSA often is of no use, because CMs are not visible on DSA. If an acute clot is seen without an obvious underlying lesion, the possibility of a high-flow vascular malformation should be evaluated with CTA and—if nothing is seen—delayed imaging often can be helpful to better visualize pathologic lesions once the clot has resorbed, often in 4 weeks to 6 weeks (**Fig. 4**).

Treatment and follow-up

Treatment of CMs either is surgical resection or observation, with data supporting excision of symptomatic lesions, lesions with recurrent hemorrhage, or lesions with high risk of neurologic deficit (such as large lesions or those located in the posterior fossa).[34,39,44] For patients with multiple CMs, resection should be limited to symptomatic lesions or lesions with documented expansion over time.[40,45] Radiation therapy is controversial and generally not indicated. Research into novel pharmacologic agents is ongoing, but to date there is no medical therapy approved for obliteration of CMs. It is common to observe lesions that are small, asymptomatic, or located in areas of high potential surgical morbidity.[1,39]

For patients treated with surgery, most return to full activity with no restrictions. Seizures are markedly reduced or cured in approximately 80% of cases after resection.[44] Follow-up typically is annual MRI studies for 5 years, then every 2 years to 3 years thereafter.[1]

Screening

Screening of first-degree relatives with genetic counseling should be considered in patients who have multiple CMs on imaging or if there is a known family history of CMs, because a germline mutation is likely, with CCM1, CCM2, or CCM3 found in greater than 90% of familial cases.1,46 If multiple intracranial lesions are seen on imaging, the likelihood of a familial form of the disease approaches 85%, whereas single lesions have only an approximately 16% likelihood of harboring a germline mutation.[46]

STRUCTURAL ARTERIOPATHIES (ANEURYSMS AND MOYAMOYA)

Intracranial Aneurysms

Pathophysiology

Intracranial aneurysms are far less common in children than in adults. Structurally abnormal areas of arterial wall can cause bleeding, mass effect, and concomitant

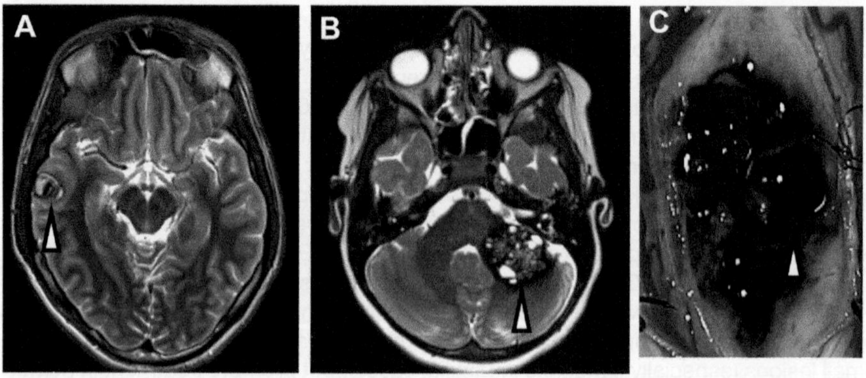

Fig. 4. (*A*) Axial T2 MRI showing right temporal lesion suggestive of hemorrhagic CM. (*B*) Axial T2 MRI of the brain showing a larger posterior fossa lesion consistent with a CM, with typical bubble popcorn–like appearance (*arrowhead*). (*C*) Intraoperative image showing lobulated appearance CM. These are the bubbles that can rupture and bleed, usually under low pressure (*arrowhead*).

neurologic deficit (**Fig. 5**). The pathophysiology of aneurysms in the pediatric population changes with increasing age.

Younger children, in particular those under 5 years of age, have predominantly dissecting, fusiform aneurysms, whereas older children more commonly have saccular aneurysms.[47–49] Saccular (berry) aneurysms result from hemodynamic stresses that often are greatest at branch points in larger intracranial arteries, whereas dissecting aneurysms are caused by intimal tears in the arterial wall, leading to a free flap pulling away from the normal lumen. This dissection has the double hit of both occluding the parent artery (possibly leading to ischemic stroke) and also creating a weakened area of the vessel at the site of the injury that can enlarge and potentially rupture to cause bleeding. Hereditary aneurysms are rare, accounting for 5% to 20% of all reported cases in children and young adults but less than 5% of prepubertal cases.[50,51]

Epidemiology and risk

Unruptured, asymptomatic intracranial aneurysms—for all age groups—are found in 3% of all people alive, with only 4% of all of these present in children.[47,52–56] Aneurysmal hemorrhage in children also is extremely rare, with only 0.6% of all aneurysmal SAH patients age 18 years or younger.[47,54,57] To put this in context, there are approximately 18,000 SAHs/year in the United States, meaning that there are approximately only 100 pediatric aneurysmal SAH cases annually in the United States.[58,59] Children are less likely than adults to have multiple aneurysms and are approximately 4 times more likely to have giant (>2.5-cm) aneurysms.[47–49,56]

Overall, etiologies of pediatric intracranial aneurysms include saccular (45%–70%), posttraumatic (dissecting aneurysms, 5%–40%), infectious (5%–15%), and genetic (polycystic kidney disease, fibromuscular dysplasia, Marfan syndrome, Ehlers-Danlos, HHT, and Klippel-Trénaunay syndrome).[60]

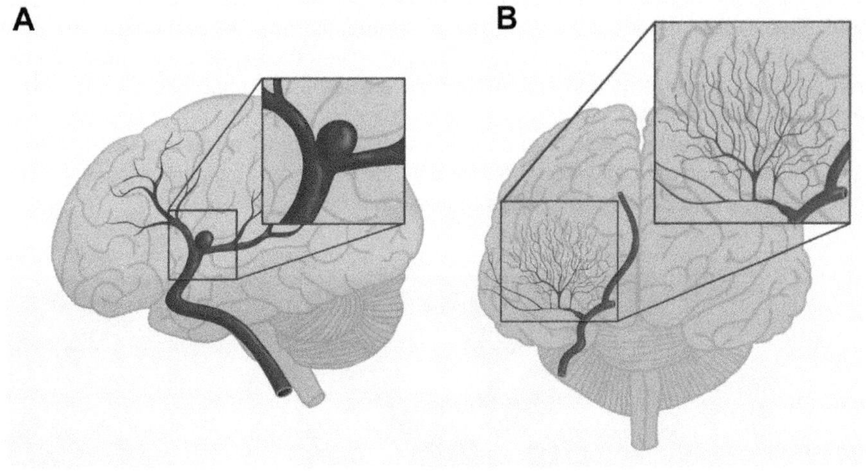

Fig. 5. Structural arteriopathies. (*A*) Intracranial aneurysms, such as the saccular aneurysm seen here, occur most commonly at branch points in large intracranial arteries, where hemodynamic stresses are highest. Hemorrhage of these lesions can have devastating consequences. Middle cerebral artery with aneurysm (inset). (*B*) Moyamoya arteriopathy is a progressive narrowing of large intracranial arteries of unknown cause but typically involving overgrowth of smooth muscle cells in the media leading to vessel occlusion and ischemic stroke in children. The slow rate of progression of disease results in the development of collateral vessels (*inset*) that on arteriography resemble a puff of smoke, the translation of moyamoya from Japanese.

Aneurysms cause problems by bleeding, with more than half of pediatric aneurysm patients presenting with SAH, approximately one-third presenting with symptoms related to mass effect (headache, seizure, and focal neurologic deficits), and approximately 10% found on imaging after severe trauma.[47] The presentation of symptomatic pediatric intracranial aneurysms includes headache (80%), loss of consciousness (25%), seizure (20%), focal deficit (20%), and vision changes (10%).[47,48,56,61]

Diagnostic evaluation

Aneurysms in children typically are found after symptomatic presentation, although increasingly incidental lesions are discovered after imaging for other reasons. Acutely ill patients ("worst headache of my life") should be evaluated emergently with a CT/CTA to identify the presence of an aneurysm (or AVM).[62] Catheter-based DSA successfully identifies pathology in 97% of patients versus 80% of the time without DSA[10] (**Fig. 6**). Practically, evaluation by the PCP consists mostly of CT/CTA in the emergent setting and MRI/MRA for nonacute presentations. MRI/MRA should be considered for screening at-risk patients (discussed later).

Treatment and follow-up

Management of pediatric aneurysms generally is straightforward, with larger (>3-mm) or symptomatic lesions referred to high-volume tertiary centers for review and treatment. If acutely symptomatic, emergent transfer is indicated, whereas incidentally found asymptomatic lesions generally can be addressed in an elective, outpatient fashion.

The rarity of pediatric aneurysms precludes firm evidence-based guidelines for treatment indications.1,62 In general, aneurysms that have ruptured or that demonstrate enlargement over time or symptomatic lesions should be considered for treatment. Depending on location and patient status, it may be reasonable to treat aneurysms greater than 3 mm in size, particularly given the expected life span of children. Mycotic aneurysms sometimes regress with effective antibiotic therapy, obviating other interventions.[1]

Follow-up frequently consists of an office visit at 1 month, a baseline MRI/MRA at 6 months and then annually thereafter for 5 years, with some centers suggesting lifetime imaging every 3 years to 5 years thereafter.[63]

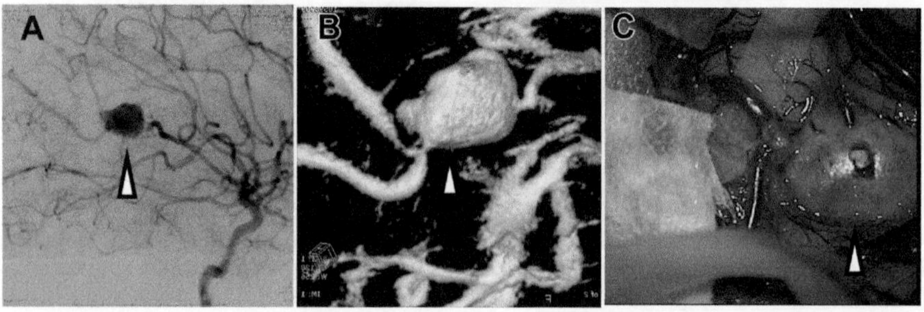

Fig. 6. (*A*) Catheter angiogram (lateral projection) showing a left temporal dissecting aneurysm of the distal middle cerebral artery. (*B*) Three-dimensional reconstruction showing narrow neck of vessels leaving dissection/aneurysm, putting downstream brain tissue at risk of stroke (*arrowhead*). (*C*) Intraoperative photo of aneurysm. Arrowhead is pointing to aneurysm.

Screening

Genetic or familial aneurysms are rare, accounting for approximately 20% of all reported cases in young adults but less than 5% of prepubertal cases.[50,51] Generally, only family members of sibling pairs or 3 first-degree relatives who harbor known intracranial aneurysms (with particular note of family members who presented with aneurysms in childhood) are recommended for screening, usually with MRI/MRA.[50,51,62,64] A single relative who presented with an aneurysm in later adulthood typically is not a reason to screen children.

Moyamoya

Pathophysiology

Moyamoya is a progressive arteriopathy of the branches of the internal carotid artery (ICA) of unknown etiology, likely comprising a heterogeneous group of genetically distinct disorders that share a common clinical presentation, typically presenting with ischemic stroke.[65] As the ICAs narrow, collateral vessels develop (just like traffic re-routes around a blockage and takes smaller roads that become congested with increased volume); these are called a *puff of smoke*, due to their appearance on an angiogram. Historically, the arteriopathy of moyamoya has distinguished between disease (without other medical conditions) and syndrome (arteriopathy found in association with a select group of other systemic disorders).[65]

Moyamoya patients of Asian ancestry are likely to have a specific RNF213 gene mutation, identified in 95% of familial cases and approximately 80% of sporadic cases; these patients have significantly earlier disease onset and severity, including posterior cerebral artery stenosis.[66] Up to 56% of Asian Americans with moyamoya may harbor mutations in RNF213, suggesting that this subset of patients may benefit from referral for genetic counseling after diagnosis.[67,68] In contrast, this same study found that no RNF213 mutations were found in any of a cohort of non-Asians with moyamoya in the United States.[67] Other genetic causes are rare, with the exception of neurofibromatosis type 1 (NF1) and Down syndrome—which are common in many pediatric practices.

Epidemiology and risk

First described in Japan, moyamoya now has been identified in patients worldwide, ranging from 3/100,000 to 1/1,000,000.[65] Demographics of pediatric moyamoya in the United States reveal a 60:40 female preponderance.[69] The average age of presentation varies from 5 years old to 8 years old, although any age patient—from infancy to adulthood—can have moyamoya.[69–71] Asian ancestry is a risk factor for moyamoya due to higher prevalence of RNF213 mutations.[67,68]

Associations exist between moyamoya and radiotherapy of the head or neck (especially for optic gliomas, craniopharyngiomas, and pituitary tumors), Down syndrome (26-fold increased likelihood of moyamoya), NF1 (with or without hypothalamic–optic pathway tumors; approximately 2.5% prevalence of moyamoya), and sickle cell anemia (up to 29% of sickle cell patients on chronic transfusion therapy for stroke may be candidates for revascularization).[65,72–75]

Moyamoya is a problem because of the risk of stroke; up to 6% of all pediatric strokes in the United States are due to moyamoya.[65] Pediatric patients with moyamoya typically present with ischemic symptoms and up to 10% of all reported transient ischemic attacks in the United States are associated with moyamoya.[71] The natural history of moyamoya is variable; however, moyamoya inevitably progresses in a majority of cases.[65,76] In general, it has been estimated that up to two-thirds of patients with moyamoya disease demonstrate symptomatic progression, which cannot be halted by medical treatment alone, with 66% to 90% experiencing symptomatic stroke within 5 years if untreated.[1,65]

Diagnostic evaluation

Most cases of moyamoya are clinically silent until presentation with stroke or transient ischemic attack. There often is nothing of note on physical examination. The evaluation of moyamoya should start with an MRI/MRA. Many patients show watershed infarcts and evidence of narrowed ICA branches, and approximately 80% of symptomatic patients have ivy sign—sulcal hyperintensity on fluid-attenuated inversion recovery (FLAIR) imaging indicative of slow blood flow[77,78] (**Fig. 7**). If suspected, then referral to a high-volume center should be done directly.

Ultimately, definitive diagnosis is made with DSA. The risk of DSA-related complications is very low (<1%) when performed in experienced centers.[18,79] If a diagnosis of moyamoya is made, typically patients are started on low-dose aspirin and planned for surgery. Acute stroke often is a contraindication to immediate surgery, with a delay of several weeks until revascularization usually is recommended to reduce the risk of secondary infarcts during recovery.

Treatment and follow-up

Evidence supports surgical revascularization as the primary therapy, even in most asymptomatic children.[72,76,80,81] Without intervention, there is an annual 13% risk of ischemic stroke coupled with a 7% risk of hemorrhage.[82] Indirect revascularization is the more common intervention in children, a surgical procedure (such as pial synangiosis), in which a pedicle of vascularized tissue is grafted to the brain and used as a source of new blood supply. Done at high-volume centers, this procedure can reduce the 5-year risk of stroke to approximately 5%; a near 15-fold reduction.[76,83]

Follow-up demonstrates durable protection from stroke, with stroke rates of approximately 5% at 5 years in 1 study and approximately 7% at 20 years postoperatively in another.[83,84] It is important to follow children, often with annual MRI/MRA, because up to 30% develop posterior circulation disease within 5 years, which can be treated with occipital revascularization.[85,86] Overall, evidence strongly supports the use of surgical revascularization at experienced centers as an effective method

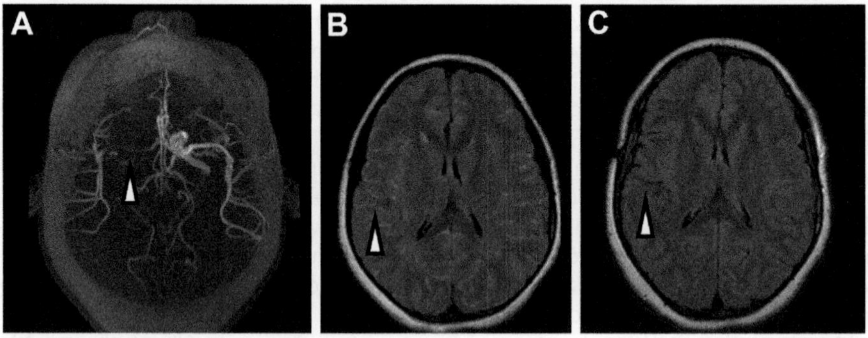

Fig. 7. (*A*) Axial MRA of the brain showing markedly narrow right middle cerebral artery suggestive of moyamoya (*arrowhead*). (*B*) Axial FLAIR images showing high signal (white curvilinear appearance) of sulci known as the ivy sign, indicative of slow blood flow downstream of moyamoya arteriopathy. (*C*) Same FLAIR images in same patient following pial synangiosis, demonstrating improved blood flow after revascularization with marked reduction in ivy sign (now a more healthy black signal in sulci). Arrowhead in B and C shows a cortical sulcus with ivy sign (bright signal) in B and resolution in C.

to reduce stroke risk significantly over decades in pediatric moyamoya patients.[76] Most of these children go on to live full, normal lives.[87]

Screening

A particularly important role for PCPs in the prevention of stroke is awareness of specific at-risk populations so that relevant signs and symptoms are not overlooked.[72,74,88,89] Recognition of at-risk populations (sickle cell disease, NF1, Down syndrome, Alagille syndrome, post–brain radiation, and HHT) can improve the likelihood of identifying pediatric moyamoya before catastrophic stroke, and screening with MRI/MRA is warranted in patients with symptoms suggestive of cerebral ischemia.

In general, screening for sickle cell patients with high intracranial doppler velocities of the middle cerebral artery that do not respond to transfusion therapy are an indication for MRI/MRA.[76] Otherwise, given the low rate of familial moyamoya in the United States (approximately 4%), current indications for screening MRI/MRA in asymptomatic individuals are limited to patients with first-degree or second-degree relatives with known diagnoses of moyamoya or identical twins in which 1 of the twins has moyamoya.[1] Absent worrisome symptoms, the MRI/MRA can be delayed until an age at which the child can tolerate imaging without the added risk of sedation.

Table 1 provides a summary of the information, discussed previously, regarding AVMs, CMs, aneurysms, and moyamoya.

INCIDENTAL FINDINGS AND DEVELOPMENTAL VARIANTS

For PCPs and parents, a major cause for concern can be a report of an unexpected finding on an intracranial imaging study. Although obvious pathology (an AVM, CM, moyamoya, and so forth) is easy to refer to neurosurgery, there are some more difficult decisions surrounding unclear diagnoses. The 3 most common incidental vascular-related findings on imaging studies that prompt referral to neurosurgery are possible aneurysms, asymmetric vessels, and developmental venous anomalies. These often do not require referral to other providers and can be addressed simply with a careful read by neuroradiology and reassurance to the family. In cases of uncertainty, it can be efficient simply to arrange for the films to be seen by a specialist (if they are willing) in order to minimize unnecessary visits. As discussed previously, it is critical for the actual images (not just the written report) to be available for review.

Aneurysm

A common finding is a small (2 mm or less) lesion that is found incidentally on an imaging study. Often these lesions are located outside the subarachnoid space (and, therefore, not likely to cause SAH) or are difficult to distinguish from an infundibulum (a normal anatomic variant of a patent vessel that simply has a trumpeted end that can look like an aneurysm). A vast majority of these findings are either not aneurysms or present a vanishingly low risk of bleeding, making routine follow-up the preferred course (many times without a need for any further imaging or perhaps with a single interval study to document stability).[52,57] It can be important to reassure families that 1 of every 30 human beings has an intracranial aneurysm, with a vast majority of no consequence. Modifiable risk factors, such as avoiding smoking (including secondary exposure from family members), hypertension, and vasoactive drug use, can minimize aneurysm development and progression. Although it may seem odd, there is a marked difference in risk between lesions less than 2 mm and those greater than 3 mm, underscoring the need for referral.

Table 1
Summary of characteristics of vascular malformations and structural arteriopathies

	General Information	Risk of Hemorrhage or Stroke	Morbidity/ Mortality	Treatment
AVM	High flow lesion with no intervening brain tissue	3%–6% annual bleed risk after hemorrhage	12%–25% death with each bleed	Surgery, radiation—sometimes with embolization Observation in complex cases
CM	Low flow lesion with no intervening brain tissue	0.3% to 18% annual	Seizure, headache, focal neurologic deficit	Surgery or observation
Aneurysm	Dysplastic arterial wall (berry or dissection)	Wide variation	Wide variation	Wide variation
Moyamoya	Overgrowth of smooth muscle of major intracranial arteries leading to ischemia (typically ICAs and branches)	Stroke risk 66%–90% over 5 y, bleeding far less likely in children	(66-90% risk of stroke [including fatality] over 5 years)	Surgery

Asymmetric Vessels

Radiology reports frequently note asymmetric calibers of intracranial vessels, in particular the vertebral arteries. A dominant (or, conversely, hypoplastic) vertebral artery has been reported in approximately 10% of all patients.[90] This is of no clinical significance unless there are elements of the history to suggest trauma or other causes of a recent vertebral dissection. In contrast, marked asymmetry of the ICAs may be suggestive of an ICA dissection or moyamoya, and review of the intracranial distal segments of the arteries, along with evaluation for stroke, is necessary.

Developmental Venous Anomalies

As discussed previously, DVAs sometimes are associated with CMs, so if a DVA is observed on a scan, review of the area should be done to look for a CM. Sometimes a special sequence to highlight previous bleeding (susceptibility-weighted images) can reveal a tiny CM that might be below the level of resolution on other sequences. DVAs exist, however, in 2.5% of all people, and absent the rare finding of a CM, DVAs are of no clinical consequence.[91]

FREQUENTLY ASKED QUESTIONS ABOUT PEDIATRIC INTRACRANIAL VASCULAR ABNORMALITIES

If a child has been screened for a vascular lesion, such as an AVM, and the imaging was normal, is a repeat interval scan needed? And—if so—when?

If the MRI/MRA does not reveal any AVM, evidence supports the practice of not needing to repeat any imaging (unless new symptoms develop) for at least 5 years.[92]

If a patient has a known vascular lesion (such as an AVM, aneurysm, or CM) that either is awaiting treatment or cannot be treated, what sort of activity restrictions (if any) should be discussed in order to reduce the risk of bleeding? ("Can my child ride amusement rides/go in a bouncy house/play football etc.?")

It appears that mild physical head and neck trauma and systemic inflammation (such as infection) do not significantly contribute as a trigger to increased likelihood of vascular malformation rupture in children.[93] Specifically, the common question to PCPs from families centered on "What might cause my child's AVM to bleed?" can be answered with some degree of confidence that there is little—other than severe trauma or major physiologic shifts (such as extreme hypertension) —that can increase the chance of hemorrhage. Repeated head trauma, however, especially with sports, such as football and boxing, may increase this risk and typically neurosurgeons who even may allow limited contact sports (such as lacrosse, ice hockey, or soccer) often prohibit football or boxing. Although the data are somewhat reassuring, many neurosurgeons markedly curtail the majority of potentially risky behaviors (including many higher-velocity amusement rides, such as roller coasters) during a relatively limited period before definitive treatment.

A child was scanned for an unrelated reason and an incidental, asymptomatic vascular lesion was found. What sorts of diagnoses merit neurosurgical referral—and how urgently?

Any new hemorrhage merits urgent neurosurgical referral, unless a known trauma exists that correlates directly with the finding. Other findings should prompt immediate discussion with the family to obtain a more focused history and physical, with questions targeted at the specific pathology identified. AVMs, CMs, and moyamoya all should be referred to neurosurgery for relatively timely evaluation (days to weeks, depending on the focused history and potential findings). Aneurysms are more complicated, with a general rule suggesting that those greater than 3 mm merit neurosurgical referral and those 2 mm or less perhaps amenable to a timely dedicated film review, as discussed previously. DVAs (without CM) and anatomic variants of asymmetric vessels (as outlined previously) often do not require neurosurgical evaluation, although consultation is always recommended if there is any question on behalf of the PCP.

Box 1
Genetic conditions associated with cerebrovascular disease

Moyamoya syndrome

HHT

Ehlers-Danlos syndrome

Alpha$_1$-antitrypsin deficiency

Marfan syndrome

Fibromuscular dysplasia

Autosomal dominant polycystic kidney disease

NF1

Multiple familial CMs

Multiple familial intracranial aneurysms

Box 2
Independent predictors of a surgical lesion

Sleep-related headache (meaning, headache that wakes a patient from sleep)

No family history of migraine (headache without any family history of migraine)

Vomiting

Absence of visual symptoms (headache without classic migraine findings, such as scotomata or fortification spectra)

Headache of <6 mo duration

Confusion

Abnormal neurologic examination findings

[a] A positive correlation exists between a larger number of predictors and higher risk of a surgical lesion ($P<.0001$).[94]

Clinics Care Points

- Identifying cerebrovascular abnormalities in children can be a challenging task for a PCP, because most are without antecedent symptoms or obvious physical findings prior to ischemic or hemorrhagic stroke.
- Regarding history, **Box 1** lists several familial or preexisting conditions that may be associated with an increased risk of cerebrovascular disease. Asking about these is helpful, but it is important to remember that normal, age-related disease likely is not of clinical consequence (adult relatives, such as grandparents with stroke, aneurysm, or ICH, are not worrisome unless these problems occurred in childhood or as very young adults). Some risk factors can be determined by identification of salient points from the history (**Box 2**).
- Moyamoya, although rare, has the largest number of known at-risk populations and the PCP can have an outsized impact in preventing stroke through increased awareness of these associations, leading to recognition of otherwise occult ischemic symptoms.
- Physical examination rarely is revealing, with the odd exception of a bruit heard on the scalp (almost never present in AVM but sometimes identified in VOGM patients) or focal neurologic deficits that might be subtle enough to be detected only on careful neurologic examination (pronator drift, numbness in a cortical distribution, or marked cognitive/behavioral decline without proximate cause). The obvious exception to this rule is an infant with a high-flow AVM or VOGM, who may have macrocephaly, failure to thrive, dilated scalp vessels, or evidence of high-flow cardiac output failure.
- When referral to a specialist is indicated, it is of the utmost importance to make sure that the actual images (if taken) are physically available for review. Reports alone are are useless and every effort should be made to have copies of the images in the office and—if possible—also in the hands of the family directly. This is important for outpatient visits—and potentially a matter of life and death in emergencies.

DISCLOSURE

None.

ACKNOWLEDGMENTS

The authors would like to thank Ms Elsa Martin for her illustrations in this article.

REFERENCES

1. Ferriero DM, Fullerton HJ, Bernard TJ, et al. Management of stroke in neonates and children: a scientific statement from the American Heart Association/American Stroke Association. Stroke 2019;50:e51–96.
2. Lawton MT, Rutledge WC, Kim H, et al. Brain arteriovenous malformations. Nat Rev Dis Primers 2015;1:15008.
3. Awad IA, Robinson JR Jr, Mohanty S, et al. Mixed vascular malformations of the brain: clinical and pathogenetic considerations. Neurosurgery 1993;33:179–88 [discussion: 88].
4. Willinsky RA, Lasjaunias P, Terbrugge K, et al. Multiple cerebral arteriovenous malformations (AVMs). Review of our experience from 203 patients with cerebral vascular lesions. Neuroradiology 1990;32:207–10.
5. Gross BA, Storey A, Orbach DB, et al. Microsurgical treatment of arteriovenous malformations in pediatric patients: the Boston Children's Hospital experience. J Neurosurg Pediatr 2015;15:71–7.
6. Fullerton HJ, Wu YW, Zhao S, et al. Risk of stroke in children: ethnic and gender disparities. Neurology 2003;61:189–94.
7. Jordan LC, Kleinman JT, Hillis AE. Intracerebral hemorrhage volume predicts poor neurologic outcome in children. Stroke 2009;40:1666–71.
8. Beslow LA, Licht DJ, Smith SE, et al. Predictors of outcome in childhood intracerebral hemorrhage: a prospective consecutive cohort study. Stroke 2010;41:313–8.
9. Adil MM, Qureshi AI, Beslow LA, et al. Factors associated with increased in-hospital mortality among children with intracerebral hemorrhage. J Child Neurol 2015;30(8):1024–8.
10. Al-Jarallah A, Al-Rifai MT, Riela AR, et al. Nontraumatic brain hemorrhage in children: etiology and presentation. J Child Neurol 2000;15:284–9.
11. Broderick J, Talbot GT, Prenger E, et al. Stroke in children within a major metropolitan area: the surprising importance of intracerebral hemorrhage. J Child Neurol 1993;8:250–5.
12. Liu J, Wang D, Lei C, et al. Etiology, clinical characteristics and prognosis of spontaneous intracerebral hemorrhage in children: A prospective cohort study in China. J Neurol Sci 2015;358:367–70.
13. Recinos PF, Rahmathulla G, Pearl M, et al. Vein of Galen malformations: epidemiology, clinical presentations, management. Neurosurg Clin N Am 2012;23:165–77.
14. Cooke D, Tatum J, Farid H, et al. Transvenous embolization of a pediatric pial arteriovenous fistula. J Neurointerv Surg 2012;4:e14.
15. Tomlinson FH, Rufenacht DA, Sundt TM Jr, et al. Arteriovenous fistulas of the brain and the spinal cord. J Neurosurg 1993;79:16–27.
16. Blauwblomme T, Bourgeois M, Meyer P, et al. Long-term outcome of 106 consecutive pediatric ruptured brain arteriovenous malformations after combined treatment. Stroke 2014;45:1664–71.
17. Riordan CP, Orbach DB, Smith ER, et al. Acute fatal hemorrhage from previously undiagnosed cerebral arteriovenous malformations in children: a single-center experience. J Neurosurg Pediatr 2018;22:244–50.

18. Lin N, Smith ER, Scott RM, et al. Safety of neuroangiography and embolization in children: complication analysis of 697 consecutive procedures in 394 patients. J Neurosurg Pediatr 2015;16(4):432–8.
19. Gross BA, Scott RM, Smith ER. Management of brain arteriovenous malformations. Lancet 2014;383:1635.
20. Mohr JP, Parides MK, Stapf C, et al. Medical management with or without interventional therapy for unruptured brain arteriovenous malformations (ARUBA): a multicentre, non-blinded, randomised trial. Lancet 2014;383:614–21.
21. Gaballah M, Storm PB, Rabinowitz D, et al. Intraoperative cerebral angiography in arteriovenous malformation resection in children: a single institutional experience. J Neurosurg Pediatr 2014;13:222–8.
22. Walkden JS, Zador Z, Herwadkar A, et al. Use of intraoperative Doppler ultrasound with neuronavigation to guide arteriovenous malformation resection: a pediatric case series. J Neurosurg Pediatr 2015;15:291–300.
23. Potts MB, Jahangiri A, Jen M, et al. Deep arteriovenous malformations in the basal ganglia, thalamus, and insula: multimodality management, patient selection, and results. World Neurosurg 2014;82:386–94.
24. Potts MB, Sheth SA, Louie J, et al. Stereotactic radiosurgery at a low marginal dose for the treatment of pediatric arteriovenous malformations: obliteration, complications, and functional outcomes. J Neurosurg Pediatr 2014;14:1–11.
25. Borcek AO, Emmez H, Akkan KM, et al. Gamma Knife radiosurgery for arteriovenous malformations in pediatric patients. Childs Nerv Syst 2014;30:1485–92.
26. Hanakita S, Koga T, Shin M, et al. The long-term outcomes of radiosurgery for arteriovenous malformations in pediatric and adolescent populations. J Neurosurg Pediatr 2015;16(2):222–31.
27. Walcott BP, Hattangadi-Gluth JA, Stapleton CJ, et al. Proton beam stereotactic radiosurgery for pediatric cerebral arteriovenous malformations. Neurosurgery 2014;74:367–73 [discussion: 74].
28. Saliou G, Eyries M, Iacobucci M, et al. Clinical and genetic findings in children with CNS arteriovenous fistulas. Ann Neurol 2017;82(6):972–80.
29. Walcott BP, Smith ER, Scott RM, et al. Dural arteriovenous fistulae in pediatric patients: associated conditions and treatment outcomes. J Neurointerv Surg 2013; 5(1):6–9.
30. Walcott BP, Smith ER, Scott RM, et al. Pial arteriovenous fistulae in pediatric patients: associated syndromes and treatment outcome. J Neurointerv Surg 2013; 5(1):10–4.
31. Thiex R, Mulliken JB, Revencu N, et al. A novel association between RASA1 mutations and spinal arteriovenous anomalies. AJNR Am J Neuroradiol 2010;31: 775–9.
32. Duran D, Karschnia P, Gaillard JR, et al. Human genetics and molecular mechanisms of vein of Galen malformation. J Neurosurg Pediatr 2018;21:367–74.
33. Faughnan ME, Palda VA, Garcia-Tsao G, et al. International guidelines for the diagnosis and management of hereditary haemorrhagic telangiectasia. J Med Genet 2011;48:73–87.
34. Gross BA, Smith ER, Scott RM. Cavernous malformations of the basal ganglia in children. J Neurosurg Pediatr 2013;12:171–4.
35. Vanaman MJ, Hervey-Jumper SL, Maher CO. Pediatric and inherited neurovascular diseases. Neurosurg Clin N Am 2010;21:427–41.
36. Gault J, Sarin H, Awadallah NA, et al. Pathobiology of human cerebrovascular malformations: basic mechanisms and clinical relevance. Neurosurgery 2004; 55:1–16 [discussion: 16–7].

37. Mottolese C, Hermier M, Stan H, et al. Central nervous system cavernomas in the pediatric age group. Neurosurg Rev 2001;24:55–71 [discussion: 2–3].
38. Rigamonti D, Hadley MN, Drayer BP, et al. Cerebral cavernous malformations. Incidence and familial occurrence. N Engl J Med 1988;319:343–7.
39. Gross BA, Du R, Orbach DB, et al. The natural history of cerebral cavernous malformations in children. J Neurosurg Pediatr 2016;17(2):123–8.
40. Zabramski JM, Wascher TM, Spetzler RF, et al. The natural history of familial cavernous malformations: results of an ongoing study. J Neurosurg 1994;80: 422–32.
41. Hang Z, Shi Y, Wei Y. [A pathological analysis of 180 cases of vascular malformation of brain]. Zhonghua Bing Li Xue Za Zhi 1996;25:135–8.
42. Barnes B, Cawley CM, Barrow DL. Intracerebral hemorrhage secondary to vascular lesions. Neurosurg Clin N Am 2002;13:289–97, v.
43. Al-Shahi R, Bhattacharya JJ, Currie DG, et al. Prospective, population-based detection of intracranial vascular malformations in adults: the Scottish Intracranial Vascular Malformation Study (SIVMS). Stroke 2003;34:1163–9.
44. Gross BA, Smith ER, Goumnerova L, et al. Resection of supratentorial lobar cavernous malformations in children: clinical article. J Neurosurg Pediatr 2013; 12:367–73.
45. Frim DM, Scott RM. Management of cavernous malformations in the pediatric population. Neurosurg Clin N Am 1999;10:513–8.
46. Merello E, Pavanello M, Consales A, et al. Genetic Screening of Pediatric Cavernous Malformations. J Mol Neurosci 2016;60:232–8.
47. Gemmete JJ, Toma AK, Davagnanam I, et al. Pediatric cerebral aneurysms. Neuroimaging Clin N Am 2013;23:771–9.
48. Garg K, Singh PK, Sharma BS, et al. Pediatric intracranial aneurysms-our experience and review of literature. Childs Nerv Syst 2014;30(5):873–83.
49. Allison JW, Davis PC, Sato Y, et al. Intracranial aneurysms in infants and children. Pediatr Radiol 1998;28:223–9.
50. Broderick JP, Sauerbeck LR, Foroud T, et al. The Familial Intracranial Aneurysm (FIA) study protocol. BMC Med Genet 2005;6:17.
51. Brown RD Jr, Huston J, Hornung R, et al. Screening for brain aneurysm in the Familial Intracranial Aneurysm study: frequency and predictors of lesion detection. J Neurosurg 2008;108:1132–8.
52. Vlak MH, Algra A, Brandenburg R, et al. Prevalence of unruptured intracranial aneurysms, with emphasis on sex, age, comorbidity, country, and time period: a systematic review and meta-analysis. Lancet Neurol 2011;10:626–36.
53. Sedzimir CB, Robinson J. Intracranial hemorrhage in children and adolescents. J Neurosurg 1973;38:269–81.
54. Locksley HB, Sahs AL, Knowler L. Report on the cooperative study of intracranial aneurysms and subarachnoid hemorrhage. Section II. General survey of cases in the central registry and characteristics of the sample population. J Neurosurg 1966;24:922–32.
55. Roche JL, Choux M, Czorny A, et al. [Intracranial arterial aneurysm in children. A cooperative study. Apropos of 43 cases]. Neurochirurgie 1988;34:243–51.
56. Gerosa M, Licata C, Fiore DL, et al. Intracranial aneurysms of childhood. Childs Brain 1980;6:295–302.
57. Unruptured intracranial aneurysms–risk of rupture and risks of surgical intervention. International Study of Unruptured Intracranial Aneurysms Investigators. N Engl J Med 1998;339:1725–33.

58. Roger VL, Go AS, Lloyd-Jones DM, et al. Executive summary: heart disease and stroke statistics–2012 update: a report from the American Heart Association. Circulation 2012;125:188–97.
59. Go AS, Mozaffarian D, Roger VL, et al. Heart disease and stroke statistics–2013 update: a report from the American Heart Association. Circulation 2013;127: e6–245.
60. Gross BA, Smith ER, Scott RM, et al. Intracranial aneurysms in the youngest patients: characteristics and treatment challenges. Pediatr Neurosurg 2015;50: 18–25.
61. Lasjaunias P, Wuppalapati S, Alvarez H, et al. Intracranial aneurysms in children aged under 15 years: review of 59 consecutive children with 75 aneurysms. Childs Nerv Syst 2005;21:437–50.
62. Roach ES, Golomb MR, Adams R, et al. Management of stroke in infants and children: a scientific statement from a Special Writing Group of the American Heart Association Stroke Council and the Council on Cardiovascular Disease in the Young. Stroke 2008;39:2644–91.
63. Tonn J, Hoffmann O, Hofmann E, et al. "De novo" formation of intracranial aneurysms: who is at risk? Neuroradiology 1999;41:674–9.
64. Aeron G, Abruzzo TA, Jones BV. Clinical and imaging features of intracranial arterial aneurysms in the pediatric population. Radiographics 2012;32:667–81.
65. Scott RM, Smith ER. Moyamoya disease and moyamoya syndrome. N Engl J Med 2009;360:1226–37.
66. Fujimura M, Sonobe S, Nishijima Y, et al. Genetics and biomarkers of moyamoya disease: significance of RNF213 as a susceptibility gene. J Stroke 2014;16: 65–72.
67. Cecchi AC, Guo D, Ren Z, et al. RNF213 rare variants in an ethnically diverse population with Moyamoya disease. Stroke 2014;45:3200–7.
68. Lee MJ, Chen YF, Fan PC, et al. Mutation genotypes of RNF213 gene from moyamoya patients in Taiwan. J Neurol Sci 2015;353:161–5.
69. Bao XY, Duan L, Yang WZ, et al. Clinical features, surgical treatment, and long-term outcome in pediatric patients with moyamoya disease in China. Cerebrovasc Dis 2015;39:75–81.
70. Jackson EM, Lin N, Manjila S, et al. Pial synangiosis in patients with moyamoya younger than 2 years of age. J Neurosurg Pediatr 2014;13:420–5.
71. Adil MM, Qureshi AI, Beslow LA, et al. Transient ischemic attack requiring hospitalization of children in the United States: kids' inpatient database 2003 to 2009. Stroke 2014;45:887–8.
72. Griessenauer CJ, Lebensburger JD, Chua MH, et al. Encephaloduroarteriosynangiosis and encephalomyoarteriosynangiosis for treatment of moyamoya syndrome in pediatric patients with sickle cell disease. J Neurosurg Pediatr 2015; 16(1):64–73.
73. Kainth DS, Chaudhry SA, Kainth HS, et al. Prevalence and characteristics of concurrent down syndrome in patients with moyamoya disease. Neurosurgery 2013; 72:210–5 [discussion: 5].
74. Koss M, Scott RM, Irons MB, et al. Moyamoya syndrome associated with neurofibromatosis Type 1: perioperative and long-term outcome after surgical revascularization. J Neurosurg Pediatr 2013;11:417–25.
75. Duat-Rodriguez A, Carceller Lechon F, Lopez Pino MA, et al. Neurofibromatosis type 1 associated with moyamoya syndrome in children. Pediatr Neurol 2014; 50:96–8.

76. Smith ER, Scott RM. Spontaneous occlusion of the circle of Willis in children: pediatric moyamoya summary with proposed evidence-based practice guidelines. A review. J Neurosurg Pediatr 2012;9:353–60.
77. Jung MY, Kim YO, Yoon W, et al. Characteristics of brain magnetic resonance images at symptom onset in children with moyamoya disease. Brain Dev 2015;37: 299–306.
78. Rafay MF, Armstrong D, Dirks P, et al. Patterns of cerebral ischemia in children with moyamoya. Pediatr Neurol 2015;52:65–72.
79. Landrigan-Ossar M, McClain CD. Anesthesia for interventional radiology. Paediatr Anaesth 2014;24:698–702.
80. Lin N, Baird L, Koss M, et al. Discovery of asymptomatic moyamoya arteriopathy in pediatric syndromic populations: radiographic and clinical progression. Neurosurg Focus 2011;31:E6.
81. Fasano RM, Meier ER, Hulbert ML. Cerebral vasculopathy in children with sickle cell anemia. Blood Cells Mol Dis 2015;54:17–25.
82. Thines L, Petyt G, Aguettaz P, et al. Surgical management of Moyamoya disease and syndrome: Current concepts and personal experience. Revue Neurol (Paris) 2015;171:31–44.
83. Kazumata K, Ito M, Tokairin K, et al. The frequency of postoperative stroke in moyamoya disease following combined revascularization: a single-university series and systematic review. J Neurosurg 2014;121:432–40.
84. Funaki T, Takahashi JC, Takagi Y, et al. Incidence of late cerebrovascular events after direct bypass among children with moyamoya disease: a descriptive longitudinal study at a single center. Acta Neurochir (Wien) 2014;156:551–9 [discussion: 9].
85. Lee JY, Choi YH, Cheon JE, et al. Delayed posterior circulation insufficiency in pediatric moyamoya disease. J Neurol 2014;261:2305–13.
86. Gross BA, Stone SS, Smith ER. Occipital pial synangiosis. Acta Neurochir (Wien) 2014;156:1297–300.
87. Riordan CP, Storey A, Cote DJ, et al. Results of more than 20 years of follow-up in pediatric patients with moyamoya disease undergoing pial synangiosis. J Neurosurg Pediatr 2019;1–7. https://doi.org/10.3171/2019.1.PEDS18457.
88. Ganesan V, Smith ER. Moyamoya: defining current knowledge gaps. Dev Med Child Neurol 2015;57(9):786–7.
89. Wang C, Roberts KB, Bindra RS, et al. Delayed cerebral vasculopathy following cranial radiation therapy for pediatric tumors. Pediatr Neurol 2014;50:549–56.
90. Eskander MS, Drew JM, Aubin ME, et al. Vertebral artery anatomy: a review of two hundred fifty magnetic resonance imaging scans. Spine 2010;35:2035–40.
91. Maher CO, Piatt JH Jr. Section on Neurologic Surgery AAoP. Incidental findings on brain and spine imaging in children. Pediatrics 2015;135:e1084–96.
92. Latino GA, Al-Saleh S, Carpenter S, et al. The diagnostic yield of rescreening for arteriovenous malformations in children with hereditary hemorrhagic telangiectasia. J Pediatr 2014;165:197–9.
93. Singhal NS, Hills NK, Sidney S, et al. Role of trauma and infection in childhood hemorrhagic stroke due to vascular lesions. Neurology 2013;81:581–4.
94. Medina LS, Pinter JD, Zurakowski D, et al. Children with headache: clinical predictors of surgical space-occupying lesions and the role of neuroimaging. Radiology 1997;202(3):819–24.

Epilepsy Surgery in Children

Luis E. Bello-Espinosa, MD[a,*], Greg Olavarria, MD[b]

KEYWORDS

- Epilepsy • Electroencephalography (EEG) • Antiepileptic drug (AED)
- Corpus callosotomy • Hemispherotomy • Vagal nerve stimulator (VNS)
- Stereoelectroencephalography (SEEG)

KEY POINTS

- The evaluation of a child with seizures involves a team of specialists at a center with expertise in treating these children, and referral to such centers should not be delayed.
- Many behaviors in infants and children can mimic seizure activity, and noninvasive studies are done first to differentiate these behaviors from seizures (electroencephalogram).
- Ideal surgical candidates have epilepsy refractory to medical management, and, importantly, absence of a tumor or lesion on MRI does not preclude the child's surgical candidacy.
- Unlike adults, children tend to have foci outside the temporal lobe for seizures, and at times, intracranial electrodes are placed to better define a seizure focus and map eloquent areas.
- Children not candidates for resection can have a vagal nerve stimulator or other such device placed to mitigate seizure activity.

DEFINITION OF EPILEPSY

In the United States, 470,000 children have active epilepsy.[1] The International League Against Epilepsy (ILAE) and the International Bureau for Epilepsy[2] define epilepsy as the occurrence of at least 1 epileptic seizure, associated with the presence of an enduring alteration in the brain capable to giving rise to recurrent epileptic seizures. A single seizure in a normal brain is not sufficient to be defined as epilepsy.[2,3] The primary care provider confronts the challenge of determining if the initial events have the characteristics of a seizure and not one of the many imitators of seizures,[4] that could lead to a false diagnosis of epilepsy.[5,6]

[a] Division Head Pediatric Neurology, Arnold Palmer Hospital for Children, Leon Neuroscience Center of Excellence, 100 West Gore Street, Orlando, FL 32806, USA; [b] Pediatric Neurosurgery, Arnold Palmer Hospital for Children, 100 West Gore Street, Suite 403, Orlando, FL 32806, USA
* Corresponding author.
E-mail address: luis.bello-espinosa@orlandohealth.com

Pediatr Clin N Am 68 (2021) 845–856
https://doi.org/10.1016/j.pcl.2021.04.016 pediatric.theclinics.com

Epilepsy Mimics

A significant number of children are brought to the primary care provider with symptoms that imitate seizure activity.

Clinics Care Points: Epilepsy Mimics

- Nonepileptic behaviors in healthy children can be categorized as behavioral (psychogenic, breath-holding, staring/inattention, daydreaming, self-stimulatory); movement related (dystonias, benign myoclonus, tics); cardiogenic (syncope, arythmias, vasovagal); and other causes (hypoglycemia, vertigo, and cataplexy). Syncope (cardiac, orthostatic, reflex) and psychogenic causes predominate.
- Dystonic and choreiform movements, and self-stimulating repetitive behaviors in the child with cerebral palsy may easily be confused with seizure activity.
- In an otherwise healthy child, benign myoclonic jerks and rapid eye movements during sleep may elicit concern in a caregiver, but are rarely associated with epilepsy.

Although it often takes a referral to a pediatric neurologist and video electroencephalogram (EEG) evaluation to make a definitive diagnosis[4] of epilepsy, a careful clinical history of episodes can be helpful. Details of import include the following:

- Precipitating factors: sleep deprivation, life stressors, anxiety, history of bullying, history of trauma (physical, emotional, sexual), or parental separation favor the events as nonepileptic
- Patient's own narrative and eyewitness observations: triggers, movements, vocalizations, eye opening or closing, tongue-biting, incontinence, amnesia among others
- The lack of a postictal period after a convulsive event, suggesting a nonepileptic event
- Duration of the event is less helpful

SEIZURE TYPES

In 2017, the ILAE introduced a modified classification of seizure types. Seizures may start as focal, generalized, or of unknown onset, with each having subcategories of motor and nonmotor features. The new terminology replaces the previous classification (**Fig. 1**). Focal seizures localize to 1 hemisphere, whereas generalized seizures have a bilateral network of generators. Tonic-clonic motor types and nonmotor absence-type events come under this classification.

FEBRILE SEIZURES

Febrile seizures are defined by the ILAE as a seizure occurring after 1 month of age associated with a febrile illness, not meeting criteria for another acute symptomatic seizure or related to a central nervous system infection. There is a familial predilection, with a risk of 1 in 5 if a sibling is affected, and 1 in 3 if both parents and a previous child were affected.[7] Children at risk for recurrent seizures, apart from family history, usually have a history of ambiguous fever, prolonged event or postictal state, and developmental delay. Reassurance is the best approach for parents, as the risk of developing epilepsy is 2.4% (complex features or status at presentation of febrile seizure is very rare).[8–10] Treatment is usually supportive; however, treatment with a benzodiazepine, such as oral or rectal diazepam during a febrile illness, has been used effectively in children at higher risk of recurrent febrile seizures.[11–13]

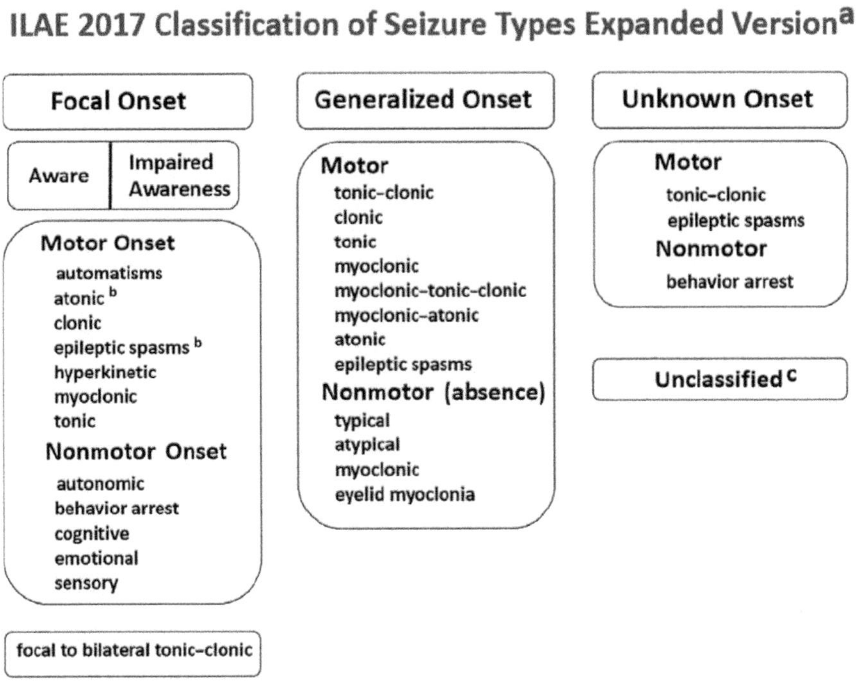

Fig. 1. ILAE classification of seizure types. The following clarifications should guide the choice of seizure type. For focal seizures, specification of level of awareness is optional. Retained awareness means the person is aware of self and environment during the seizure, even if immobile. A focal aware seizure corresponds to the prior term simple partial seizure. A focal impaired awareness seizure corresponds to the prior term complex partial seizure, and impaired awareness during any part of the seizure renders it a focal impaired awareness seizure. Focal aware or impaired awareness seizures optionally may further be characterized by one of the motor-onset or nonmotor-onset symptoms, reflecting the first prominent sign or symptom in the seizure. Seizures should be classified by the earliest prominent feature, except that a focal behavior arrest seizure is one for which cessation of activity is the dominant feature throughout the seizure. A focal seizure name also can omit mention of awareness when awareness is not applicable or unknown and thereby classify the seizure directly by motor onset or nonmotor-onset characteristics. Atonic seizures and epileptic spasms would usually not have specified awareness. Cognitive seizures imply impaired language or other cognitive domains or positive features, such as déjà vu, hallucinations, illusions, or perceptual distortions. Emotional seizures involve anxiety, fear, joy, other emotions, or appearance of affect without subjective emotions. An absence is atypical because of slow onset or termination or significant changes in tone supported by atypical, slow, generalized spike and wave on the EEG. A seizure may be unclassified because of inadequate information or inability to place the type in other categories. [a]Definitions, other seizure types, and descriptors are listed in Fisher and colleagues. From Fisher RS, Boas W van E, Blume W, et al. Epileptic Seizures and Epilepsy: Definitions Proposed by the International League Against Epilepsy (ILAE) and the International Bureau for Epilepsy (IBE). *Epilepsia*. 2005;46(4):470-472. [b]Degree of awareness usually is not specified. [c]Because of inadequate information or inability to place in other categories.

CAUSES OF EPILEPSY IN CHILDREN

Causes of the epilepsies have been identified in several epidemiologic studies.[1] A recent population-based study claims that among all children with epilepsy, genetic causes account for 34% of cases. Structural causes account for 26% of cases, which includes perinatal events, malformations of brain development, tumors, hemorrhage, leukomalacia, and tubers of tuberous sclerosis. A cause could not be found in up to 40% of children with epilepsy, and this pertains mostly to children more than 5 years of age. Infectious, traumatic, and metabolic causes are rare, probably because of the effectiveness of preventative measures. A detailed discussion of age-related epilepsy syndromes and their treatment is beyond the scope of this article.

MANAGEMENT AND TREATMENT OF CHILDREN WITH EPILEPSY

Clinics Care Points, the Evaluation of Epilepsy

- Referral to a pediatric neurologist can help differentiate abnormal movements or behaviors as epileptic in origin, but an awake and sleep EEG is often essential to make this distinction.[14]
- If routine EEG fails to delineate the condition, video-EEG monitoring is recommended.[15]
- Neuroimaging is recommended (computed tomographic scan is often done on an emergent basis), preferably a detailed MRI of the brain, to exclude a structural cause for seizure.[16]
- Once the diagnosis is confirmed, treatment options include anticonvulsant medication, dietary regimens, immunomodulation agents,[17,18] and surgery.

Evaluation of Potential Candidates for Epilepsy Surgery

Candidates for epilepsy surgery should be identified by a multidisciplinary group of specialists. *Intractable epilepsy* is defined as failure of adequate trials of 2 tolerated and appropriately chosen antiepileptic drugs. In a review on the topic, only 13% of children were controlled on a second anticonvulsant medication after the first failed.[19] Intractability with medical management can occur in up to 15% to 30% of children; however, less than 1% of patients with drug-resistant epilepsy is referred to full-service epilepsy centers annually. Access and timely referrals to life-changing epilepsy surgery remain a challenge worldwide and even in the United States.[20,21]

In children with structural abnormalities on MRI causing seizures, removal of the offending lesion can lead to seizure freedom.[22] Children without a lesion or with multifocal onset of seizures present more of a challenge but should not be ruled out as surgical candidates. Causes of brain abnormalities causing epilepsy include tumors, brain damaged by trauma, stroke, or infection, cortical dysplasia, and syndromes such as Sturge-Weber or tuberous sclerosis. The areas of the brain involved can include 1 lobe or area, multiple lobes, or the whole cerebral hemisphere.

Evaluation of the surgical candidate proceeds in stages, starting with noninvasive (video EEG, MRI, neuropsychological testing, single-photon emission computed tomography, and PET) tests, then more invasive monitoring if needed.[23,24] Ideal candidates with the best chance for seizure freedom have concordant or matching diagnostic studies pointing to 1 specific area of the brain, and preferably a clear lesion on MRI. These patients can undergo 1 surgery (1 stage) for resection of the focus or lesion.

Patients with no lesion on MRI, multiple abnormal areas, or a lesion near eloquent cortex will often require an invasive study to locate the seizure focus (also known as 2-stage surgery).[25] A simplified flow chart for the workup and decision making is provided (**Fig. 2**). Success is defined as seizure freedom, complete resection, or disconnection of the seizure focus, with preservation of eloquent function.

Invasive Studies to Determine Seizure Focus: Subdural Grids and Stereoelectroencephalography

Invasive recording is recommended in patients without a focal lesion on imaging, multiple abnormalities, or a lesion near eloquent (motor, language) cortex that requires mapping of these functional areas before resection. Mapping of epileptogenic foci and subsequent decision making regarding respective surgery are among the most challenging aspects of surgical epilepsy. The traditional method of recording seizure activity directly from the brain involves placing electrodes in a sheet, grid, or strips directly on the brain surface (subdural electrodes) with a craniotomy, also known as ECOG or electrocorticography (**Fig. 3**). Grids and strips can be used during resection of a lesion in the operating room to ensure all the seizure generating area is resected. The surgeon can also implant a grid, strip, or depth electrodes for several days to a week, allowing for mapping of the seizure focus and eloquent areas (motor function and speech), then remove them, and a resection can be performed. This procedure comes with a risk of infection because of the electrode array sitting in both the subdural space and tunneled outside the child's head and connected to the recording device (both intracranial and extracranial).[26,27]

Many centers have moved to insertion of an array of depth electrodes rather than grids (stereoelectroencephalography [SEEG]). The electrodes are inserted into specific targets using navigation or MRI guidance (stereotactic placement) and can offer an alternative that is less invasive and covers a larger area of brain tissue (**Fig. 4**). Deeper areas of cortex can be accessed without the need for a larger craniotomy used for grids, and an extensive map of the seizure focus can be developed, and later

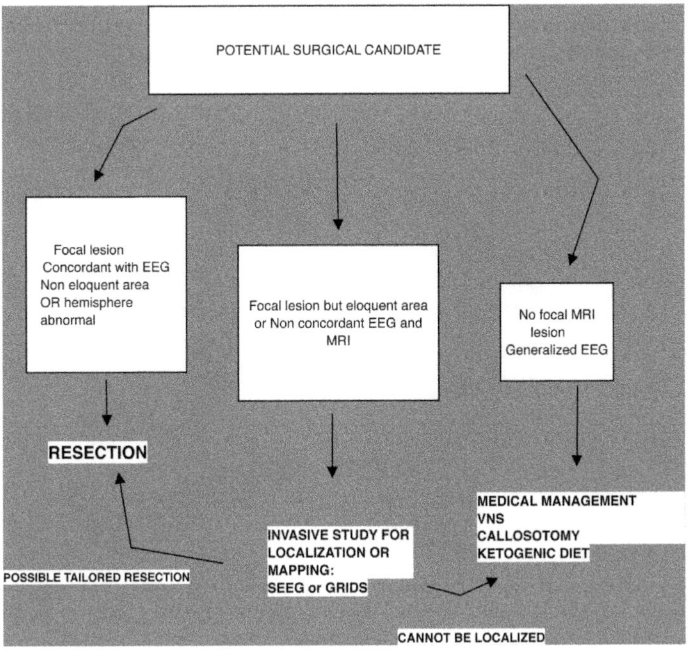

Fig. 2. Epilepsy surgery flowchart. The evaluation of a potential surgical candidate.

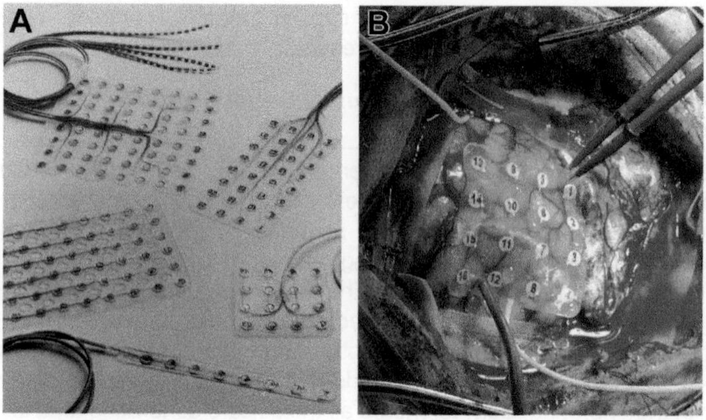

Fig. 3. Subdural grid electrodes. (*A*) Examples of implantable grids used for invasive localization and/or mapping of the patient with refractory epilepsy. (*B*) Intraoperative view at the time of subdural grid placement.

resection can be planned.[28–31] Difficult-to-access brain areas, such as the insular cortex, can also be targeted by intracranial depth electrodes.[32]

RESECTIVE AND DISCONNECTIVE SURGERY: FOCAL AND LOBAR RESECTIONS, HEMISPHERECTOMY AND HEMISPHEROTOMY, AND CORPUS CALLOSOTOMY

A focal lesion on MRI with concordant EEG localization presents the team with the ideal candidate for surgical resection. The temporal lobe remains the most common source of epilepsy in older children and adults, and the inner part of the temporal lobe or hippocampus is a common seizure generator. Outcomes in adults have shown excellent results with complete resection with low complication rates; literature supports surgical resection over continued medical management.[33]

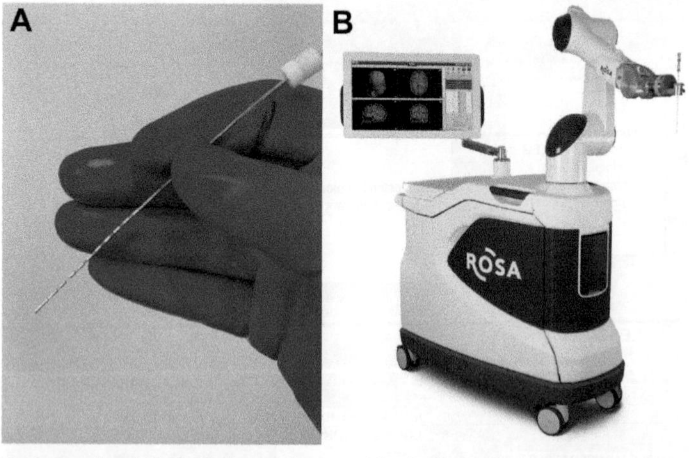

Fig. 4. SEEG electrodes. (*A*) SEEG electrodes provide similar information to surface grids, but can be inserted in a minimally invasive fashion. (*B*) SEEG electrodes are placed using computer-assisted navigation, often with robotic guidance, such as the ROSA system shown here. (*Courtesy of* Zimmer Biomet Robotics.)

A variety of resective surgeries in children have shown similar success.[34] Tumors are commonly associated with seizures in children, and they are usually low grade. Complete resection offers long-term seizure freedom in most.[35,36] Like tumors, areas of cortical dysplasia (malformed brain architecture) are common generators of seizures in children, and, when focal, resection can be highly effective. Predictors of surgical success, as with tumors, are short preoperative seizure duration, focal abnormality on MRI, and complete resection[37,38] (**Fig. 5**). Resections outside the temporal lobe are generally less effective. In some cases, complete resection is not possible because of the presence of essential neurologic function within the volume of epileptogenic cortex.[39–41] Expectations of caregivers must be tempered by the epilepsy team in such challenging cases.

The surgical strategy of disconnecting an epileptogenic focus can be used with success in specific pathologic circumstances. Sometimes a whole hemisphere has pathologic condition that generates seizures. Examples include stroke, trauma, infection, and malformations to include hemimegalencephaly and Rasmussen encephalitis. Surgery that once required removal of the entire abnormal hemisphere has evolved to disconnection surgery, whereby white matter tracts connecting 1 side with the other are transected, including the corpus callosum[42–46] (**Fig. 6**). The corpus callosum, which connects the 2 hemispheres in the midline, can be divided to prevent spread of seizures to include dangerous atonic seizures or drop attacks. Recent reports have described hemispherotomy and callosotomy done endoscopically.[47] An important reminder for the primary care physician is that a child may seize in the postoperative period secondary to the intervention itself. Reassurance is essential, as early postoperative seizures do not portend a lack of surgical success or long-term seizure freedom.

OTHER INTERVENTIONS: LASER ABLATION, VAGAL NERVE STIMULATION, RESPONSIVE NEUROSTIMULATION, AND DEEP BRAIN STIMULATION

- In cases whereby the seizure focus is deep-seated or difficult to reach through an open surgical approach, a target can also be ablated using a focused laser delivered through an intracranial catheter.[48] This has been used in pediatric cases of

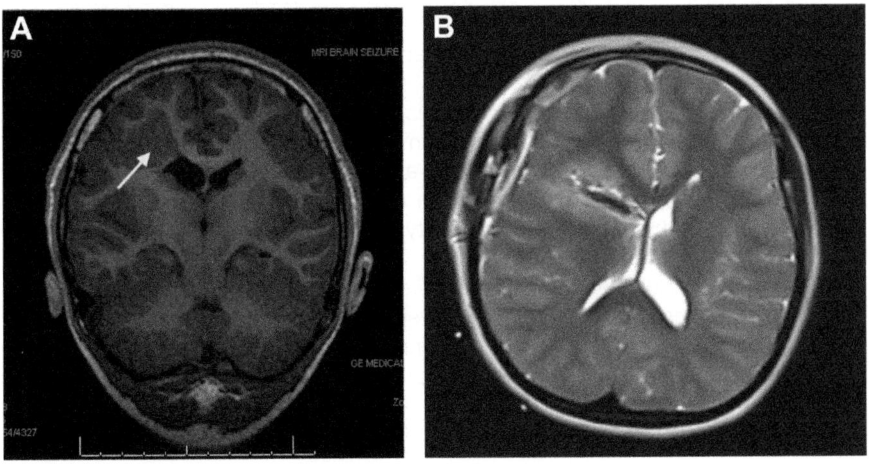

Fig. 5. Cortical dysplasia as an epileptogenic focus. (*A*) Preoperative axial T2-weighted MRI demonstrating a small nodular focus of cortical dysplasia abutting the right lateral ventricle (*arrow*). (*B*) Postoperative axial T2-weighted MRI following resection of cortical dysplasia. Complete resection in this case resulted in outstanding seizure control.

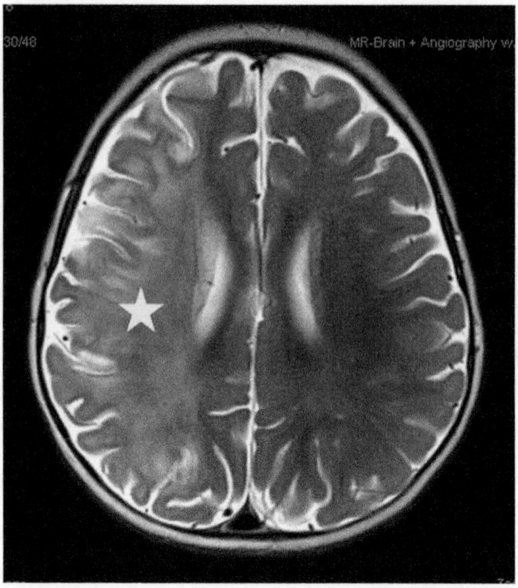

Fig. 6. The patient with unilateral hemispheric pathologic condition (T2 axial MRI shown) and refractory epilepsy may be a candidate for disconnection surgery.

hypothalamic hamartoma, malformations, or heterotopias, and cases of hippocampal pathologic condition with some success.

- For children without a lesion on MRI, nonlocalizing findings, or an eloquent area focus not amenable to resection, implantable devices have been developed to mitigate seizure activity. Vagal nerve stimulation (VNS) uses electrical current generated by a small pulse generator that is connected to an electrode placed on the left vagus nerve to send signals to widespread areas of the brain (**Fig. 7**). VNS can offer a 50% to 75% reduction in seizure frequency and is well tolerated.[49,50] Complications of VNS are infrequent and include infection and equipment malfunction. Stimulation typically occurs on a programmed cycle; however, newer models have a feature that activates the device based on physiologic changes predictive of impending seizure to include changes in patient heart rate.
- Responsive neurostimulation or RNS is a closed-loop system (EEG feedback measured by the device initiates a stimulus) with a component of intracranial electrode recording brain activity and a generator implanted on the skull. The generator responds to abnormal brain activity by delivering a stimulus to the electrode interrupting the seizure activity. Very few cases of RNS in pediatric patients are reported.[51]
- Deep brain stimulation is an open-loop system of stimulation (runs on a continuous programmed cycle without physiologic feedback) of the thalamus for intractable epilepsy. A generator delivers a programmed stimulus to an intracranial electrode implanted with MRI guidance. A 2018 review of pediatric cases showed some promising results.[52]

Summary

At some point, the primary care physician or provider will undoubtedly have patients with seizures or epilepsy in their practice. A fluency with the concepts of epilepsy and

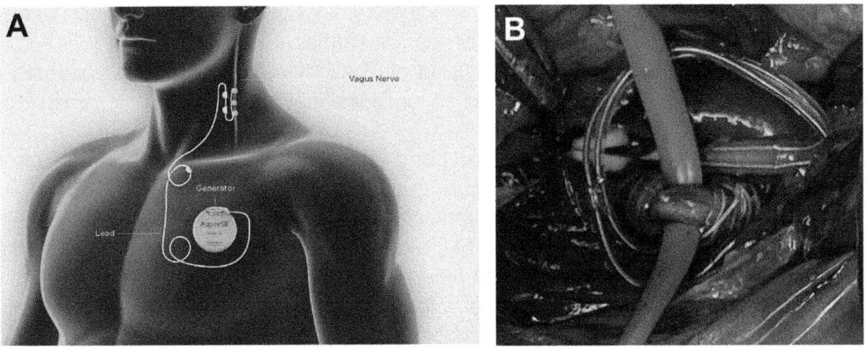

Fig. 7. VNS. (*A*) The patient with nonlocalizing epilepsy may be a candidate for VNS. This technique involves placement of an electrode array on the left vagus nerve in the neck connected to a pulse generator placed under the skin on the upper chest. This technique is indicated for adjunctive therapy in reducing the frequency of seizures in patients 4 years of age and older with partial onset seizures refractory to antiepileptic medications. (*B*) Intraoperative view of vagal nerve stimulator electrode applied to the left vagus nerve. (*Courtesy of* Liva Nova USA, Inc.)

epilepsy surgery can inform the provider when to reassure parents and when to ask for help. Success with treatment is defined as seizure freedom, but even adequate seizure control can improve quality of life and prevent sudden death.

Clinics Care Points, Surgical Workup, and Management for Children with Epilepsy

- Medical intractability occurs in 15% to 30% of children with epilepsy.
- Diagnosis involves EEG, MRI, and other studies, reviewed by a team specializing in identifying candidates for surgery.
- Absence of a lesion or tumor on MRI does *not* preclude a child's surgical candidacy.
- Some children will need more invasive monitoring (subdural grids or SEEG) to pinpoint a seizure focus for resection.
- Options for surgical intervention include resection, disconnection, and neurostimulation.

DISCLOSURE

None to report.

REFERENCES

1. Zack MM, Kobau R. National and state estimates of the numbers of adults and children with active epilepsy - United States, 2015. *MMWR Morb Mortal Wkly Rep* 2017;66(31):821–5.
2. Stuijvenberg M, Vos S de, Tjiang GCH, et al. Parents' fear regarding fever and febrile seizures. *Acta Paediatr* 1999;88(6):618–22.
3. Fisher RS, Boas WE, Blume W, et al. Epileptic seizures and epilepsy: definitions proposed by the International League Against Epilepsy (ILAE) and the International Bureau for Epilepsy (IBE). *Epilepsia* 2005;46(4):470–2.
4. Brodtkorb E. Common imitators of epilepsy. *Acta Neurol Scand Suppl* 2013;196:5–10.

5. Xu Y, Nguyen D, Mohamed A, et al. Frequency of a false positive diagnosis of epilepsy: a systematic review of observational studies. *Seizure* 2016;41:167–74.
6. Scheffer IE, Berkovic S, Capovilla G, et al. ILAE classification of the epilepsies: position paper of the ILAE Commission for Classification and Terminology. *Epilepsia* 2017;58(4):512–21.
7. Neligan A, Bell GS, Giavasi C, et al. Long-term risk of developing epilepsy after febrile seizures: a prospective cohort study. *Neurology* 2012;78(15):1166–70.
8. Berg AT, Shinnar S. Complex febrile seizures. *Epilepsia* 1996;37(2):126–33.
9. Seinfeld SA, Pellock JM, Kjeldsen MJ, et al. Epilepsy after febrile seizures: twins suggest genetic influence. *Pediatr Neurol* 2016;55:14–6.
10. Le Gal F, Lebon S, Ramelli GP, et al. When is a child with status epilepticus likely to have Dravet syndrome? *Epilepsy Res* 2014;108(4):740–7.
11. Berg AT, Shinnar S, Hauser WA, et al. Predictors of recurrent febrile seizures: a metaanalytic review. J *Pediatr* 1990;116(3):329–37.
12. Epilepsy - NICE Pathways. Available at: https://pathways.nice.org.uk/pathways/epilepsy#path=view%3A/pathways/epilepsy/treating-prolonged-or-repeated-seizures-and-convulsive-status-epilepticus.xml%26content=view-index. Accessed September 20, 2020.
13. Offringa M, Newton R, Cozijnsen MA, et al. Prophylactic drug management for febrile seizures in children. *Cochrane Database Syst Rev* 2017;(2):CD003031.
14. Wilmshurst JM, Gaillard WD, Vinayan KP, et al. Summary of recommendations for the management of infantile seizures: Task Force Report for the ILAE Commission of Pediatrics. *Epilepsia* 2015;56(8):1185–97.
15. Yu HJ, Lee CG, Nam SH, et al. Clinical and ictal characteristics of infantile seizures: EEG correlation via long-term video EEG monitoring. *Brain Dev* 2013; 35(8):771–7.
16. Gaillard WD, Chiron C, Cross JH, et al. Guidelines for imaging infants and children with recent-onset epilepsy. *Epilepsia* 2009;50(9):2147–53.
17. Bello-Espinosa LE, Rajapakse T, Rho JM, et al. Efficacy of intravenous immunoglobulin in a cohort of children with drug-resistant epilepsy. *Pediatr Neurol* 2015;52(5):509–16.
18. Sethi NK, Nitin K, Sethi NY. Immunotherapy for pharmacoresistant epilepsy. 2020. Available at: http://n.neurology.org/content/immunotherapy-pharmacoresistant-epilepsy. Accessed September 21, 2020.
19. Kwan P, Brodie MJ. Early identification of refractory epilepsy. N Engl J Med 2000; 342(5):314–9.
20. Englot DJ, Ouyang D, Garcia PA, et al. Epilepsy surgery trends in the United States: 1990-2008. Neurology 2012;78:1200–6.
21. Ibrahim GM, Barry BW, Fallah A, et al. Inequities in access to pediatric epilepsy surgery: a bioethical framework. Neurosurg Focus 2012;32(3):E2.
22. Berg AT, Mathern GW, Bronen RA, et al. Frequency, prognosis, and surgical treatment of structural abnormalities seen with magnetic resonance imaging in childhood epilepsy. Brain 2009;132(Pt 10):2785–97.
23. Perry MS, Duchowny M. Evaluation of intractable epilepsy in children. In: Albright AL, Pollack IF, Adelson DP, editors. Principles and practice of pediatric neurosurgery. 3rd edition. New York, NY: Thieme Medical Publishers; 2015. p. 932–9.
24. Ryvlin P, Cross JH, Rheims S. Epilepsy surgery in children and adults. Lancet Neurol 2014;13:1114–26.
25. Jayakar P, Gaillard WD, Tripathi M, et al. Diagnostic test utilization in evaluation for resective epilepsy surgery in children. Epilepsia 2014;55(4):507–18.

26. Vakharia VN, Duncan JS, Whit JA, et al. Getting the best outcomes from epilepsy surgery. Ann Neurol 2018;83(4):676–90.
27. Roth J, Carlson C, Devinsky O, et al. Safety of staged epilepsy surgery in children. Neurosurgery 2014;74:154–62.
28. Onal C, Otsubo H, Araki T, et al. Complications of invasive subdural grid monitoring in children with epilepsy. J Neurosurg 2003;98:1017–26.
29. Mullin JP, Shriver M, Alomar S, et al. Is SEEG safe? A systematic review and meta-analysis of stereo-electroencephalography-related complications. Epilepsia 2016;57(3):386–401.
30. McGovern RA, Knight EP, Gupta A, et al. Robot-assisted stereoelectroencephalography in children. J Neurosurg Pediatr 2019;23:288–96.
31. Goldstein HE, Youngerman BE, Shao B, et al. Safety and efficacy of stereoelectroencephalography in pediatric focal epilepsy: a single-center experience. J Neurosurg Pediatr 2018;22:444–52.
32. Gonzalez-Martinez J, Mullin J, Vadera S, et al. Stereotactic placement of depth electrodes in medically intractable epilepsy. J Neurosurg 2014;120:639–44.
33. Tomycz LD, Hale AT, Haider AS, et al. Invasive insular sampling in pediatric epilepsy: a single-institution experience. Oper Neurosurg (Hagerstown) 2018;15: 310–7.
34. Wiebe S, Blume WT, Girvin JP, et al. A randomized, controlled trial of surgery for temporal-lobe epilepsy. N Engl J Med 2001;345:311–8.
35. Dwivedi R, Ramanujam B, Chandra PS, et al. Surgery for drug-resistant epilepsy in children. N Engl J Med 2017;377:1639–47.
36. Fallah A, Weil AG, Sur S, et al. Epilepsy surgery related to pediatric brain tumors: Miami Children's Hospital experience. J Neurosurg Pediatr 2015;16:675–80.
37. Khan RB, Boop FA, Onar A, et al. Seizures in children with low-grade tumors: outcome after tumor resection and risk factors for uncontrolled seizures. J Neurosurg 2006;104:377–82.
38. Bourgeois M, Sainte-Rose C, Lellouch-Tubiana A, et al. Surgery of epilepsy associated with focal lesions in childhood. J Neurosurg 1999;90:833–42.
39. Hamiwka L, Jayakar P, Resnick T, et al. Surgery for cortical malformations in childhood: ten-year follow up. Epilpesia 2005;46(4):556–60.
40. Martinez-Lizana E, Fauser S, Brandt A, et al. Long-term seizure outcome in pediatric patients with focal cortical dysplasia undergoing tailored and standard surgical resections. Seizure 2018;62:66–73.
41. Choi SA, Kim SY, Kim H, et al. Surgical outcome and predictive factors of epilepsy surgery in pediatric isolated focal cortical dysplasia. Epilepsy Res 2018; 139:54–9.
42. Ansari SF, Maher CO, Tubbs RS, et al. Surgery for extratemporal nonlesional epilepsy in children: meta-analysis. Childs Nerv Syst 2010;26(7):945–51.
43. Dorward IG, Titus JB, Limbrick DD, et al. Extratemporal, nonlesional epilepsy in children: postsurgical clinical and neurocognitive outcomes. J Neurosurg Pediatr 2011;7:179–88.
44. Enlgot DJ, Breshears JD, Sun PP, et al. Seizure outcomes after resective surgery for extra-temporal lobe epilepsy in pediatric patients. J Neurosurg Pediatr 2013; 12:126–33.
45. Handler MH, O'Neill B. Hemispherotomy and hemispherectomy. In: Cohen AR, editor. Pediatric neurosurgery: tricks of the trade. New York: Thieme Medical Publishers, Inc.; 2016. p. 703–11.
46. Jea A, Vachhrajani S, Widjaja E, et al. Corpus callosotomy in children and the disconnection syndromes: a review. Childs Nerv Syst 2008;24:685–92.

47. Roland JL, Smyth MD. Recent advances in the neurosurgical treatment of pediatric epilepsy. J Neurosurg Pediatr 2019;23:411–21.
48. Elliott RE, Rodgers SD, Bassani L, et al. Vagus nerve stimulation for children with treatment-resistant epilepsy: a consecutive series of 141 cases. J Neurosurg Pediatr 2011;7:491–500.
49. Thompson KM, Wozniak SE, Roberts CM, et al. Vagus nerve stimulation for partial and generalized epilepsy from infancy to adolescence. J Neurosurg Pediatr 2012;10:200–5.
50. North RY, Raskin JS, Curry DJ. MRI-guided laser interstitial thermal therapy for epilepsy. Neurosurg Clin North Am 2017;28:545–57.
51. Kokoszka MA, Panov F, La Vega-Talbott M, et al. Treatment of medically refractory seizures with responsive neurostimulation: 2 pediatric cases. J Neurosurg Pediatr 2018;21:421–7.
52. Yan H, Toyota E, Anderson M, et al. A systematic review of deep brain stimulation for the treatment of drug-resistant epilepsy in childhood. J Neurosurg Pediatr 2019;23(3):261–410.

Mild Traumatic Brain Injury in Children

Aaron M. Yengo-Kahn, MD, Rebecca A. Reynolds, MD,
Christopher M. Bonfield, MD*

KEYWORDS

• Pediatric • mTBI • Concussion • Sport-related concussion • Return-to-play
• Return-to-learn

KEY POINTS

- Children with a suspected head injury should be removed immediately from activity and monitored closely for red flag signs and symptoms, the appearance of which should necessitate further evaluation.
- Concussion, or mild traumatic brain injury, is defined as a head injury with a Glasgow Coma Scale between 13 and 15 and neuroimaging, if performed, does not demonstrate an acute abnormality.
- Initial management includes 24 to 48 hours of physical and cognitive rest. A period of strict rest beyond 48 to 72 hours may prolong recovery.
- Graded return to learn and play protocols should be followed, and children should first return to school and then to sports.
- The vast majority of children recover in 2 to 4 weeks. Only a small percentage have prolonged symptoms (>1 month).

BACKGROUND

Traumatic brain injury (TBI) encompasses a spectrum of disease that is, based on the Glasgow Coma Scale (GCS) at initial presentation (**Table 1**).[1] The annual incidence of pediatric TBI is estimated to be between 1 to 6 million cases worldwide, of which mild TBI (mTBI) accounts for the vast majority.[2] The diagnosis of mTBI is often synonymously used with concussion. Concussion, or mTBI, is defined as a head injury with a GCS between 13 and 15 and neuroimaging, if performed, does not demonstrate an acute abnormality.[3] The underlying mechanism of injury is transient rotational and/or linear acceleration of the head that induces mechanical forces on the brain, resulting in neuronal dysfunction. Although the mechanism is often a direct blow to the head, an impact to the body with a subsequent "whiplash" motion of the head

Department of Neurosurgery, Vanderbilt University Medical Center, Medical Center North, Suite T-4224, 1161 21st Avenue South, Nashville, TN 37232, USA
* Corresponding author.
E-mail address: chris.bonfield@vumc.org

Pediatr Clin N Am 68 (2021) 857–874
https://doi.org/10.1016/j.pcl.2021.04.011
pediatric.theclinics.com

Table 1 The Glasgow Coma Scale		
Eyes (4)	**Verbal (5)**	**Motor (6)**
4 - Opens eyes spontaneously	5 - Oriented, appropriate	6 - Follows commands
3 - Opens eyes to voice	4 - Confused, conversational	5 - Localizes to pain
2 - Opens eyes to stimulation	3 - Inappropriate words	4 - Withdraws to pain
1 - Does not open eyes	2 - Incomprehensible sounds	3 - Flexor posturing
	1 - No response	2 - Extensor posturing
	1T - Intubated	1 - No movement

GCS = Eyes + Verbal + Motor.
A GCS of 15 is the maximum. A GCS of 3 is the minimum.
Produced with data from Teasdale and Jennett, 1974.[1]

and neck may also transmit the necessary forces for a symptomatic mTBI.[3,4] Twenty-nine percent of pediatric mTBIs are diagnosed in the outpatient setting,[5] and an outpatient provider's early diagnosis and implementation of graded return to school and sport guidelines are fundamental keys to management.[6]

DISCUSSION

Prevalence and Incidence

Pediatric TBI is a global phenomenon, with mTBI constituting more than 80% of cases.[2] More children are affected with mTBI than adults, largely owing to different activity and behaviors of children and adolescents. For example, in the United States, there are 35 million child athletes, compared with 400,000 and 20,000 athletes at the collegiate and professional levels, respectively.[7] When pediatric mTBI is assessed by mechanism of injury in the United States, the predominant mechanism changes according to age group. For children under the age of 4, falls are the predominant mechanism of injury (70%). For children 5 to 14 years old, falls and being struck by an object are equally frequent (35%). For teenagers and young adults aged 15 to 24 years, falls, being struck by an object, motor vehicle collision, and assault comprise 20% of injuries each.[8] Although commonly associated with sports, pediatric mTBI can result from many different mechanisms of injury.

Because sport-related concussion (SRC) comprises a significant portion of pediatric mTBI (70%), it warrants further scrutiny.[9] Sport- and recreation-related TBI equates to approximately 283,000 injured children annually in the United States, and its incidence is increasing, particularly in the adolescent age group.[5] Contact sports are the most common etiology with football at the top of the list.[9–11] In general, the incidence of SRC is higher for males than females.[12] However, when analyzed on a high school, gender-stratified, sport-by-sport basis in the United States, the highest rate of concussions were witnessed in men's football followed by women's soccer, men's ice hockey, men's lacrosse, and women's basketball.[11] One systematic international review that included both high school-aged and younger children indicated that rugby presented the highest rate of concussion, followed by hockey and American football.[13] Although the epidemiologic study of high school sports injuries has improved immensely through the national High School Reporting Information Online registry,[11] youth sports before the high school years have not been extensively studied owing to a lack of available documentation.[14] One study about American youth football showed that 33,000 TBI-related visits to the emergency room are for children aged 5 to 14 year old, which equates to 12% of all sport-related TBI across all age groups.[9]

However, more comprehensive analyses focused on elementary and middle school-aged children are needed. In the setting of the surge in SRC research and news media coverage in recent years, the rates of concussion diagnoses have generally increased,[5] but the rate of recurrent concussions and practice-related concussions has generally decreased.[11] The reassuring downtrend suggests heightened awareness of the condition by health care providers, athletic coaches, and organizational leaders and implementation of best practice prevention and treatment recommendations for children who are at risk for or sustain an SRC.

Evaluation

Appropriate treatment for mTBI is contingent on early recognition of the condition. Although frequently performed, imaging is not required to diagnose an mTBI. The diagnosis relies largely on clinical acumen by assimilating a patient's history of present illness, a comprehensive review of systems, and thorough physical examination. There are numerous available assessment tools to aid in diagnosis, such as the Sport Concussion Assessment Tool (SCAT), now in its fifth edition,[15] and the associated Child SCAT5 (for use from age 5–12 years).[16] These tools may be used on the sideline or in the clinic to support or refute the diagnosis of concussion. The instrument includes brief neurologic, neurocognitive and symptom evaluations.[17] Symptom burdens are commonly assessed (both on the SCAT5 and independently) using the Post-Concussion Symptom Scale (PCSS). Although these basic tools may provide decisional support, they are neither essential nor definitive for diagnosing mTBI.[18] The PCSS is helpful for classifying mTBI symptoms into symptom domains (**Fig. 1**),

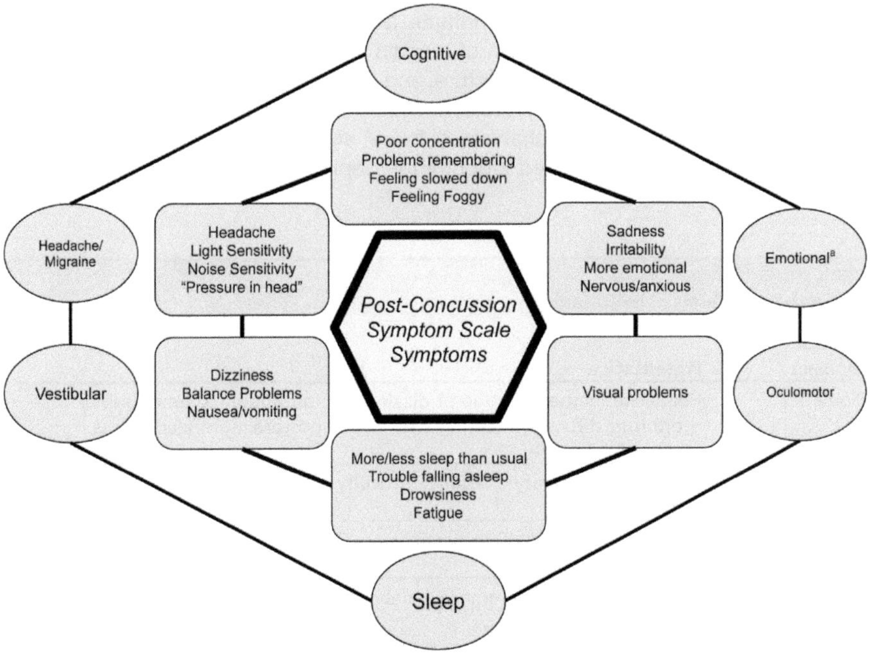

Fig. 1. Mapping symptoms from the PCSS to concussion subtypes. Inner ring includes symptoms from the PCSS mapped to major concussion subtypes (outer ring) based on classifications in Lumba-Brown et al. 2019.[20] [a]Note: The "emotional" symptom domain often used interchangeably with "mood/anxiety" domain.

which include headaches, cognitive changes, mood/emotional changes, oculomotor difficulty, vestibular issues, sleep aberration, and cervical strain.[19,20] The constellation of reported symptoms varies from patient to patient, but headaches, fatigue, and sleepiness are most common (**Table 2**).[18] Although symptoms vary, there are key features that should trigger further workup in the emergency room or transfer to a higher level of care at a designated pediatric trauma center. These red flag symptoms include worsening confusion, increasing drowsiness, refractory headaches, asymmetric pupils, focal neurologic deficit, refractory vomiting, seizures, and loss of consciousness (**Box 1**).[21,22] Patients demonstrating these signs and symptoms warrant an imaging workup and should not be managed in the outpatient setting. A thorough understanding of normal versus red flag symptoms after mTBI is critical to providing safe and effective care for these patients.

Red flag symptoms are a clear indication for neuroimaging; however, opinions have varied over the years as to indications for neuroimaging for patients without red flag symptoms. Recent high-quality research as well as recommendations from the Centers for Disease Control and Prevention (CDC) have helped to clarify this issue. In 2009, the Pediatric Emergency Care Applied Research Network group published validated guidelines that identified children who present with GCS 14 or 15 and are at low risk for clinically important TBI.[23] The appropriate identification of this low-risk subgroup of pediatric patients with mTBI enabled evidence-based recommendations to guide providers in safely deferring an imaging workup. Children with clinically important TBI were defined for the purposes of the study as death from TBI, neurosurgical intervention, intubation after 24 hours from time of injury, or hospital admission longer than 2 nights. The criteria were stratified according to children who were younger or older than 2 years of age, and the sensitivities were 100% and 97% for each age group, respectively. Salient data for infants and toddlers (<2 years old) included mental status, presence and location of a scalp hematoma, loss of consciousness, mechanism of injury, palpable skull fracture, and acting at baseline per the child's parents. For children 2 years and older, relevant information included mental status, loss of consciousness, vomiting, mechanism of injury, signs of basilar skull fracture, and headache severity. Their validated algorithm is depicted in **Fig. 2**.[23] This study has

Table 2
Signs and symptoms of concussion in sport

Clinical Domain	Presentation
Somatic	Headache, nausea, vertigo or dizziness, photophobia, phonophobia, tinnitus, difficulty focusing with vision, postural lightheadedness, anosmia, fatigue
Cognitive	Mental fog, memory difficulty, difficulty concentrating, word-finding difficulty
Behavioral	Mood lability, irritability, hypersomnia, insomnia, anxiety, depression, personality changes
Physical signs	Loss of consciousness, amnesia, neurologic deficit
Sleep/wake disturbance	Somnolence, drowsiness
Balance impairment	Gait unsteadiness

From Ahluwalia et al. 2020[21]; used with permission.

Box 1
Concussion red flag symptoms

Unequal pupils

Progressive headache

Progressive nausea/vomiting

Prolonged or delayed loss of consciousness

Focal neurologic deficit (1-sided facial droop, weakness, numbness)

Significantly altered mental status

Progressive alteration in behavior or mental status

Delayed seizure

From Ahluwalia et al.,[21] 2020; used with permission.

since been reviewed as Level B evidence and integrated into the CDC guidelines for evaluation of pediatric mTBI.[21]

Once the decision is made to pursue neuroimaging, the computed tomography (CT) scan is considered the gold standard in pediatric mTBI evaluation. This imaging modality carries the risks of ionizing radiation, high doses of which have been known to be associated with delayed malignancy. The long-standing concern about early exposure to ionizing radiation has prompted assessments of the usefulness of MRI in the evaluation of TBI, particularly with the advent of rapid sequence MRIs.[24] Standard brain MRIs have higher sensitivity in detecting intracranial structural abnormalities, which adds to their appeal.[25] Yet, MRI usefulness has historically been limited owing to length of scan, common need for sedation in pediatrics, and high cost. The advent of rapid sequence MRI decreased the time of the standard scan from 65 minutes to 5 to 15 minutes to improve its usefulness in the acute setting[26,27]; however, the shortened study time also undermines the ability to detect less obvious abnormalities. The major issue cited against using MRI in acute TBI evaluation, rapid sequence or otherwise, is the lower sensitivity it displays in assessing bony anatomy.[27] The sensitivity of the MRI for skull fracture detection is comparable to that of a skull radiograph whose sensitivity of 63% for single fractures obviates its usefulness.[21,28] Therefore, CT scan remains the preferred imaging modality by health care providers and the CDC owing to its expediency and accuracy, despite the risk of ionizing radiation.[21] In general, CT scans are readily available, and newer generations of scanners have lower doses of radiation, as well.

In addition to the SCAT,[15–17] a number of adjuncts have been developed to assist in diagnosing concussion.[29–31] The usefulness of most of these tools is typically beyond the scope of the average pediatric outpatient provider's clinic and more relevant to sideline staff (eg, athletic trainers) and the detailed interviews of concussion clinics and practicing neuropsychologists. The PCSS has been demonstrated to be useful in tracking symptoms over time and defining the need for symptom-specific therapies should long-term problems persist.[19,20] Given the variable complexity in clinical adjuncts, outpatient providers should routinely rely on the patient's reported clinical history of head trauma and symptomatology to make their diagnosis.[19,20]

Last, it is important to note that, despite a substantial amount of research devoted to mTBI serum biomarkers, there is no current evidence or guidelines to suggest the use of serum biomarkers for mTBI.[3,21,32]

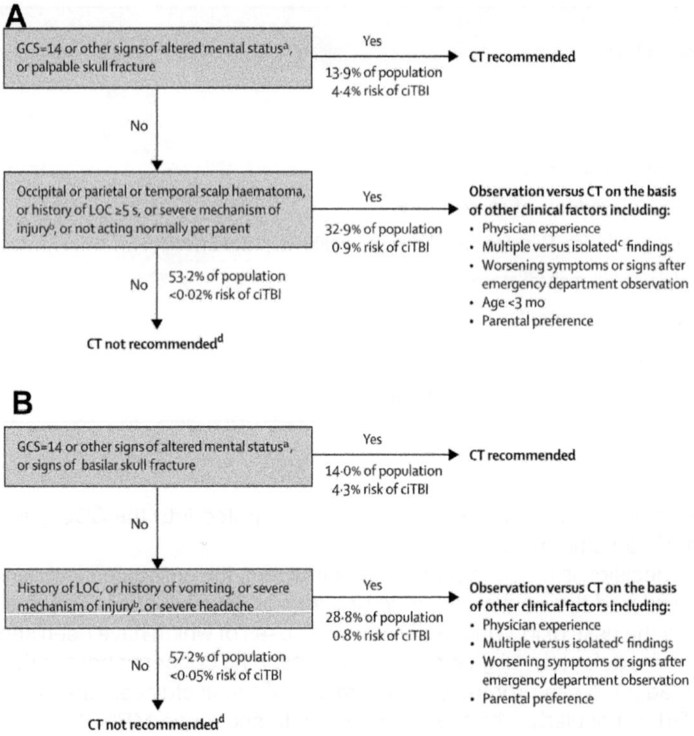

Fig. 2. Algorithm for determining the need for neuroimaging after head injury in children with GCS scores of 14 to 15. (*A*) Suggested CT algorithm for children younger than 2 years. (*B*) Suggested CT algorithm for children older than 2 years. ciTBI, clinically important traumatic brain injury; LOC, loss of consciousness. [a]Other signs of altered mental status: agitation, somnolence, repetitive questioning, or slow response to verbal communication. [b]Severe mechanism of injury: motor vehicle crash with patient ejection, death of another passenger, or rollover; pedestrian or bicyclist without helmet struck by a motorized vehicle; falls of more than 0.9 m (3 feet) (or >1.5 m [5 feet] for *B*); or head struck by a high-impact object. [c]Patients with certain isolated findings (ie, with no other findings suggestive of TBI), such as isolated LOC, isolated headache, isolated vomiting, and certain types of isolated scalp hematomas in infants older than 3 months, have a risk of ciTBI substantially lower than 1%. [d]Risk of ciTBI exceedingly low, generally lower than risk of CT-induced malignancies. Therefore, CT scans are not indicated for most patients in this group. (*From* Kupperman et al., Pediatric Emergency Care Applied Research Network (PECARN). Identification of children at very low risk of clinically-important brain injuries after head trauma: a prospective cohort study. Lancet. 2009 Oct 3;374(9696):1160-70. doi: 10.1016/S0140-6736(09)61558-0. Epub 2009 Sep 14. Erratum in: Lancet. 2014 Jan 25;383(9914):308. Reproduced with permission of Elsevier, Inc.)

Approach

Initial physical and cognitive rest

Once the diagnosis of a concussion or mTBI has been made, management and treatment is largely supportive, hinging on appropriate counseling with regard to rest and activity. Immediately after the postinjury evaluation, physical and cognitive rest for 1 to 3 days remains a mainstay of management consistent across mTBI guidelines.[32] Most important, children with a suspected concussion should not be returned to activity on the same day as injury.[3,32] Historically, the slight risk of second impact syndrome, or diffuse cerebral edema related to 2 head impact injuries in close temporal proximity, drove these recommendations.[33] Recent evidence has suggested that those who continue to participate in activity after a concussion, especially in sports, actually may suffer longer recovery times and ultimately miss more days of activity.[34] At present, all 50 states have passed legislation forbidding the return to organized physical education class or sports until cleared by a provider trained in concussion management (although the required credentials vary state to state).[3,35] At the earliest, this clearance can be obtained 24 hours after the injury.

Once symptoms have stabilized or improved after the initial period of rest, children may gradually resume normal daily activity as tolerated. Notably, extensive rest may paradoxically lead to more symptoms and a longer recovery.[36] Thus, typical initial recommendations include cognitive rest for 1 to 2 days and return to school as symptoms are tolerated, followed by a graded return to full school and activity.[3,37,38] Children and adolescents should return to school first then sport,[6] but can also proceed nearly in parallel.

Graded return to learn

Typically, children and adolescents can return to some level of academics in 2 to 5 days.[37] A graduated return-to-learn progression commences once the individual has resumed typically daily activities without increasing symptoms such as reading and screen time.[3] The progression described within the most recent Concussion in Sport Group Consensus Guidelines is presented in **Table 3**.[3]

Adolescents (ie, high school students) may take longer to return to school than younger children and are simultaneously more concerned about negative academic effects.[6,39] Accommodations are necessary for 17% to 73%[37] of students and those with medical letters from providers are more likely to get these.[40] Thus, providing the patient with a letter to the school describing symptoms, expected required short-term accommodations, and/or absence excuse is an important aspect of care that can improve the return to learning process and communication between health care providers and schools.[21,37] A template for such a letter is available from the CDC Heads Up website (https://www.cdc.gov/headsup/providers/discharge-materials.html).

Graded return to play

Following a graded return-to-play (or sport) protocol is most applicable for those children and adolescents aiming to return to an organized sport; however, much of the concept can be applied to all children and adolescents simply looking to return to activities. The progression described within the most recent Concussion in Sport Group Consensus Guidelines is presented in **Table 4**.[3] The CDC recognizes a similar graded approach.[21] Each step requires 24 hours and therefore at least 6 days are required between injury and return to normal gameplay. If symptoms recur at a given stage, the

Table 3
Stages of return to learn

Stage	Activity
Stage 1 (activities at home)	Typical activities as tolerated in 5- to 15-minute intervals
Stage 2 (school activities)	Cognitive activities, such as homework, outside of the classroom
Stage 3 (return to school part time)	Partial school day or full day with increased breaks Introduction of schoolwork should be gradual
Stage 4 (return to school full time)	Gradually increased school activities until return to normal school day

From McCrory et al. 2017.[3] Reproduced by permission of BMJ Publishing Group Ltd.

Table 4
Stages of return to play

Stage	Activity
Stage 1 (symptom limited activity)	Slow return and exposure to work/school activity
Stage 2 (light aerobic exercise)	Increase in heart rate by walking or stationary cycling
Stage 3 (sport-specific exercise)	Increase movement; note, this cannot include activities in which head impact is possible
Stage 4 (noncontact training drills)	Increase in coordination, thinking tasks, and overall exercise In this stage, resistance training may begin
Stage 5 (full contact practice)	Assess functional skills If medically cleared, the athlete may return to baseline training regimen
Stage 6 (return to sport)	Resume normal play, no restrictions

From McCrory et al. 2017.[3] Reproduced by permission of BMJ Publishing Group Ltd.

athlete should repeat the previous step. For those children and adolescents not involved in organized sports and who be potentially less motivated to participate in the graduated activity protocol, it is important to note that earlier return to aerobic exercise is increasingly recognized to be associated with a faster recovery.[41–43]

When to refer: specialty concussion clinic

Current guidelines suggest waiting 1 month before referral to a specialty concussion center for children and adolescents.[3,21,32] However, for those with a substantial symptom burden, risk factors for prolonged recovery (discussed elsewhere in this article), or those unable to progress with return to activity, earlier referral should be considered.[32,44] Despite these guidelines, evidence is mounting for early referral (<1 week from symptom onset) and its association with quicker recovery, so a lower threshold for referral may be beneficial.[44–46] A concussion or mTBI clinic provides comprehensive care by a multidisciplinary team that typically includes sports medicine physicians, physiotherapists, behavioral health specialists, and others.[32] The reasons for referral and the recommended timing for referrals are presented in **Table 5**.

When to refer: therapy

Physical therapy should be considered if the child is struggling to progress through graduated return to activity at 1 to 2 weeks. For competitive athletes and those highly motivated to return to activity, early subthreshold aerobic activity starting around 72 hours after injury, has been shown to improve recovery by about 4 days in a randomized controlled trial.[41] Determining a patient's exercise threshold requires a physical therapy consultation for exercise tolerance testing.[41,47] If athletes are able to complete exercise tolerance testing without worsening of their symptoms, this factor may indicate physiologic recovery from the concussion, whereas those who demonstrate worsening of symptoms may benefit from a subthreshold aerobic exercise regimen.[48] Exercise tolerance testing, subthreshold aerobic exercise, and multimodal physical therapy have been shown to be safe both in acute injuries (<72 hours after injury) and for those who have persistent symptoms.[41,47,49–52]

Vestibular therapy is appropriate for the vestibular subtype of concussion, which is characterized by dizziness, nausea, vertigo, disequilibrium, and fogginess.[19] On physical examination, these children may demonstrate abnormal vestibular ocular reflexes, visual motion sensitivity, nystagmus, imbalance, and gait dysfunction.[19,53] The

Table 5
Where, when, and why to refer

Referral to	Reason to Refer	When	Purpose
Multidisciplinary concussion clinic[a]	1. High initial symptom burden 2. Risk factors for prolonged recovery (ADHD, prior concussions, headache or psychiatric history etc.) 3. Prolonged symptoms (>1 mo) 4. When considering additional therapy referrals to centralize care	1/2. Within 1–2 wk if high risk 3. At 1 mo if symptoms persistent and no high risk factors 4. If considering physical, vestibular or vision therapy	1/2/3/4. Connect patient with multidisciplinary care team for more comprehensive concussion care
Physical therapy	1. Patient is struggling to progress through graduated activity protocols 2. Highly motivated or competitive athletes for consideration of subthreshold aerobic activity programs 3. Exercise tolerance testing	1. Failure to progress activity within 1–2 wk of injury 2. Within 72 h for early subthreshold aerobic activity programs 3. If athlete suspected recovered but mild symptoms persist	1. Provide structure and regimen to break recovery plateaus 2. Attempt to minimize physiologic recovery time 3. Exercise tolerance testing may determine physiologic recovery
Vestibular therapy and vision therapy	1. Vestibular concussion subtype (see **Fig. 1**) 2. Oculomotor signs or symptoms (double vision/blurry vision)	1/2. Symptoms persist >2 wk or highly symptomatic	1/2. Specific intervention for vestibular and vision symptoms, prevent prolonged disability
Neurology	1. Persistent headache	1. >2 wk of new or worsened headache after injury	1. Focused headache treatment
Psychiatry	1. High emotional PCSS subscores (see **Fig. 1**) 2. Worsened psychiatric symptoms in those with family or personal psychiatric histories	1/2. 1–2 wk after injury if symptoms persisting or worsening	1/2. Focused psychiatric care, consideration of pharmaceutical interventions
Neuropsychology	1. Persistent cognitive symptoms	1. Symptoms > 1 mo	1. Formal neuropsychological testing to identify areas for cognitive therapy 2. Results may aid in clinical decision-making

Abbreviation: ADHD, attention deficit hyperactivity disorder.
[a] Referral to a multidisciplinary concussion clinic is recommended as the first stop to centralize care and referrals to other specialists with experience in brain injury rehabilitation.

presence of these signs and symptoms substantially increase the risk of prolonged recovery[53] and suggest the need for vestibular therapy. Vestibular therapy may be conducted by either physical or occupational therapists, is patient specific, and can include targeted gaze stability training, graded exposure to visually stimulating environments, or dynamic balance treatment.[54] There is some limited evidence that earlier treatment may be beneficial and short interval follow-up to assess for persistent vestibular complaint is useful to make a timely referral.[55–58]

Similarly, vision therapy is helpful for patients with significant vision complaints, including persistent light sensitivity, blurry vision, and diplopia, which are associated with double the risk of a prolonged recovery.[59,60] Vision therapy could be computer based or conducted in person by a therapist. Specific exercises vary, but aim to retrain the oculomotor system by addressing fixation, accommodation, version, vergence, pursuit, or even with reading protocols.[60,61] Vision rehabilitation may be performed in conjunction with vestibular therapy or may involve optical modifications such as prisms, tinted lenses, or filters.[59] There is limited evidence for vision therapy in pediatric mTBI, and evaluation within the concussion clinic should precede a direct referral to neuro-ophthalmology for these complaints.

When to refer: neurology, psychiatry, and neuropsychology

The most common pediatric concussion/mTBI subtype is headache/migraine.[19,62] About 10% of children continue to have persistent headaches at 2 weeks after an mTBI, and 8% continue to have headaches at 3 months.[63] Those patients who continue to have persistent headaches often have a personal or family history of migraine or other headaches requiring treatment.[62,64,65] Referral to neurology for persistent headache is recommended at 2 weeks after injury at the earliest given the majority of patients have resolution at this point. Empirically re-imaging a patient for continued headache or other persistent symptoms 2 weeks or more after injury is low yield and cost ineffective.[66] New or acutely worsening symptoms and new neurologic deficits several days to weeks after concussion should be evaluated as potentially unrelated and require the standard clinical and imaging evaluation.

As many as 5% to 12% of adolescents and children who suffer an mTBI may go on to develop a temporary postinjury psychiatric disorder.[67–70] A family or personal history of psychiatric disorders preceding the injury increase the subsequent risk of worsened or new psychiatric symptoms, the most common of which is personal change.[68,70] Those patients scoring high on the PCSS emotional subscore[69] and those at increased risk based on medical history who are exhibiting new or worsened psychiatric symptoms should be referred for psychiatric evaluation.

A referral to neuropsychological assessment is generally restricted to those with persistent cognitive symptoms for 1 month or more.[21,32] A neuropsychological assessment may consist of written testing with a neuropsychologist or a computerized assessment administered by a team doctor, sports medicine physician, or athletic trainer in the case of athletes with SRC. Although neuropsychological testing may aid in clinical decision-making, management decisions, such as returning to sport or school, should not be solely based on these test results.[3]

Medications

Most children require supportive care with over-the-counter medications such as acetaminophen or antiemetics in the acute injury period. Care should be taken when recommending aspirin or nonsteroidal anti-inflammatory drugs for 48 to 72 hours after injury owing theoretic increased risk of intracranial hemorrhage.[32,71] Notably, these risks have been extrapolated from limited studies and the actual risk of hemorrhage related to these medications is low.[72]

There is limited evidence to support any specific medication regimens that may improve outcomes in pediatric mTBI.[32,63,73–75] Nonsteroidal anti-inflammatory drug and acetaminophen (Tylenol) use should be limited to 2 to 3 uses per week owing to the potential for overuse headaches.[32,63] There is limited evidence to support the use of amitriptyline for persistent headache, and this condition is best managed by a headache specialist or psychiatrist.[63,75] Melatonin has been promoted for its palliative effects for sleep disturbances and headache.[63,73] A recent randomized controlled trial of melatonin for persistent postconcussion symptoms did not find any substantial improvement in symptoms[74]; however, melatonin is low risk and low cost and may provide symptomatic relief in the more acute period. Otherwise, there is no substantial evidence for the use of other supplements or vitamins to improve mTBI symptoms or outcomes.[73,76]

Clinical Outcomes

Typical recovery

Clinical recovery from mTBI or concussion is typically defined as resolution of symptoms.[77] For children, mTBI recovery rates have been studied after a SRC. Clinical

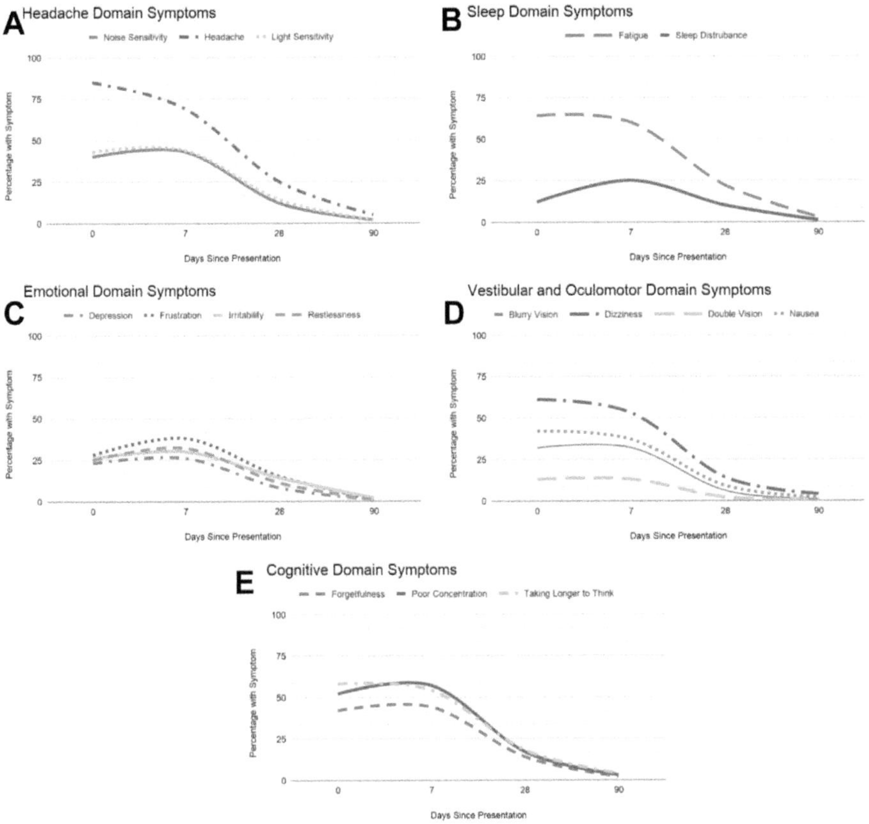

Fig. 3. (*A–E*) Resolution of various concussion symptoms by symptom domain. In general, symptoms improve dramatically between days 7 and 28. Only a small portion of patients remain symptomatic 90 days after presentation. (*Data from* Eisenberg, Meehan and Mannix. Pediatrics, 2014.[83])

recovery may be present at rest, but patients may experience exercise- or activity-induced relapse of symptoms.[77,78] This nuance likely underlies why most young athletes seem to demonstrate clinical recovery within 7 to 14 days but take closer to a month to return to competition.[79] Most recent studies have found that complete recovery is likely 3 to 4 weeks,[6,77,80] despite peak recovery within 1 to 2 weeks after the injury.[81] By week 4 (28 days) after an injury, approximately 80% of pediatric patients with an mTBI have recovered fully.[81,82] Specific symptoms may resolve at vary rates (**Fig. 3**).[83] Symptoms persist longer than a month in 10% to 20% of children and generally more than 1 symptom for more than 1 month is considered postconcussion syndrome (PCS).[84,85] In school-aged children, 13% are likely to be symptomatic at 3 months after injury and 2% at 1 year after injury.[86]

Risk factors for prolonged recovery

Given the potential for prolonged recovery to affect a child's quality of life, substantial scientific and investigative energies have been directed at accurately identifying those children for early intervention. Over the past 20 years, a substantial number of risk factors have been proposed, many with literature both supporting and refuting their existence.[84,87] Important preinjury factors that increase PCS risk include family[88] or personal[89–91] migraine or headache history, family or personal history of psychiatric illness.[88,92] and prior concussion history.[88,89,91] Although amnesia[93–95] and loss of consciousness[89,93,94] have been advocated as important injury-related risk factors for PCS, these injuries are likely inter-related with the broader finding that a greater initial symptom burden is strongly associated with an increased PCS risk.[93] More detailed accounting of risk factors can be found in 2 recent review articles on the subject (Iverson and colleagues[87] and Zuckerman and colleagues[84]). Further research in this area is still necessary to identify other risk factors and confirm prior finding studies on a larger scale.

SUMMARY

Mild TBI, or concussion, is a common diagnosis in the United States and around the world. Children carry the largest disease burden. Health care providers can diagnose mTBI in children with a history of head trauma who have an initial GCS of 13 to 15, and neuroimaging, if performed, is negative for acute findings. Symptoms typically resolve in days to weeks with 80% of children reporting symptom resolution by 4 weeks after injury. The core acute management includes 24 to 72 hours of physical and cognitive rest with graded return to learn and return to sport guidelines. The 10% to 20% of patients who report 1 or more symptoms extending beyond 1 month meet criteria for a diagnosis of PCS and should be referred to a multidisciplinary concussion clinic, if not already completed. Concussion clinics can create a tailored approach to the management of mTBI sequelae, with options for neuropsychiatric evaluation for academic or behavioral issues, neurology evaluation for seizures, headaches, or sleep problems, ophthalmologic evaluation for vision issues, and physical and occupational therapy. Pediatric outpatient providers are the foundation for the diagnosis and conservative symptomatic management of children with acute mTBI.

Clinics Care Points

- If any suspicion exists for a symptomatic mTBI or concussion, the child should be removed from the offending activity and monitored for symptoms.
- A prolonged period of physical and cognitive rest, that is, cocoon therapy, is not recommended and may prolong symptoms.

- Clinical recovery for most children and adolescents occurs by 4 weeks after mTBI.
- Early referrals to specialty, multidisciplinary concussion clinics should be considered for those with clear risk factors for prolonged recovery, including a history of 1 or more prior concussions and those with significant initial symptom burdens.
- For school-aged children, education accommodations are often necessary and students with medical letters are more likely to receive appropriate accommodations. Templates are available at https://www.cdc.gov/headsup/providers/discharge-materials.html
- Both physical and occupational or vestibular-ocular therapy may be helpful for those children with significant symptom burdens or no improvement in symptoms by 2 to 4 weeks.
- Referrals to neurology or other provider specializing in headache management may be considered 2 weeks after mTBI if the patient is experiencing persistent headaches or has an existing headache history.
- There is no significant evidence to support the use of any medication to improve outcomes in pediatric mTBI.

DISCLOSURE

Dr C.M. Bonfield serves as an unaffiliated neurotrauma consultant for the National Football League. The remaining authors have no financial or commercial conflicts of interest to disclose.

REFERENCES

1. Teasdale G, Jennett B. Assessment of coma and impaired consciousness. A practical scale. Lancet 1974;2(7872):81–4.
2. Dewan MC, Mummareddy N, Wellons JC 3rd, et al. Epidemiology of global pediatric traumatic brain injury: qualitative review. World Neurosurg 2016;91:497–509.e1.
3. McCrory P, Meeuwisse W, Dvorak J, et al. Consensus statement on concussion in sport—the 5th international conference on concussion in sport held in Berlin, October 2016. Br J Sports Med 2017;51(11):838–47.
4. Giza CC, Hovda DA. The new neurometabolic cascade of concussion. Neurosurgery 2014;75(Suppl 4):S24–33.
5. Zhang AL, Sing DC, Rugg CM, et al. The rise of concussions in the adolescent population. Orthop J Sports Med 2016;4(8). 2325967116662458.
6. Davis GA, Anderson V, Babl FE, et al. What is the difference in concussion management in children as compared with adults? A systematic review. Br J Sports Med 2017;51(12):949–57.
7. McCarthy MT, Kosofsky BE. Clinical features and biomarkers of concussion and mild traumatic brain injury in pediatric patients. Ann N Y Acad Sci 2015;1345:89–98.
8. Percent distributions of TBI-related emergency department visits by age group and injury mechanism — United States, 2006–2010 | Concussion | Traumatic Brain Injury | CDC Injury Center. 2019. Available at: https://www.cdc.gov/traumaticbraininjury/data/dist_ed.html. [Accessed 17 April 2020].
9. Sarmiento K, Thomas KE, Daugherty J, et al. Emergency department visits for sports- and recreation-related traumatic brain injuries among children - United States, 2010-2016. MMWR Morb Mortal Wkly Rep 2019;68(10):237–42.

10. Waltzman D, Womack LS, Thomas KE, et al. Trends in emergency department visits for contact sports-related traumatic brain injuries among children - United States, 2001-2018. MMWR Morb Mortal Wkly Rep 2020;69(27):870–4.
11. Kerr ZY, Chandran A, Nedimyer AK, et al. Concussion incidence and trends in 20 high school sports. Pediatrics 2019;144(5):e20192180.
12. Yue JK, Winkler EA, Burke JF, et al. Pediatric sports-related traumatic brain injury in United States trauma centers. Neurosurg Focus 2016;40(4):E3.
13. Pfister T, Pfister K, Hagel B, et al. The incidence of concussion in youth sports: a systematic review and meta-analysis. Br J Sports Med 2016;50(5):292–7.
14. Kerr ZY, Cortes N, Caswell AM, et al. Concussion rates in U.S. middle school athletes, 2015-2016 school year. Am J Prev Med 2017;53(6):914–8.
15. Echemendia RJ, Meeuwisse W, McCrory P, et al. The Sport Concussion Assessment Tool 5th edition (SCAT5): background and rationale. Br J Sports Med 2017; 51(11):848–50.
16. Davis GA, Purcell L, Schneider KJ, et al. The child Sport Concussion Assessment Tool 5th edition (Child SCAT5): background and rationale. Br J Sports Med 2017; 51(11):859–61.
17. Yengo-Kahn AM, Hale AT, Zalneraitis BH, et al. The Sport Concussion Assessment Tool: a systematic review. Neurosurg Focus 2016;40(4):E6.
18. Lovell MR, Iverson GL, Collins MW, et al. Measurement of symptoms following sports-related concussion: reliability and normative data for the post-concussion scale. Appl Neuropsychol 2006;13(3):166–74.
19. Lumba-Brown A, Teramoto M, Bloom OJ, et al. Concussion guidelines step 2: evidence for subtype classification. Neurosurgery 2020;86(1):2–13.
20. Lumba-Brown A, Ghajar J, Cornwell J, et al. Representation of concussion subtypes in common postconcussion symptom-rating scales. Concussion 2019; 4(3):CNC65.
21. Lumba-Brown A, Yeates KO, Sarmiento K, et al. Centers for Disease Control and Prevention guideline on the diagnosis and management of mild traumatic brain injury among children. JAMA Pediatr 2018;172(11):e182853.
22. Ahluwalia R, Mummareddy N, Bonfield CM, et al. Sport-related traumatic brain injury. 1st edition. Hoboken (NJ): Wiley and Sons; 2020.
23. Kuppermann N, Holmes JF, Dayan PS, et al. Identification of children at very low risk of clinically-important brain injuries after head trauma: a prospective cohort study. Lancet 2009;374(9696):1160–70.
24. Young JY, Duhaime A-C, Caruso PA, et al. Comparison of non-sedated brain MRI and CT for the detection of acute traumatic injury in children 6 years of age or less. Emerg Radiol 2016;23(4):325–31.
25. Currie S, Saleem N, Straiton JA, et al. Imaging assessment of traumatic brain injury. Postgrad Med J 2016;92(1083):41–50.
26. Pan J, Quon JL, Johnson E, et al. Rapid-sequence brain magnetic resonance imaging for Chiari I abnormality. J Neurosurg Pediatr 2018;22(2):158–64.
27. Lindberg DM, Stence NV, Grubenhoff JA, et al. Feasibility and accuracy of fast MRI versus CT for traumatic brain injury in young children. Pediatrics 2019; 144(4):e20190419.
28. Mulroy MH, Loyd AM, Frush DP, et al. Evaluation of pediatric skull fracture imaging techniques. Forensic Sci Int 2012;214(1–3):167–72.
29. Okonkwo DO, Tempel ZJ, Maroon J. Sideline assessment tools for the evaluation of concussion in athletes: a review. Neurosurgery 2014;75(Suppl 4):S82–95.

30. Mummareddy N, Brett BL, Yengo-Kahn AM, et al. Sway balance mobile application: reliability, acclimation, and baseline administration. Clin J Sport Med 2020; 30(5):451–7.
31. Legarreta AD, Mummareddy N, Yengo-Kahn AM, et al. On-field assessment of concussion: clinical utility of the King-Devick test. Open Access J Sports Med 2019;10:115–21.
32. Silverberg ND, Iaccarino MA, Panenka WJ, et al. Management of concussion and mild traumatic brain injury: a synthesis of practice guidelines. Arch Phys Med Rehabil 2020;101(2):382–93.
33. McLendon LA, Kralik SF, Grayson PA, et al. The controversial second impact syndrome: a review of the literature. Pediatr Neurol 2016;62:9–17.
34. Asken BM, Bauer RM, Guskiewicz KM, et al. Immediate removal from activity after sport-related concussion is associated with shorter clinical recovery and less severe symptoms in collegiate student-athletes. Am J Sports Med 2018;46(6): 1465–74.
35. Rose SC, Weber KD, Collen JB, et al. The diagnosis and management of concussion in children and adolescents. Pediatr Neurol 2015;53(2):108–18.
36. Thomas DG, Apps JN, Hoffmann RG, et al. Benefits of strict rest after acute concussion: a randomized controlled trial. Pediatrics 2015;135(2):213–23.
37. Purcell LK, Davis GA, Gioia GA. What factors must be considered in "return to school" following concussion and what strategies or accommodations should be followed? A systematic review. Br J Sports Med 2019;53(4):250.
38. DeMatteo C, Bednar ED, Randall S, et al. Effectiveness of return to activity and return to school protocols for children postconcussion: a systematic review. BMJ Open Sport Exerc Med 2020;6(1):e000667.
39. Ransom DM, Vaughan CG, Pratson L, et al. Academic effects of concussion in children and adolescents. Pediatrics 2015;135(6):1043–50.
40. Grubenhoff JA, Deakyne SJ, Comstock RD, et al. Outpatient follow-up and return to school after emergency department evaluation among children with persistent post-concussion symptoms. Brain Inj 2015;29(10):1186–91.
41. Leddy JJ, Haider MN, Ellis MJ, et al. Early subthreshold aerobic exercise for sport-related concussion: a randomized clinical trial. JAMA Pediatr 2019; 173(4):319–25.
42. Lawrence DW, Richards D, Comper P, et al. Earlier time to aerobic exercise is associated with faster recovery following acute sport concussion. PLoS One 2018;13(4):e0196062.
43. Grool AM, Aglipay M, Momoli F, et al. Association between early participation in physical activity following acute concussion and persistent postconcussive symptoms in children and adolescents. JAMA 2016;316(23):2504–14.
44. Kontos AP, Jorgensen-Wagers K, Trbovich AM, et al. Association of time since injury to the first clinic visit with recovery following concussion. JAMA Neurol 2020;77(4):435–40.
45. Eagle SR, Puligilla A, Fazio-Sumrok V, et al. Association of time to initial clinic visit with prolonged recovery in pediatric patients with concussion. J Neurosurg Pediatr 2020;1–6.
46. Desai N, Wiebe DJ, Corwin DJ, et al. Factors affecting recovery trajectories in pediatric female concussion. Clin J Sport Med 2019;29(5):361–7.
47. Haider MN, Johnson SL, Mannix R, et al. The buffalo concussion bike test for concussion assessment in adolescents. Sports Health 2019;11(6):492–7.

48. Cordingley D, Girardin R, Reimer K, et al. Graded aerobic treadmill testing in pediatric sports-related concussion: safety, clinical use, and patient outcomes. J Neurosurg Pediatr 2016;25(6):693–702.
49. Grabowski P, Wilson J, Walker A, et al. Multimodal impairment-based physical therapy for the treatment of patients with post-concussion syndrome: a retrospective analysis on safety and feasibility. Phys Ther Sport 2017;23:22–30.
50. Leddy J, Hinds A, Sirica D, et al. The role of controlled exercise in concussion management. PM R 2016;8(3 Suppl):S91–100.
51. Leddy J, Baker JG, Haider MN, et al. A physiological approach to prolonged recovery from sport-related concussion. J Athl Train 2017;52(3):299–308.
52. Leddy JJ, Willer B. Use of graded exercise testing in concussion and return-to-activity management. Curr Sports Med Rep 2013;12(6):370–6.
53. Ellis MJ, Cordingley D, Vis S, et al. Vestibulo-ocular dysfunction in pediatric sports-related concussion. J Neurosurg Pediatr 2015;16(3):248–55.
54. Park K, Ksiazek T, Olson B. Effectiveness of vestibular rehabilitation therapy for treatment of concussed adolescents with persistent symptoms of dizziness and imbalance. J Sport Rehabil 2018;27(5):485–90.
55. Murray DA, Meldrum D, Lennon O. Can vestibular rehabilitation exercises help patients with concussion? A systematic review of efficacy, prescription and progression patterns. Br J Sports Med 2017;51(5):442–51.
56. Schneider KJ, Meeuwisse WH, Nettel-Aguirre A, et al. Cervicovestibular rehabilitation in sport-related concussion: a randomised controlled trial. Br J Sports Med 2014;48(17):1294–8.
57. Alsalaheen BA, Mucha A, Morris LO, et al. Vestibular rehabilitation for dizziness and balance disorders after concussion. J Neurol Phys Ther 2010;34(2):87–93.
58. Ellis MJ, Leddy JJ, Willer B. Physiological, vestibulo-ocular and cervicogenic post-concussion disorders: an evidence-based classification system with directions for treatment. Brain Inj 2015;29(2):238–48.
59. Simpson-Jones ME, Hunt AW. Vision rehabilitation interventions following mild traumatic brain injury: a scoping review. Disabil Rehabil 2019;41(18):2206–22.
60. Kapoor N, Ciuffreda KJ, Han Y. Oculomotor rehabilitation in acquired brain injury: a case series. Arch Phys Med Rehabil 2004;85(10):1667–78.
61. Scheiman MM, Talasan H, Lynn Mitchell G, et al. Objective assessment of vergence after treatment of concussion-related CI. Optom Vis Sci 2017;94(1):74–88. https://doi.org/10.1097/opx.0000000000000936.
62. Seifert T. The relationship of migraine and other headache disorders to concussion. Handb Clin Neurol 2018;158:119–26.
63. Kuczynski A, Crawford S, Bodell L, et al. Characteristics of post-traumatic headaches in children following mild traumatic brain injury and their response to treatment: a prospective cohort. Dev Med Child Neurol 2013;55(7):636–41.
64. Seifert TD, Evans RW. Posttraumatic headache: a review. Curr Pain Headache Rep 2010;14(4):292–8.
65. Seifert TD. Sports concussion and associated post-traumatic headache. Headache 2013;53(5):726–36.
66. Morgan CD, Zuckerman SL, King LE, et al. Post-concussion syndrome (PCS) in a youth population: defining the diagnostic value and cost-utility of brain imaging. Childs Nerv Syst 2015;31(12):2305–9.
67. Max JE. Neuropsychiatry of pediatric traumatic brain injury. Psychiatr Clin North Am 2014;37(1):125–40.

68. Max JE, Koele SL, Castillo CC, et al. Personality change disorder in children and adolescents following traumatic brain injury. J Int Neuropsychol Soc 2000;6(3): 279–89.
69. Ellis MJ, Ritchie LJ, Koltek M, et al. Psychiatric outcomes after pediatric sports-related concussion. J Neurosurg Pediatr 2015;16(6):709–18.
70. Emery CA, Barlow KM, Brooks BL, et al. A systematic review of psychiatric, psychological, and behavioural outcomes following mild traumatic brain injury in children and adolescents. Can J Psychiatry 2016;61(5):259–69.
71. Ungprasert P, Matteson EL, Thongprayoon C. Nonaspirin nonsteroidal anti-inflammatory drugs and risk of hemorrhagic stroke. Stroke 2016;47(2):356–64.
72. Esquivel AO, Sherman SS, Bir CA, et al. The interaction of intramuscular ketorolac (toradol) and concussion in a rat model. Ann Biomed Eng 2017;45(6):1581–8.
73. Ashbaugh A, McGrew C. The role of nutritional supplements in sports concussion treatment. Curr Sports Med Rep 2016;15(1):16–9.
74. Barlow KM, Brooks BL, Esser MJ, et al. Efficacy of melatonin in children with post-concussive symptoms: a randomized clinical trial. Pediatrics 2020;145(4): e20192812.
75. Cushman DM, Borowski L, Hansen C, et al. Gabapentin and tricyclics in the treatment of post-concussive headache, a retrospective cohort study. Headache 2019;59(3):371–82.
76. Trojian TH, Wang DH, Leddy JJ. Nutritional supplements for the treatment and prevention of sports-related concussion-evidence still lacking. Curr Sports Med Rep 2017;16(4):247–55.
77. Haider MN, Leddy JJ, Pavlesen S, et al. A systematic review of criteria used to define recovery from sport-related concussion in youth athletes. Br J Sports Med 2018;52(18):1179–90.
78. Silverberg ND, Iverson GL, McCrea M, et al. Activity-related symptom exacerbations after pediatric concussion. JAMA Pediatr 2016;170(10):946–53.
79. Valovich McLeod TC, Kostishak N Jr, Anderson BE, et al. Patient, injury, assessment, and treatment characteristics and return-to-play timelines after sport-related concussion: an investigation from the athletic training practice-based research network. Clin J Sport Med 2019;29(4):298–305.
80. Henry LC, Elbin RJ, Collins MW, et al. Examining recovery trajectories after sport-related concussion with a multimodal clinical assessment approach. Neurosurgery 2016;78(2):232–41.
81. Ledoux A-A, Tang K, Yeates KO, et al. Natural progression of symptom change and recovery from concussion in a pediatric population. JAMA Pediatr 2019; 173(1):e183820.
82. Hung R, Carroll LJ, Cancelliere C, et al. Systematic review of the clinical course, natural history, and prognosis for pediatric mild traumatic brain injury: results of the International Collaboration on Mild Traumatic Brain Injury Prognosis. Arch Phys Med Rehabil 2014;95(3 Suppl):S174–91.
83. Eisenberg MA, Meehan WP 3rd, Mannix R. Duration and course of post-concussive symptoms. Pediatrics 2014;133(6):999–1006.
84. Zuckerman SL, Brett BL, Jeckell AS, et al. Prognostic factors in pediatric sport-related concussion. Curr Neurol Neurosci Rep 2018;18(12):104.
85. Rose SC, Fischer AN, Heyer GL. How long is too long? The lack of consensus regarding the post-concussion syndrome diagnosis. Brain Inj 2015;29(7–8): 798–803.
86. Barlow KM, Crawford S, Stevenson A, et al. Epidemiology of postconcussion syndrome in pediatric mild traumatic brain injury. Pediatrics 2010;126(2):e374–81.

87. Iverson GL, Gardner AJ, Terry DP, et al. Predictors of clinical recovery from concussion: a systematic review. Br J Sports Med 2017;51(12):941–8.
88. Morgan CD, Zuckerman SL, Lee YM, et al. Predictors of postconcussion syndrome after sports-related concussion in young athletes: a matched case-control study. J Neurosurg Pediatr 2015;15(6):589–98.
89. Zemek R, Barrowman N, Freedman SB, et al. Clinical risk score for persistent postconcussion symptoms among children with acute concussion in the ED. JAMA 2016;315(10):1014–25.
90. Terry DP, Huebschmann NA, Maxwell BA, et al. Preinjury migraine history as a risk factor for prolonged return to school and sports following concussion. J Neurotrauma 2018. https://doi.org/10.1089/neu.2017.5443.
91. Tator CH, Davis HS, Dufort PA, et al. Postconcussion syndrome: demographics and predictors in 221 patients. J Neurosurg 2016;125(5):1206–16.
92. Legarreta AD, Brett BL, Solomon GS, et al. The role of family and personal psychiatric history in postconcussion syndrome following sport-related concussion: a story of compounding risk. J Neurosurg Pediatr 2018;22(3):238–43.
93. Meehan WP 3rd, Mannix R, Monuteaux MC, et al. Early symptom burden predicts recovery after sport-related concussion. Neurology 2014;83(24):2204–10.
94. Heyer GL, Schaffer CE, Rose SC, et al. Specific factors influence postconcussion symptom duration among youth referred to a sports concussion clinic. J Pediatr 2016;174:33–8.e2.
95. Miller JH, Gill C, Kuhn EN, et al. Predictors of delayed recovery following pediatric sports-related concussion: a case-control study. J Neurosurg Pediatr 2016;17(4):491–6.

Cervical Spine Injury in Children and Adolescents

Andrew Jea, MD[a,*], Ahmed Belal, MD[b], Mohamed A. Zaazoue, MD[b], Jonathan Martin, MD, FAAP, FACS, FANS[c]

KEYWORDS

- Pediatric • Cervical spine injury • Return to play • Clinical decision-making tools

KEY POINTS

- Cervical spinal cord injuries are rare but catastrophic injuries in pediatric practice.
- Other cervical spine injuries, including myofascial/"whiplash" injuries, stingers, cervical cord neuropraxia, and fractures without spinal column instability are more commonly encountered by the practicing pediatrician.
- Physical examination and existing clinical decision-making tools can assist the primary care provider with determining the need for radiographs, consultation by a specialist, and return to play.

BACKGROUND AND EPIDEMIOLOGY

Injury is the leading cause of death and disability in children. Every year, 1 in 6 children in the United States requires emergency department care for the treatment of injuries.[1] Cervical spine injuries are among the most feared and serious consequences of pediatric trauma. The bimodal age distribution of cervical spine injuries in children reflects differences in spinal characteristics and pathophysiology. The first peak occurs between the ages of 3 and 5 years, and injury most commonly occurs at the craniocervical junction (between the occiput and C2). The second peak occurs between 14 and 16 years of age, and an injury in this older age group most commonly involves the middle to lower cervical spine, resembling an adult injury pattern.[2]

Spinal cord injuries are fortunately rare, with an incidence of 1.2 per 100,000 per year in children younger than 11 years, and 13.2 per 100,000 per year in children 11 or older.[3] The peak months for injury are June through August during the summer vacation, and late December to early January during winter vacation.[4]

[a] Department of Neurosurgery, University of Oklahoma College of Medicine, 1000 North Lincoln Boulevard, Suite 4000, Oklahoma City, OK 73104, USA; [b] Department of Neurological Surgery, Indiana University School of Medicine, 355 West 16th Street, Suite 5100, Indianapolis, IN 46202, USA; [c] Division of Neurosurgery, Connecticut Children's Medical Center, 282 Washington Street, Hartford, CT 06106, USA
* Corresponding author.
E-mail address: Andrew-Jea@ouhsc.edu

Pediatr Clin N Am 68 (2021) 875–894
https://doi.org/10.1016/j.pcl.2021.04.012
0031-3955/21/

The most common cause of cervical spine trauma is motor vehicle accidents, accounting for 48% to 61%[2,5] of injuries in all age groups. Falls are more common in children younger than 8, accounting for 18% to 30% of cervical spine injuries in this population. Sports-related injuries are more frequent in older children and adolescents where they account for 20% to 38%[6] of injuries. It has been reported that approximately 5 to 15 children will suffer sports-related spine injuries for every 100,000 participants.[7] Most of these children will be evaluated and treated by hospital-based providers, including subspecialty spine specialists.

In contrast, a substantial number of pediatric patients present with relatively low-acuity complaints of neck pain. In the United States, there are more than 30 million children participating in organized athletics.[1] A recent review of the prevalence of neck pain among athletes cited a 1-year prevalence of 38% to 73%.[8] This juxtaposition of a high volume of patient complaints and low incidence of serious injury results in a quandary for the primary care provider. Familiarity with the evaluation and management of these patients is of great utility to the primary care provider.

BIOMECHANICS AND ANATOMIC CONSIDERATIONS

The cervical spinal column consists of 7 vertebrae (C1-7) with intervertebral disks starting below C2, and ligaments extending from the occiput to C7 and beyond. The cervical spine serves as a conduit for the spinal cord and cervical nerve roots as well as the vertebral arteries (**Fig. 1**). Normal physiologic range of motion for flexion, extension, rotation, and lateral bending[9] is illustrated in **Fig. 2**.

The cervical spine of a child differs structurally and qualitatively from that of the adult (**Table 1**). These anatomic differences impact both the patterns and types of injuries seen in pediatric patients.[10]

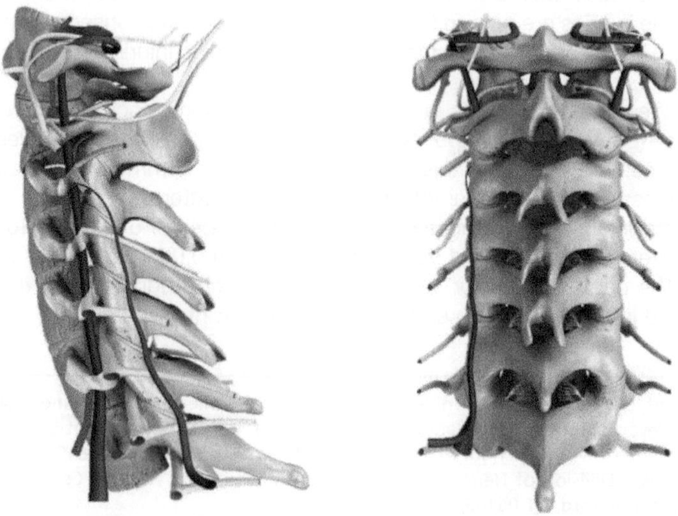

Fig. 1. The cervical spine is composed of 7 bony vertebrae extending from the skull base to thoracic spine/chest. It serves as a conduit for the spinal cord, cervical nerve roots, and vertebral arteries. In addition to the vertebral bodies and lateral pillars created by facet joints, stability is provided by intervertebral disks, capsular ligaments, longitudinal ligaments, and muscles that support the spine.

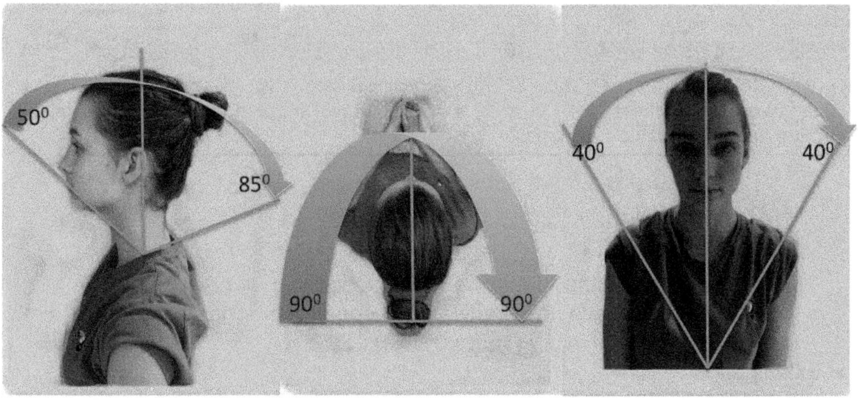

Fig. 2. Range of motion of the cervical spine includes 50° of cervical flexion, 85° of extension, 90° of lateral rotation, and 40° of lateral flexion.

CLINICAL EVALUATION

Clinical evaluation of the child presenting with complaints related to neck trauma begins with a directed history and physical examination. Evaluation of the preverbal child presents challenges that are beyond the scope of this text. We focus on the evaluation of the awake and cooperative child likely to be encountered in a primary care setting.

- History:
  - Understanding the mechanism of injury is essential for the purpose of both evaluation and triage. For an injury that was witnessed or that can be recalled by the patient,
    - Were forces applied compressive on the top of the head, flexing the neck forward, extending the neck backward, or flexing the neck to the side?
    - Was the injury a result of a high-risk mechanism[11,12] (**Table 2**)?
    - Does the patient manifest any low-risk criteria for significant spinal injury[12] (**Box 1**)?
  - A clear picture of quality, location, and nature of pain symptoms assists the examiner with assembly of an appropriate differential diagnosis.
    - Was the pain immediate or delayed in onset?
    - Is the pain constant, or intermittent?
    - Does the pain radiate? If so where? To the shoulder? To the arm?
    - Where is the pain worst? Neck, arm, shoulder?
    - What is the nature of the pain? Sharp? Dull/aching? Burning?
    - Is the pain impacted by position or movement?
  - Does the patient report any neurologic complaints, including

Table 1
The pediatric cervical spine

Disproportionately large head for body size	Large proportion of bone is cartilaginous
Underdeveloped neck musculature	Anterior wedging of vertebra
Relative ligamentous laxity	Unfused ossification centers
Horizontal facet orientation	Underdeveloped uncinate processes

Table 2
High-risk injury mechanisms

• Fall greater than 3 feet or 5 stairs	• Bicycle collision
• Diving/axial load to head	• Accident involving motorized all-terrain vehicle
• High-speed motor vehicle accident	

    - Sensory loss/numbness?
    - Weakness?
    - Headache, vomiting, dizziness, vertigo, diplopia, or confusion?
  - Does the patient have any predisposing conditions[13] that would place him or her at risk for spinal injury (**Table 3**)?
- Examination
  - Inspection: The normal contour of the cervical spine is lordotic, a gentle curvature with a ventral apex (**Fig. 3**A). Injury to the spinal column or its supporting structures can lead to protective muscle spasm with straightening/reversal of lordosis (**Fig. 3**B), or torticollis (**Fig. 4**).
  - Palpation
    - Palpation of the spinous processes and posterior cervical musculature should be conducted.
      - Midline tenderness has been identified as an independent risk factor for spinal column injury.[11,12,14]
      - Tenderness of the paraspinal musculature, either generalized or in specific trigger point locations should be noted.
    - Palpation of landmarks on the anterior and posterior shoulder to include the sternoclavicular joint, clavicle, acromion and acromion-clavicular joint, coracoid process, as well as the supporting musculature, is performed to exclude primary shoulder pathology.
  - Range of motion
    - Active range of motion of the cervical spine is assessed for maximal flexion, extension, and lateral rotation. Passive range of motion by the examiner should be avoided if painful for the patient.
    - Shoulder range of motion should be assessed and exacerbation of pain with movement noted.
  - Provocative tests
    - The application of axial compression with or without extension and lateral flexion of the neck (Spurling test)[15] is useful in identifying nerve root compression at the neural foramen provided instability is not suspected (**Fig. 5**).

Box 1
Low-risk criteria for significant spinal injury

- Simple rear-end motor vehicle accident
- Sitting position of patient in the office
- Patient ambulatory in the office
- Delayed onset of neck pain
- Absence of midline cervical spine tenderness

Table 3
Conditions predisposing patients to potential spinal injury with minor trauma

Category	Examples
• Connective tissue disorders:	Examples: Down syndrome or Ehlers-Danlos
• Genetic or metabolic bone disease:	Examples: Osteogenesis imperfecta or hypophosphatemic rickets
• Congenital spinal stenosis:	Example: Achondroplasia
• Reduced mobility:	Example: Klippel-Feil
• Other conditions:	Examples: infectious, inflammatory, or neoplastic disease

- Neurologic assessment
  - Cranial nerve evaluation: Evaluation of cranial nerve function is prudent in the patient presenting with neck pain and associated complaints concerning for craniocervical arterial dissection, including headache, nausea/vomiting, dizziness/vertigo, diplopia, and confusion.[16] Involvement of the extracranial carotid artery can produce Horner syndrome on the affected side (unilateral miosis, ptosis, and facial anhidrosis) (**Fig. 6**).
  - Focused motor, sensory, and reflex examinations targeting myotomes and dermatomes of the upper extremity provide a targeted assessment of function of the spinal cord and cervical roots contributing to the brachial plexus (C5-T1). A simplified screening examination is suggested in **Fig. 7**.
  - Additional testing, including assessment of gait,[17] lower extremity reflexes, or pathologic reflexes, can be helpful in further characterizing upper motor neuron (spinal cord level) versus lower motor neuron (nerve root or peripheral nerve) level problems. Synthesis of the neurologic examination allows for categorization of deficits at the level of the peripheral nerves, cervical nerve root, or spinal cord (**Fig. 8**, **Table 4**).

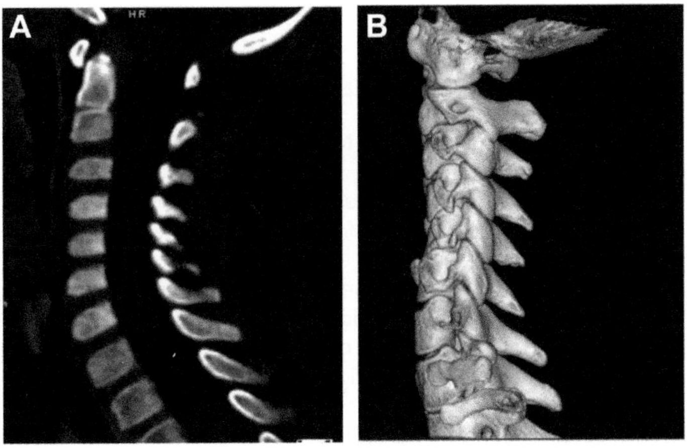

Fig. 3. (*A*) Computed tomography reconstructed images demonstrating normal cervical lordosis. (*B*) Injury of the neck can result in muscular spasm with resultant straightening of the cervical spine.

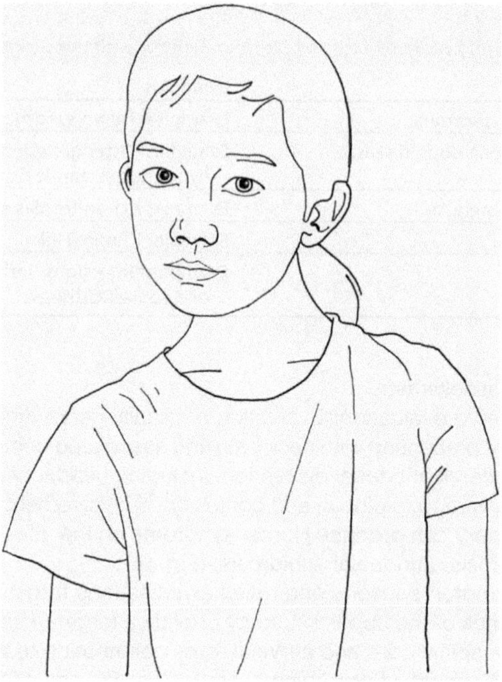

Fig. 4. Classic "cock robin" posture of spasmodic torticollis with axial rotation to the right and lateral flexion to the left. Patients manifesting this head position may harbor injury or instability at the atlanto-axial level.

CLINICAL CONDITIONS

Following completion of the history and physical examination, the primary care provider (PCP) assembles a differential diagnosis for the patient before consideration of diagnostic testing and treatment options. Familiarity with historical features, examination, and management of key diagnoses can facilitate next steps for the PCP.

Myofascial Strain/"Whiplash" Injury

- Description:
  - Paramedian pain, typically limited to the neck with local radiation to the head and/or shoulder
    - Common in setting of injury. An estimated 1-year prevalence of neck pain in children and adolescents is 20% to 40%.[18]
- Historical features
  - Clinical decision-making tools have identified several historical/observational criteria for patients at low risk for significant spinal injury (see **Box 1**). Reassuring features include delayed onset of pain and/or patients who are ambulatory and appear comfortable when upright.
- Examination features
  - Active range of motion can typically be accomplished with mild discomfort
  - Trigger points are common
  - Notably, point tenderness over bone *should be absent*
  - Radicular pain, sensory/motor signs *should be absent*

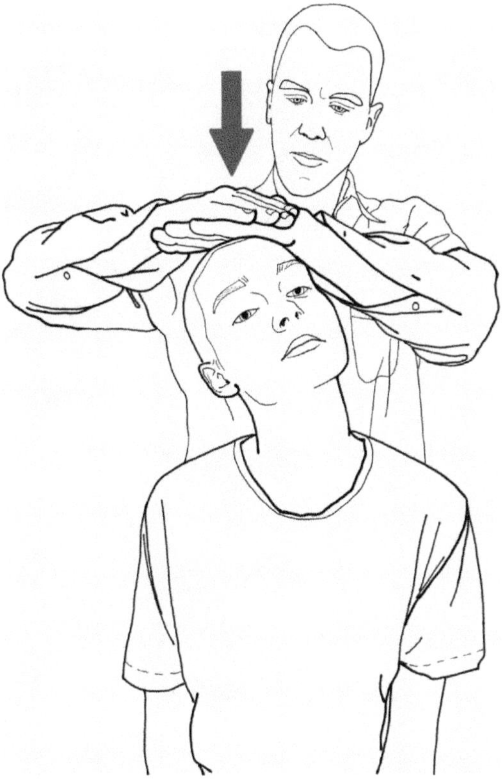

Fig. 5. Spurling test, with neck extension, compression, and lateral flexion toward the symptomatic side. Reproduction of radicular pain with this maneuver strongly suggests compression of a cervical nerve root at its exiting foramen.

- Management
  - Managed with exercise, massage, heat, nonsteroidal anti-inflammatory drugs, acupuncture, and trigger point injection

Cervical Radiculopathy

- Description:
  - Signs and symptoms result from irritation of an exiting nerve root within the neural foramen
    - Degenerative cervical radiculopathy is uncommon in children[19]
    - Radiculopathy is more common in older athletes participating in impact sports[20]

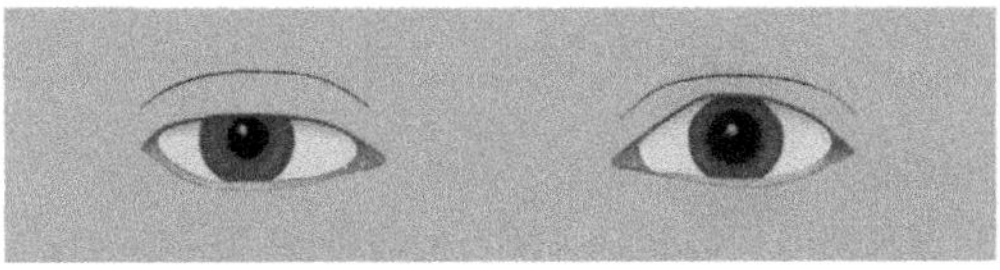

Fig. 6. Eye findings in Horner syndrome, with miosis (smaller pupil) and subtle ptosis on the affected right eye. Interruption of the sympathetic plexus in the setting of carotid artery dissection can produce this finding.

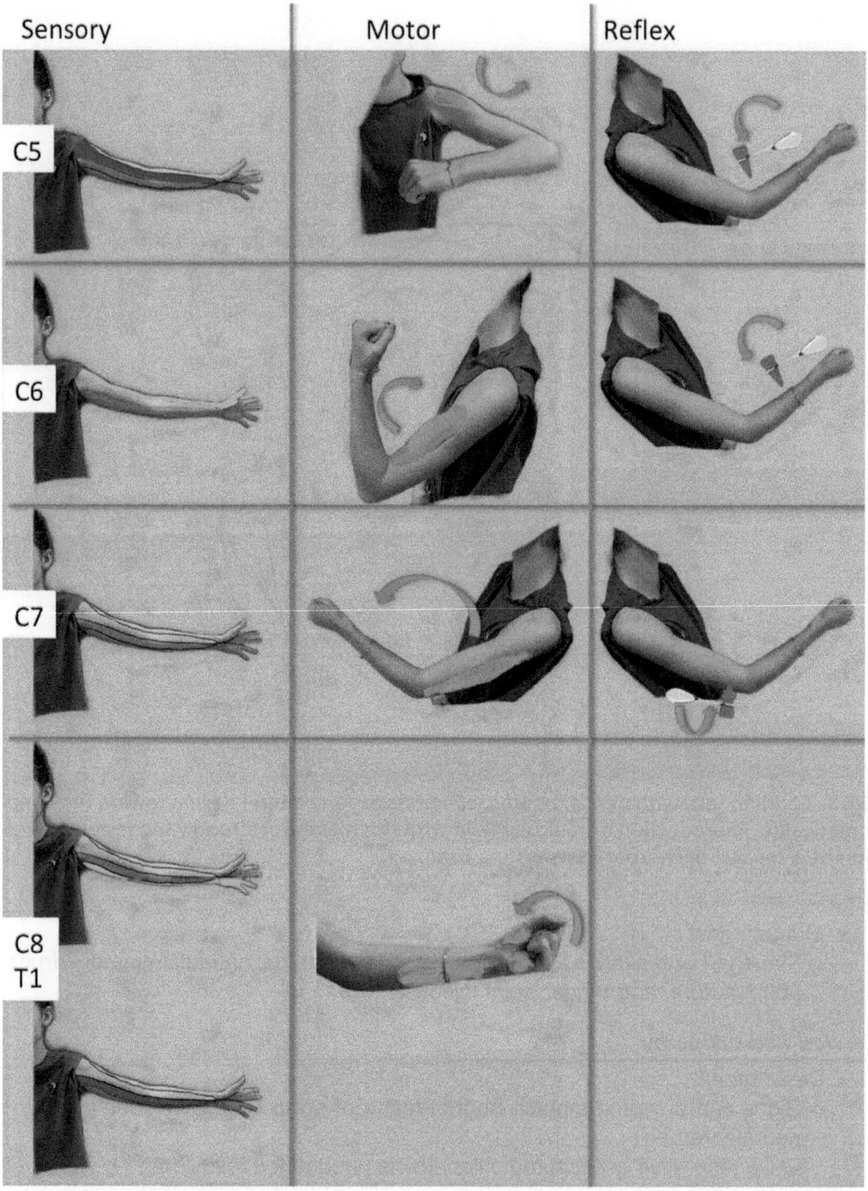

Fig. 7. Screening neurologic examination for the patient with suspected cervical spine injury. Basic knowledge of cervical dermatomes, myotomes, and reflex arcs allows for an anatomic assessment of the patient's neurologic status.

- Historical features
  - Pain traveling down the neck into the arm of the patient (**Fig. 9**)
  - Qualitatively varies from sharp to dull, aching pain
  - Pain exacerbated by neck extension
- Examination features

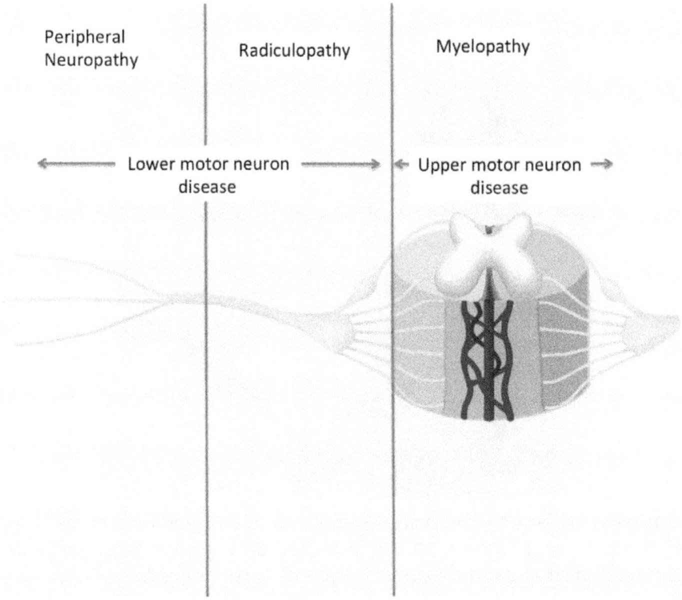

Fig. 8. Synthesis of information gathered from neurologic assessment. Data gathered through the history and physical examination enable determination of upper motor neuron (typically myelopathy) versus lower motor neuron (radiculopathy or peripheral neuropathy) pathology, and can assist with determining both the need for imaging and initial management of these patients.

- ○ Unilateral dermatomal sensory loss
- ○ Unilateral myotomal weakness
- ○ Absent reflex concordant to myotome/dermatome
- ○ Exacerbation of symptoms with Spurling's test (see **Fig. 5**)

Table 4
History and examination features allowing for discrimination of myelopathy, radiculopathy, and peripheral neuropathy

Finding	Peripheral Neuropathy	Radiculopathy	Myelopathy
Pain • Quality • Location	"Electric" Radiates either proximally or distally from injury site	Sharp, aching Radiates distally from the neck	Typically painless
Weakness	Variable, usually present	Variable, usually present	Variable, may be present
Sensory loss	Sharply demarcated borders	Indistinct borders	Indistinct borders, typically extends beyond single extremity
Tone/reflexes	Decreased	Decreased	Increased

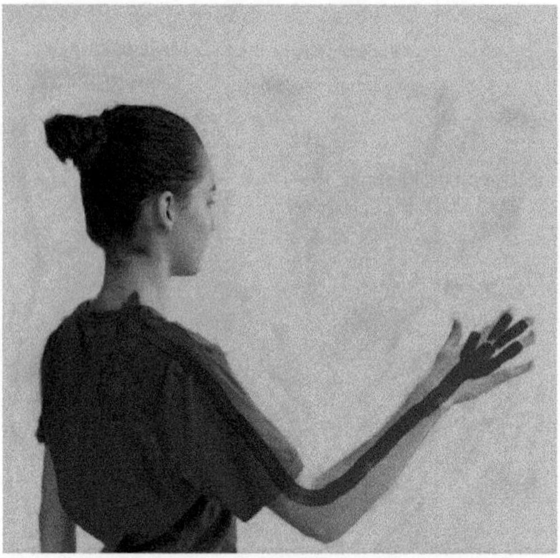

Fig. 9. Illustration representing the pain experienced in a C7 radiculopathy. Note that pain originates in the neck and extends to the impacted dermatome. Scapular pain, although outside of the dermatomal distribution, is frequently experienced.

- Management
  - Escalating regimen beginning with rest and progressing through nonsteroidal anti-inflammatory medications, physical therapy, oral steroid pulse, epidural steroid injection, and decompressive surgery for refractory patients.[21]

Stinger

- Description:
  - Set of transient symptoms that involve pain, burning/warm, or tingling down an arm, occasionally accompanied by localized weakness
  - Common in impact sports such as football, rugby, hockey, wrestling, and lacrosse, with 30% to 50% of athletes experiencing a stinger over the course of their career.[22]
- Historical features
  - Mechanism of injury: Lateral blow to head resulting in traction on the brachial plexus or nerve root impingement at the foramen (**Fig. 10**).
  - Athlete typically exits field of play shaking the affected arm, often with the arm hanging limply to the side.[23]
  - Time course variable; usually present for seconds to minutes, but can on occasion last from days up to 2 weeks.[7]
  - Does not involve contralateral arm or either leg.
- Examination features
  - Usually purely sensory in C5-6 dermatomes
  - Weakness rare; when present involves shoulder abductors, shoulder external rotators, and elbow flexors
- Management
  - Typically no treatment required
  - Athlete cannot return to play until symptoms completely resolved (see Special considerations, 'return to play criteria' later in this article).

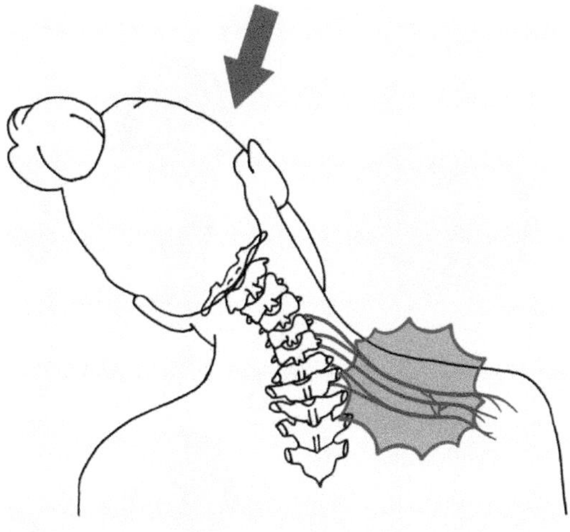

Fig. 10. "Stingers" are a result of a stretch injury of the brachial plexus. Contralateral neck flexion with ipsilateral shoulder depression is the most common mechanism for this injury.

 - Additional protective gear to limit lateral neck flexion/extension can be considered in patients to reduce the risk of repeat episodes

Cervical Cord Neuropraxia

- Description:
  - Set of transient signs/symptoms, including pain, sensory loss, and weakness attributable to the spinal cord
  - Some investigators have noted differences between pediatric and adult cervical cord neuropraxia (CCN) due to the relative absence of spinal canal stenosis in pediatric CCN.[24] CCN in pediatric patients is theorized to occur due to increased laxity in these patients, with transient deficits being the mildest form of an entity known as "spinal cord injury without radiographic abnormality" or SCIWORA.[25]
- Historical features
  - Mechanism typically involves axial loading with or without a flexion or extension moment. Can occur with "spear tackling."
  - Signs/symptoms present in more than 1 extremity simultaneously. Combination may include both arms, arms and legs, or all extremities (**Fig. 11**).
  - Symptoms typically resolve in minutes. Can persist for up to 48 hours and still be considered CCN
- Examination features
  - Variable loss of sensory and motor function
- Management
  - Initial management occurring at site of injury in accordance with field management of suspected spinal cord injury[26]
  - Patients require hospital-based evaluation following injury and involvement of a spine specialist.
  - Return to play discussion for these patients is controversial (see Special considerations, "return to play criteria" later in this article).

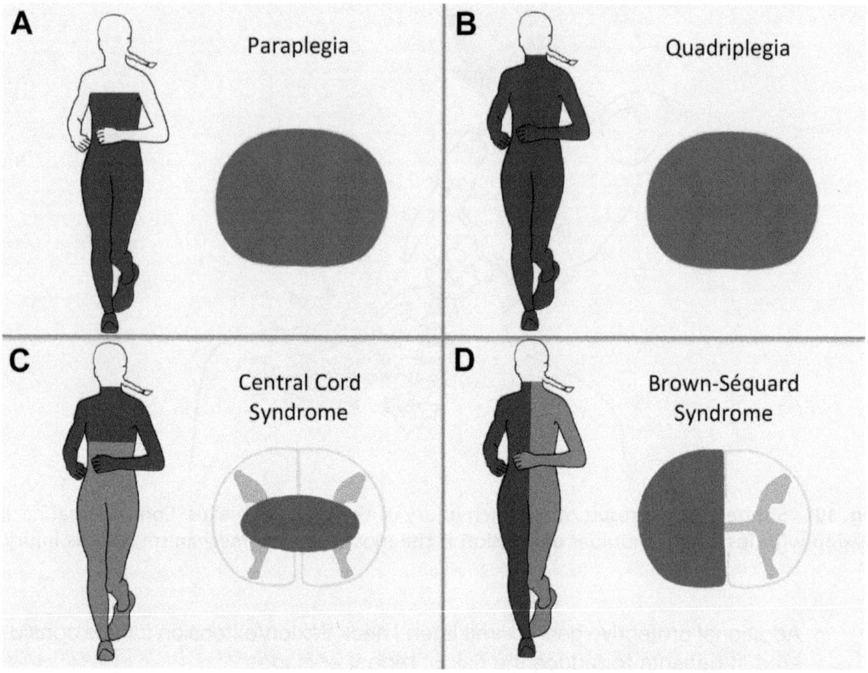

Fig. 11. Patterns of spinal cord injury. Note the contrast between these syndromes and peripheral nerve/radicular injuries based on the distribution of motor and/or sensory loss beyond the affected extremity. (*A*) *Paraplegia* and (*B*) *quadriplegia*: complete loss of motor and sensory function below the level of injury resulting in loss of function of the leg only, or arms and legs, respectively. (*C*) *Central cord syndrome*: injury of the central spinal cord resulting in functional greater impact of arm motor function than legs. Sensory deficits in this injury are variable. (*D*) *Brown-Séquard syndrome*: injury to one-half of the spinal cord resulting in ipsilateral motor weakness with contralateral sensory loss below the level of the lesion.

Cervical Spine Fractures

A detailed review of evaluation and management of the patient with cervical spine fracture is beyond the scope of this review. As patients may present in a delayed fashion with stable fracture patterns, a basic understanding of the evaluation and management may be of utility to the PCP.

- Description:
  - Minor fractures impacting neither function nor stability of the spinal column may present in a delayed fashion to the PCP. These include mild compression fractures, spinous process fractures, and laminar fractures.
    - Fractures resulting in compression of neurologic elements or spinal instability typically result in hospital-based evaluation of the patient
    - These patients may have undergone prior evaluation with plain radiographs. This radiographic technique can miss minor fractures, though rarely fractures of clinical significance[27]
- Historical features
  - Mechanism of injury may include hyperflexion, hyperextension, direct blow to the posterior neck, and rotational/torsional injures. High-risk mechanisms (see **Table 2**) increase the probability of resultant fracture.

- Location of the fracture within the spinal column impacts historical features of patient presentation
  - Fractures of weight-bearing members of the spine (vertebral body, facet complex) are worsened by upright posture and relieved by supine positioning.
- Examination features:
  - Fixed cervical rigidity or torticollis
  - Midline tenderness to palpation (spinous process/laminar fractures)
  - Inability to perform active range of motion
- Management
  - Clinical decision-making tools (see "Diagnostic evaluation" later in this article) can assist with imaging decisions.
  - Although many "stable" cervical fractures can be managed with a soft or rigid collar and oral medications, consultation with a neurosurgical or orthopedic consultant is recommended.

Spinal Cord Injury

A detailed review of evaluation and management of the patient with spinal cord injury is beyond the scope of this review. However, a basic understanding of management principles may be of utility to the PCP to facilitate aftercare and communication with the family.

- Description:
  - Set of signs/symptoms, including pain, sensory loss, and weakness attributable to the spinal cord and persisting more than 48 hours postinjury.
- Historical features
  - Mechanism variable, and similar to CCN can include axial loading injuries with or without a flexion or extension moment.
  - Signs/symptoms present in more than 1 extremity simultaneously. Combination may include both arms, arms and legs, or all extremities (see **Fig. 11**).
- Examination features
  - Variable, depending on the severity of injury. The American Spinal Injury Association (ASIA) impairment scale[28] describes functional deficits present ranging from normal motor and sensory function to complete injuries with no motor or sensory function below the level of injury (**Box 2**).
- Management:
  - Field stabilization and transport, optimally to a verified pediatric trauma center
  - Hospital-based evaluation in accordance with Advanced Trauma Life Support guidelines[29]

Box 2
American Spinal Injury Association impairment scale

- A: Complete injury
- B: Incomplete injury, sensory preserved below injury level
- C: Incomplete injury, motor preserved at less than antigravity below injury
- D: Incomplete injury, motor preserved at greater than antigravity below injury
- E: Normal examination

- Medical support in an intensive care setting may include spinal immobilization, blood pressure augmentation and deep venous thrombosis prophylaxis, as well as diligent skin and bladder care.
- Surgical intervention, when required, is performed with the following goals in mind:
  - Decompression of neurologic elements
  - Restoration of normal anatomic alignment
  - Provide stable internal fixation to allow for early weight bearing

DIAGNOSTIC EVALUATION

The intersection of the high volume of pediatric trauma patients and low frequency of pediatric cervical spine injuries creates a dilemma for pediatric providers. Clinical assessment of the pediatric trauma patient presents unique challenges, particularly in the preverbal patient. When imaging is required, selection of an appropriate diagnostic imaging technique must balance diagnostic accuracy, risk of radiation exposure, potential need for sedation, and cost. In some circumstances, multiple modalities may be required to appropriately evaluate a patient (**Box 3**).

For a more detailed discussion of diagnostic imaging, the reader can refer to the Jonathan R Wood and colleagues' article "Neuroimaging for the Primary Care Provider: A Review of Modalities, Indications, and Pitfalls," elsewhere in this issue.

Clinical decision-making (CDM) tools have been widely accepted to reduce use of radiographs in alert and stable adult trauma patients. CDM tools are derived from original research and incorporate 3 or more variables from history, physical examination, or simple tests to guide patient management.

Three CDM tools have heavily influenced cervical spine evaluation of the awake and alert pediatric trauma patient over the past 2 decades (**Fig. 12**[30]).

- The National Emergency X-Radiography Utilization Study (NEXUS) prospectively assessed the negative predictive value of 5 low-risk criteria for the detection of clinically significant cervical spine injuries. The study achieved 99.6% sensitivity but only 12.9% specificity for cervical spine injury. The study included more than 3000 patients younger than 18 years, but fewer than 1000 patients younger than 8 years and fewer than 100 children younger than 2.[14]
- The Canadian C-Spine Rule (CCSR) was a prospective study of adults that incorporated 9 independent variables in 3 categories, demonstrating a negative

Box 3
Considerations in selecting an imaging modality for the evaluation of spinal injury

- *Plain radiographs:* Plain radiographs are rapidly obtainable and low in cost. They lack the sensitivity of computed tomography (CT) for the detection of fractures. They do expose the patient to ionizing radiation. They can be obtained either as *static films* to evaluate anatomy or as *dynamic films* to assess stability
- *CT:* CT has the highest sensitivity for fracture detection, but has disadvantages of both higher cost and radiation exposure when compared with plain radiographs
- *MRI:* MRI is the standard of care for the patient with neurologic deficit, as it is the only modality capable of demonstrating the spinal cord and nerve roots. High cost and lack of specificity for instability (when ligamentous injury is detected) are disadvantages of this modality

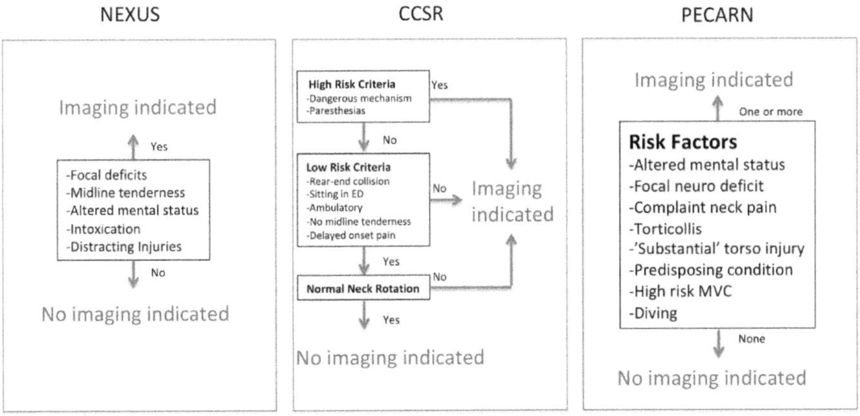

Fig. 12. Visual summary of CDM rules for cervical spine imaging in trauma patients. Reprinted with permission, AAP News June 2018.

predictive value of 100% and specificity of 42.5% for significant cervical spine injury.[12]

- The Pediatric Emergency Care Applied Research Network (PECARN) used case-control study design to develop an 8-risk factor model with 98% sensitivity and 26% specificity for the *absence* of cervical spine injury.[11]

Prospective studies of CDM for cervical spine clearance in children are unlikely to be undertaken given the challenges with designing a study of adequate power. However, existing CDMs make a compelling case for clearance of the awake and cooperative verbal child given the combination of normal neurologic examination, historical exclusion of high-risk mechanisms, absence of midline tenderness, and active range of motion as assessed by active neck rotation by the patient.

In the event that a PCP has concerns for spinal stability, options to include provision of a cervical collar or a request for emergency medical services transport to an acute care facility can be considered.

SPECIAL CONSIDERATIONS

Anticipatory Guidance

Counseling regarding injury prevention is a key role for the PCP. Familiarity with epidemiology and mechanisms of cervical spine injuries in children can inform the approach used by the provider.

- Car seats[31]
  - All infants and toddlers should ride in a rear-facing car seat as long as possible, until they reach the highest weight or height allowed by their car safety seat manufacturer.
  - All children who have outgrown their rear-racing car seat should use a front-facing car seat with harness as long as possible, until they reach the highest weight or height allowed by their car safety seat manufacturer.
- Falls[32]
  - General guidance regarding safety surrounding windows, stairs, and outdoor play equipment, such as trampolines, is suggested for toddlers and young children.

- Sports-related injuries
  - Emphasis of the importance of proper technique and adhering to coaching guidance to avoid injuries (eg, avoiding head-down tackling[33] in football).
- Teenage drivers
  - Sources such as the Centers for Disease Control and Prevention[34] have several suggestions to include 30 to 50 hours of parent-supervised driving, night-time driving restrictions, and creation of a parent-teen driving agreement to establish clear expectations and limits.

Return to Play Criteria

For most patients with symptoms referable to the neck, guidance regarding return to play is quite straightforward. Most authors[3] endorse return to play when the athlete meets defined criteria (**Box 4**).

For patients with specific sports-related injury syndromes, return to play will typically be guided by sports medicine or spine subspecialty consultants.

- Stingers[22]
  - For patients with self-resolving initial episodes, patients can return to play in the same game/match using the preceding criteria.
  - For patients experiencing 2 (or more) episodes, imaging is indicated, and return to play is made on a case-by-case basis.
- Cervical cord neuropraxia[35]
  - There remain no established guidelines for return to play for athletes following an episode of CCN.
  - Imaging with MRI and consultation with a spine provider is mandatory for these patients.
  - In the pediatric athlete with normal MRI and absent cervical canal stenosis, the risk of returning to play appears to be low.[24]

Athletic Participation and the Child with Down Syndrome

There are numerous psychological and physical benefits of competitive sports to the development and wellbeing of children, especially those with Down syndrome (DS).[36] Laxity of the upper cervical (also known as atlanto-axial instability or AAI) is known to be present in 10% to 40% of these children, although symptomatic instability is uncommon, occurring in fewer than 1% of patients.[37] Concern for potential neurologic injury with sports participation due to asymptomatic hypermobility in the patient with DS is understandable.

Recommendations for radiographic screening of patients with DS before sports participation have evolved over time. Beginning in 1983, all athletes with DS were required to undergo a screening lateral cervical radiograph before participation in the Special Olympics. If findings suggestive of instability were found, these individuals

Box 4
Suggested criteria for return to play

- Free of neck and arm pain
- Full strength and sensation in affected extremity
- Full range of neck motion without discomfort or spasm
- Neck strength in flexion, extension, and lateral bending has returned to preinjury

Box 5
Signs/symptoms concerning myelopathy in the patient with Down syndrome

- Neck pain/torticollis
- Progressive lower cranial nerve dysfunction to include worsened swallowing/phonation
- Motor regression to include worsened gait or clumsy hands
- Hyperreflexia

were banned from certain sports that put increased stress on the neck.[38] In 1984, the American Academy of Pediatrics (AAP) published a statement supporting the screening radiograph introduced by the Special Olympics.[39] However, in 2011, the AAP proposed new guidelines that recommended radiographic evaluation only in the presence of clinical evidence of AAI.[40] In 2015, the Special Olympics replaced the radiographic screening requirement with a neurologic evaluation focused on the presence of AAI symptoms and myelopathy.[41] This change was based on the lack of evidence that radiographic findings of AAI in asymptomatic children were predictive of future sports-related spinal cord injury.[42]

Current recommendations[40] regarding health care screening before sports participation for the child with DS include the following:

- Routine screening radiographs of the cervical spine are not recommended for asymptomatic children.
- For the patient with DS with symptoms related to the cervical spine and/or possible myelopathy (**Box 5**), prompt referral for evaluation by a spine specialist is recommended.

SUMMARY

Cervical spine complaints are common in pediatric practice. Familiarity and comfort with history taking, examination, and CDM tools can facilitate diagnosis and minimize the need for unnecessary radiographic evaluation. Neurosurgical consultation is prudent when concerns for neurologic impairment or spinal instability are present. Basic familiarity with anticipatory guidance to avoid spinal injuries in children as well as recommendations for return to play for the injured athlete and sports participation for children with DS allows the pediatrician to appropriately address most family questions on these topics.

Clinics care points

- Cervical spine complaints are common in pediatric practice.
- History and examination alone can safely be used to evaluate and direct treatment in most patients presenting to the PCP.
- Familiarity with cervical spine CDM tools, including NEXUS, CCSR, and PECARN can reduce the need for radiographic evaluation.
- Prompt consultation is prudent in the setting of suspected neurologic deficit or spinal instability.
- Return to play criteria for student athletes and atlanto-axial instability in DS are common sources of family questions that can be addressed by the PCP.

ACKNOWLEDGMENTS

The authors thank Ms Elsa Martin for her assistance in producing the figures.

DISCLOSURE

The authors have no disclosures.

REFERENCES

1. McCarthy MT, Kosofsky BE. Clinical features and biomarkers of concussion and mild traumatic brain injury in pediatric patients. Ann N Y Acad Sci 2015;1345: 89–98.
2. Brown RL, Brunn MA, Garcia VF. Cervical spine injuries in children: a review of 103 patients treated consecutively at a level 1 pediatric trauma center. J Pediatr Surg 2001;36(8):1107–14.
3. Weber AD, Nance ML. Clearing the pediatric cervical spine. Curr Trauma Rep 2016;2:210–5.
4. Hill SA, Miller CA, Kosnik EJ, et al. Pediatric neck injuries. A clinical study. J Neurosurg 1984;60(4):700–6.
5. Eleraky MA, Theodore N, Adams M, et al. Pediatric cervical spine injuries: report of 102 cases and review of the literature. J Neurosurg 2000;92(1 Suppl):12–7.
6. Patel JC, Tepas JJ, Mollitt DL, et al. Pediatric cervical spine injuries: defining the disease. J Pediatr Surg 2001;36(2):373–6.
7. Proctor MR, Cantu RC. Head and neck injuries in young athletes. Clin Sports Med 2000;19(4):693–715.
8. Noormohammadpour P, Farahbakhsh F, Rostami M, et al. Prevalence of neck pain among athletes: a systematic review. Asian Spine J 2018;12(6):1146–53.
9. Neumann DA. Axial skeleton: osteology and arthrology. In: Neumann DA, Kelly ER, Kiefer CL, et al, editors. Kinesiology of the musculoskeletal system : foundations for rehabilitation. Third edition. Elsevier, Inc.; 2017. p. 319–91, chap 9.
10. Kokoska ER, Keller MS, Rallo MC, et al. Characteristics of pediatric cervical spine injuries. J Pediatr Surg 2001;36(1):100–5.
11. Leonard JC, Kuppermann N, Olsen C, et al. Factors associated with cervical spine injury in children after blunt trauma. Ann Emerg Med 2011;58(2):145–55.
12. Stiell IG, Wells GA, Vandemheen KL, et al. The Canadian C-spine rule for radiography in alert and stable trauma patients. JAMA 2001;286(15):1841–8.
13. Leonard JC, Browne LR, Ahmad FA, et al. Cervical spine injury risk factors in children with blunt trauma. Pediatrics 2019;144(1):e20183221.
14. Hoffman JR, Mower WR, Wolfson AB, et al. Validity of a set of clinical criteria to rule out injury to the cervical spine in patients with blunt trauma. National Emergency X-Radiography Utilization Study Group. N Engl J Med 2000;343(2):94–9.
15. Viikari-Juntura E, Porras M, Laasonen EM. Validity of clinical tests in the diagnosis of root compression in cervical disc disease. Spine (Phila Pa 1976) 1989;14(3): 253–7.
16. Stence NV, Fenton LZ, Goldenberg NA, et al. Craniocervical arterial dissection in children: diagnosis and treatment. Curr Treat Options Neurol 2011;13(6):636–48.
17. Sutherland DH, Olshen R, Cooper L, et al. The development of mature gait. J Bone Joint Surg Am 1980;62(3):336–53.
18. Haldeman S, Carroll L, Cassidy JD. Findings from the bone and joint decade 2000 to 2010 task force on neck pain and its associated disorders. J Occup Environ Med 2010;52(4):424–7.
19. Jones HR, Ryan MM, Levin KH. Radiculopathies and plexopathies. In: Darras BT, Jones HR, Ryan MM, et al, editors. Neuromuscular disorders of infancy,

childhood, and adolescence: a clinician's approach. 2nd ed. Elsevier/Academic Press; 2015. p. 199–224, chap 12.
20. Zmurko MG, Tannoury TY, Tannoury CA, et al. Cervical sprains, disc herniations, minor fractures, and other cervical injuries in the athlete. Clin Sports Med 2003; 22(3):513–21.
21. Buchowski JM, Kelly MP, Barth BM. Axial neck pain, radiculopathy, and myelopathy: recognition and treatment. Available at: https://nam03.safelinks.protection.outlook.com/?url=https%3A%2F%2Fwww.practicalpainmanagement.com%2Fpain%2Fspine%2Fradiculopathy%2Faxial-neck-pain-radiculopathy-myelopathy-recognition-treatment&data=04%7C01%7Cr.mayakrishnan%40elsevier.com%7C71a8ef76cd604f1a1d2a08d919bfc4cb%7C9274ee3f94254109a27f9fb15c10675d%7C0%7C0%7C637569133702137423%7CUnknown%7CTWFpbGZsb3d8eyJWIjoiMC4wLjAwMDAiLCJQIjoiV2luMzIiLCJBTiI6Ik1haWwiLCJXVCI6Mn0%3D%7C1000&sdata=W1UxyueF2ojmroUWyRYf2Up6auvNMDU2eLEn1TGbF0k%3D&reserved=0. Accessed January 3, 2021.
22. Kasow DB, Curl WW. "Stingers" in adolescent athletes. Instructional Course Lectures 2006;55:711–6.
23. Dorshimer GW, Kelly M. Cervical pain in the athlete: common conditions and treatment. Prim Care 2005;32(1):231–43.
24. Clark AJ, Auguste KI, Sun PP. Cervical spinal stenosis and sports-related cervical cord neurapraxia. Neurosurg Focus 2011;31(5):E7.
25. Pang D. Spinal cord injury without radiographic abnormality in children, 2 decades later. Neurosurgery 2004;55(6):1325–42, discussion 1342-3.
26. Ahn H, Singh J, Nathens A, et al. Pre-hospital care management of a potential spinal cord injured patient: a systematic review of the literature and evidence-based guidelines. J Neurotrauma 2011;28(8):1341–61.
27. Nguyen GK, Clark R. Adequacy of plain radiography in the diagnosis of cervical spine injuries. Emerg Radiol 2005;11(3):158–61.
28. Roberts TT, Leonard GR, Cepela DJ. Classifications in brief: American Spinal Injury Association (ASIA) impairment scale. Clin Orthop Relat Res 2017;475(5): 1499–504.
29. Advanced trauma life support: student course manual. 10th Edition. American College of Surgeons. Committee on Trauma; 2018.
30. Martin JE. Protocols for cervical spine clearance can provide roadmap for patient care. AAP News: American Academy of Pediatrics; 2018.
31. Durbin DR, Hoffman BD, COUNCIL ON INJURY VIO, A. N. D. POISON PREVENTION. Child Passenger Safety. Pediatrics 2018;142(5):e20182460.
32. Cronan KM. Household safety: preventing injuries from falls, climbing, and grabbing. Available at: https://kidshealth.org/en/parents/safety-falls.html. Accessed January 3, 2021.
33. Heck JF, Clarke KS, Peterson TR, et al. National Athletic Trainers' Association Position Statement: head-down contact and spearing in tackle football. J Athl Train 2004;39(1):101–11.
34. Keep Teen Drivers Safe. Centers for Disease Control and Prevention. Available at: https://nam03.safelinks.protection.outlook.com/?url=https%3A%2F%2Fwww.cdc.gov%2Finjury%2Ffeatures%2Fteen-drivers%2Findex.html&data=04%7C01%7Cr.mayakrishnan%40elsevier.com%7C71a8ef76cd604f1a1d2a08d919bfc4cb%7C9274ee3f94254109a27f9fb15c10675d%7C0%7C0%7C637569133702147415%7CUnknown%7CTWFpbGZsb3d8eyJWIjo

iMC4wLjAwMDAiLCJQIjoiV2luMzIiLCJBTiI6Ik1haWwiLCJXVCI6Mn0%3D%7C1000&sdata=XU9p%2BjokyY5sXijecrCm2ahdD72Lxt59Nd6aqgUoVvQ%3D&reserved=0. Accessed January 3, 2021.
35. Vaccaro AR, Klein GR, Ciccoti M, et al. Return to play criteria for the athlete with cervical spine injuries resulting in stinger and transient quadriplegia/paresis. Spine J 2002;2(5):351–6.
36. Murphy NA, Carbone PS, Disabilities AAoPCoCW. Promoting the participation of children with disabilities in sports, recreation, and physical activities. Pediatrics 2008;121(5):1057–61.
37. Brockmeyer D. Down syndrome and craniovertebral instability. Topic review and treatment recommendations. Pediatr Neurosurg 1999;31(2):71–7.
38. Atlantoaxial instability in Down syndrome: subject review. American Academy of Pediatrics Committee on Sports Medicine and Fitness. Pediatrics 1995;96(1 Pt 1): 151–4.
39. American Academy of Pediatrics. Committee on Sports Medicine. Atlantoaxial instability in Down syndrome. Pediatrics 1984;74(1):152–4.
40. Bull MJ, Genetics Co. Health supervision for children with Down syndrome. Pediatrics 2011;128(2):393–406.
41. Hengartner AC, Whelan R, Maj R, et al. Evaluation of 2011 AAP cervical spine screening guidelines for children with Down syndrome. Childs Nerv Syst 2020; 36(11):2609–14.
42. Davidson RG. Atlantoaxial instability in individuals with Down syndrome: a fresh look at the evidence. Pediatrics 1988;81(6):857–65.

Cutaneous Stigmata of the Spine

A Review of Indications for Imaging and Referral

Mandana Behbahani, MD, Sandi K. Lam, MD, MBA,
Robin Bowman, MD*

KEYWORDS

• Skin stigmata • Occult spinal dysraphism • Spinal ultrasound • Spinal MRI

KEY POINTS

- Presence of a soft tissue lesion or skin stigmata overlying the spinal midline increases the likelihood of underlying dysraphic pathology.
- MRI is the gold standard of imaging workup in evaluation for an underlying spinal cord or column abnormality in association with cutaneous stigmata.
- Controversy exists regarding the timing of surgical intervention for tethering spinal cord lesions; however, the goal remains preservation or improvement of orthopedic, neurologic, and urologic function.

INTRODUCTION

Background

Spinal dysraphism refers to a spectrum of congenital spinal anomalies that involves the skin, posterior spinal elements, and underlying neuronal tissue. Open spinal dysraphism, or myelomeningocele, occurs when the underlying spinal cord is exposed at the skin level through a bifid spinal column. All skin-covered forms of spinal dysraphism are known as occult spinal dysraphism (OSD). There are various forms of OSD, which may present with different skin stigmata. These anomalies can produce a variety of neurologic, orthopedic, and/or urologic symptoms due to tethering of the spinal cord, which may occur when there is an abnormal band of tissue intermittently creating tension on the conus, or bottom of the spinal cord; this intermittent tension results in abnormalities in oxidative metabolism, which may eventually produce neuronal dysfunction.[1]

Division of Pediatric Neurosurgery, Lurie Children's Hospital and Northwestern University Feinberg School of Medicine, 225 East Chicago Avenue, Box 28, Chicago, IL 60611, USA
* Corresponding author.
E-mail address: Rbowman@luriechildrens.org

Pediatr Clin N Am 68 (2021) 895–913
https://doi.org/10.1016/j.pcl.2021.04.017
pediatric.theclinics.com

An experienced pediatric neurosurgeon is often able to accurately predict the type of tethering lesion based on the cutaneous stigmata. For most of the patients with OSD, the skin and/or soft tissue lesion is the only clinical abnormality noted on the neonatal examination. When a suspicion exists for possible OSD, a spinal ultrasound or MRI may be obtained to further delineate the child's anatomy.

In most of the cases, the initial detection of cutaneous stigmata, worrisome for underlying OSD, is made by the newborns' pediatrician, which prompts further investigation. Understanding the embryology of the cutaneous abnormality aids in the understanding of the potential pathology present. There is a variable risk of tethering of the spinal cord with differing types of cutaneous stigmata. For an infant with a dorsal appendage associated with a midline, soft tissue lipoma, nearly all patients will have an associated lipomyelomeningocele, whereas an otherwise healthy newborn with a dimple overlying the coccyx has a much lower risk of a tethered spinal cord.[2–4] As such, controversy exists regarding the need for imaging based on the type of cutaneous stigmata present, especially with patients harboring sacrococcygeal dimples.[5] Those who argue against spinal imaging for patients with coccygeal dimples note that radiographic tethering of the spinal cord can occur in approximately 4.8% of patients with no midline cutaneous markers.[6,7] Consequently, they do not feel that the risk of having an associated tethered cord is higher than the general population with no midline cutaneous stigmata, and hence no further evaluation is warranted. Conversely, other investigators have noted a much higher association of tethering with what has previously been called the "benign sacral dimple" and hence would advocate for imaging.[2–4] Unfortunately, no natural history or randomized, long-term study is available to objectively instruct parents as to the best course of action. Given the risk of possible neurologic, orthopedic, or urologic issues associated with tethering of the spinal cord, the authors recommend a low threshold for imaging in any patient with a potential concern.

Embryology

Spinal dysraphism occurs due to errors in embryonic development between gestational weeks 2 to 6.[8] These abnormalities in spinal cord development may be classified based on their embryologic origin and timing in development (**Table 1**). The embryonic stages may be classified as follows: (1) disorders of gastrulation (weeks 2–3); (2) disorder of primary neurulation (weeks 3–4); and (3) disorders of secondary neurulation or regression (weeks 5–6).[9]

Gastrulation is the process by which the bilaminar embryo composed of the epiblast and hypoblast is converted to a trilaminar disk, giving rise to the mesoblast layer and notochord (**Fig. 1**). Defects in gastrulation can be divided into disorders of notochord formation or integration.

- Disorders of notochord formation encompass caudal regression syndrome and segmental spinal dysgenesis.
- Disorders of notochord integration include neurenteric cyst and dorsal enteric fistula, as well as diastematomyelia, or split cord malformation, which will be discussed further later.[10]

Primary neurulation occurs during gestational weeks 3 to 4. The notochord signals the overlying ectoderm to form the neural plate. As the ectoderm folds and the edges meet, it allows for closure of the neural tube. The neuroectoderm then separates from the overlying cutaneous ectoderm. The neural tube forms the primitive brain and spinal cord to the sacral (S2) level.[8] Abnormalities of primary neurulation can be divided into premature dysjunction versus nondysjunction (**Fig. 2**). The dysjunction theory

Table 1
Summary of spinal dysraphism based on their embryologic origin

	Embryology in Spinal Dysraphism	
Gastrulation	Notochord formation	Caudal regression syndrome Segmental spinal dysgenesis
	Notochord integration	Neurenteric cyst Dorsal enteric fistula Diastematomyelia
Primary neurulation	Premature dysjunction	Lipomyelomeningocele Lipomyelocele Intradural lipoma
	Nondysjunction	Dorsal dermal sinus tracts Meningocele manque Myelomeningocele
Secondary neurulation	Caudal cell mass	Terminal myelocystocele Sacrococcygeal teratoma
	Regression	Lipoma of the filum terminale Tight filum terminale

implicates the neuroectoderm in releasing the superficial ectoderm prematurely, which allows the mesoderm (future lipoma) access to the neural tube.

- Pathologies associated with premature dysjunction include lipomyelomeningocele, lipomyelocele, and intradural lipoma.
- Pathologies associated with nondysjunction or an adhesion between the neuroectoderm and the superficial ectoderm include dorsal dermal sinus tracts, meningocele manqué, and myelomeningocele (or open spina bifida).[10]

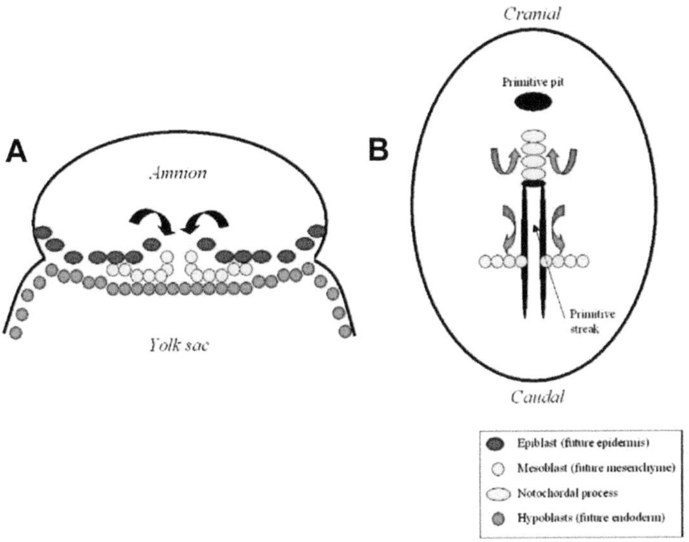

Fig. 1. Gastrulation. (*A*) Axial and (*B*) coronal view of enfolding of epiblast cells, which results in production of future mesenchymal cells. (*From* Martin, Jonathan & Keating, Robert. (2005). Atypical etiologies of tethered spinal cord syndrome for the general neurosurgeon. Seminars in Spine Surgery. 17. 30-39.)

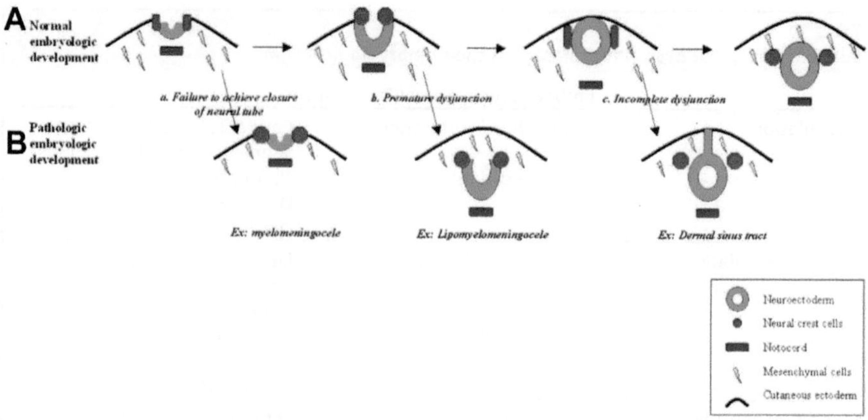

Fig. 2. Normal and pathologic neurulation. (*A*) Primary neurulation with induction of cutaneous ectoderm to neuroectoderm, enfolding of the neuroectoderm to form a closed neural tube, and dysjunction of the completed neural tube from the overlying ectoderm. (*B*) Pathologic embryologic development, due to errors in neural tube closure or abnormal dysjunction. (*From* Martin, Jonathan & Keating, Robert. (2005). Atypical etiologies of tethered spinal cord syndrome for the general neurosurgeon. Seminars in Spine Surgery. 17. 30-39.)

In secondary neurulation, which occurs during gestational weeks 5 to 6, the caudal pluripotent cell mass forms a solid medullary cord, which cavitates by retrograde dedifferentiation, a poorly understood process by which the conus medullaris, filum terminale, and distal sacrum and coccyx are formed[8] (**Fig. 3**).

- Disorders of secondary neurulation consist of tethered cord syndrome, persistent terminal ventricle, fatty filum, and intrasacral/anterior sacral meningocele.[11]

It is prudent to note that all of these disorders are part of the spectrum of embryologic development, and pathologies may occur in combination depending on timing and extent of developmental disruption.

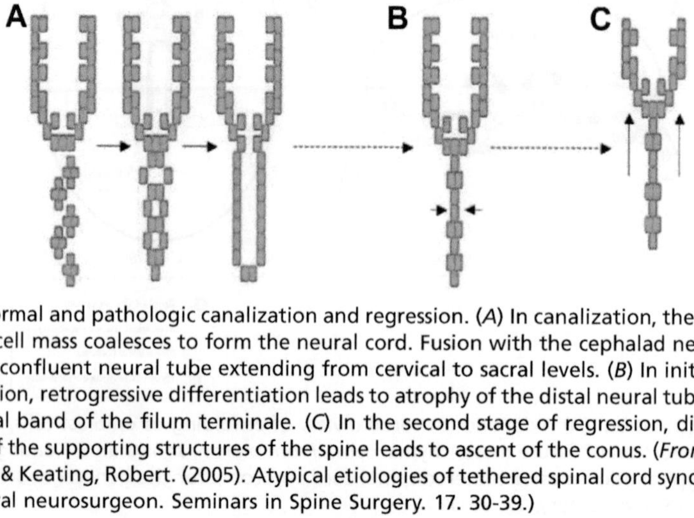

Fig. 3. Normal and pathologic canalization and regression. (*A*) In canalization, the undifferentiated cell mass coalesces to form the neural cord. Fusion with the cephalad neural tube produces confluent neural tube extending from cervical to sacral levels. (*B*) In initial stages of regression, retrogressive differentiation leads to atrophy of the distal neural tube to form atretic pial band of the filum terminale. (*C*) In the second stage of regression, differential growth of the supporting structures of the spine leads to ascent of the conus. (*From* Martin, Jonathan & Keating, Robert. (2005). Atypical etiologies of tethered spinal cord syndrome for the general neurosurgeon. Seminars in Spine Surgery. 17. 30-39.)

Causes with Cutaneous Marker

Most children with spinal dysraphism present with some form of cutaneous manifestation, as the skin and underlying nervous system both originate in the embryonic ectodermal layer. In patients with open spina bifida, the spinal cord is exposed at the skin level at birth. For further discussion of open spina bifida, the reader is referred to Chapter 15 in this volume. Most patients with an OSD and tethering lesion have an apparent cutaneous abnormality overlying the spinal midline, many having more than one skin finding.[12] Rarely, a patient will have an OSD and tethering with no midline cutaneous marker.[6,13]

OSD is divided into those with a midline spinal, soft tissue mass versus those without a visible mass (**Table 2**). The mass is most commonly of lipomatous origin, as seen in lipomyelomeningocele, terminal myelocystocele (MCC), and meningocele. Defects without an associated dorsal spinal mass may be diastematomyelia (split cord malformation), dermal sinus tract, meningocele manqué, intradural lipoma, filar lipoma, tight filum terminale, low-lying conus medullaris, neurenteric fistula/cyst, caudal regression syndrome, or segmental spinal dysgenesis.[14]

Clinical Manifestation

There is a wide range of variability in the symptomatology profile associated with spinal dysraphism. In cases of fatty filum or tethered cord, the presentation may be completely asymptomatic. However, in case of more complex spinal dysraphic deformities, patients can experience gross musculoskeletal deformities of spinal axis or lower extremities, paralysis, urinary and fecal incontinence, recurrent urinary tract infection, central nervous system infections, and pain. These symptoms may present in isolation or in combination, depending on the pathology.

Clinical symptoms associated with spinal dysraphism

- Pain: back pain, claudicating leg pain
- Musculoskeletal asymmetry: scoliosis, asymmetric foot/leg deformity
- Neurologic signs/symptoms
  - Weakness, to include regression of motor milestones
  - Sensory loss
  - Autonomic dysfunction: delayed/regression of toilet training, recurrent urinary tract infection, urgency

Table 2
Types of spinal dysraphism associated with midline spinal soft tissue mass

Appearance	Type of Dysraphism
Presence of midline mass/not covered with skin	Myelocele Myelomeningocele
Presence of midline mass/covered with skin	Lipomyelomeningocele Meningocele Myelocystocele
No midline mass present	Anterior sacral meningocele Caudal regression syndrome Diastematomyelia Dorsal dermal sinus Hydromyelia Intradural lipoma Tight filum terminale

EVALUATION

Cutaneous stigmata, as an indication of OSD, is well known in the pediatric population, and patients are screened for such findings at birth. In prior studies, 50% to 80% of patients evaluated for cutaneous stigmata were found to have underlying OSD.[11,15] OSD can be observed overlying the neuroaxis from the nasion or occiput to the sacral region. Pathologic spinal anomalies occur with increased frequency as one descends the spinal column into the lumbosacral region.[16]

Cutaneous Manifestation

Subcutaneous mass (skin tags, appendages, and lipomyelomeningocele) may be present in the midline lumbosacral region (**Fig. 4**). Although some investigators refer to these as an embryonic tail, the details related to their embryogenesis are debated. Some investigators purport that the dorsal appendage is a distal remnant of the embryonic tail containing adipose, connective, muscle, and nerve tissue representing a superficial resemblance to a vestigial tail,[17] whereas yet other researchers contend that the true tail is likely a cutaneous marker of spinal dysraphism with spinal cord tethering and are not remnants of an embryonic human tail.[18] The presence of these cutaneous markers are highly correlated with underlying pathology of spinal dysraphism.[1,2,10,17,19–22] In most of the cases, dorsal appendages or skin tags occur in conjunction with other cutaneous stigmata. Accordingly, in the case of subcutaneous lipomas, they present as a palpable mass in the lumbosacral region and may occur with concurrent associated skin stigmata.[23] Lipomas commonly attach to the spinal cord, or tether the cord, after entering the spinal column through bifid lamina. Lipomyelomeningoceles account for up to 18.8% of OSD.[22] Although spinal lipomas account for 5% of the tumors of the spinal cord, their presence is commonly associated with some forms of underlying dysraphism. Lipomas without bony involvement

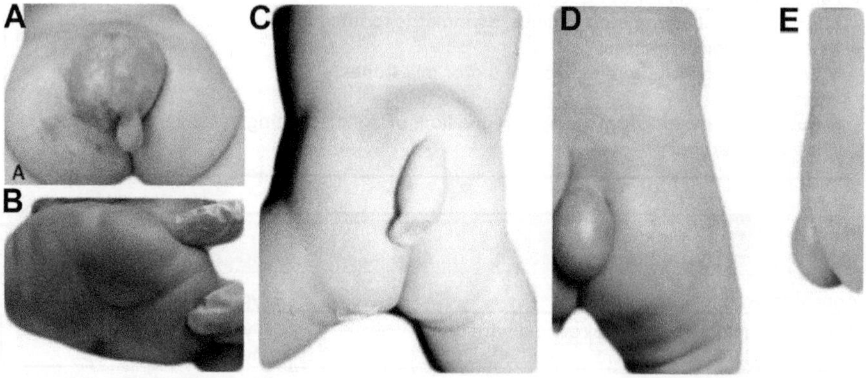

Fig. 4. Subcutaneous masses are highly associated with spinal dysraphism. (*A*) displays a large lipomatous mass with an associated appendage. In addition, subcutaneous vascular lesion of the overlying skin is also noted. The appearance of gluteal crease is not clearly able to be evaluated; however, there is clear asymmetry. (*B*) Lipomatous mass involving the lumbosacral region associated with an overlying dimple and abnormal gluteal crease. Minimal skin changes are noted in this patient. (*C*) Lipomatous lumbar region mass with a dorsal appendage, which can be referred to as tail in this case, arising from the inferior aspect of the mass. (*D* and *E*) Anterior/posterior and lateral visualization of a lumbosacral lipomatous mass. Deviation of the gluteal crease due to the location and morphology of the mass. Vascular cutaneous changes over the mass are visible.

are considered dysembriogenetic lesions.[24] The likelihood of a dorsal lipoma being associated with an underlying OSD, or tethered spinal cord, is high compared with other types of cutaneous stigmata.[10,25–27]

Myelocystocele

Constituting 4% to 8% of occult dysraphism, an myelocystocele (MCC) presents as a fluid-filled, skin-covered sac overlying the newborn's spinal column, most commonly in the lumbosacral region, although cervical and thoracic lesions have rarely been reported[19,28–32] (**Fig. 5**). The original description of MCC consisted of skin-covered spina bifida, with arachnoid-lined meningocele continuous with spinal subarachnoid space, and terminal cyst bulging into the extra-arachnoid compartment caudal to the meningocele.[20] Commonly, the hydromyelic spinal cord expands either at its terminus or dorsolaterally into an ependymal-lined cyst that pushes beyond the confines of the bifid spine and dural sac.[19] It has been proposed that terminal MCC and lipomyelomeningoceles seem to be part of the same embryologic continuum of skin-covered spina bifida, with varying degrees of lipomatous tissue.[19,20] Commonly neural tube defects such as MCC are associated with omphalocele, bladder exstrophy, imperforate anus, and spinal defects complex.[19,33–36] MCC may also occur de novo without associated congenital anomalies.[19,34,35]

Hypertrichosis refers to a prominent patch of hair that is present over the midline spine at birth (**Fig. 6**). Although variable in size, texture, color, and location, its presence is distinguishable from physiologic hair patches in each individual. Physiologic lumbosacral hypertrichosis is seen in patients of African, Asian, and Hispanic descent. Pathologic hypertrichosis is somewhat diffuse in nature and can have a V-shaped appearance. In select cases, hypertrichosis can be associated with a faun tail nevus. Presence of hypertrichosis is highly associated with an underlying split cord spinal dysraphism, or diastematomyelia.[10,25,37,38]

Dermal sinus tract is another common and ominous midline skin stigma among the newborn population that has correlation with underlying OSD (**Fig. 7**). Dermal sinus tracts have an incidence of 1 in 2500 live births.[21] They appear as a midline pit above the gluteal cleft and advance in the soft tissues in a cephalad direction toward the underlying neuronal structures. Furthermore, they are unique in their presentation, as

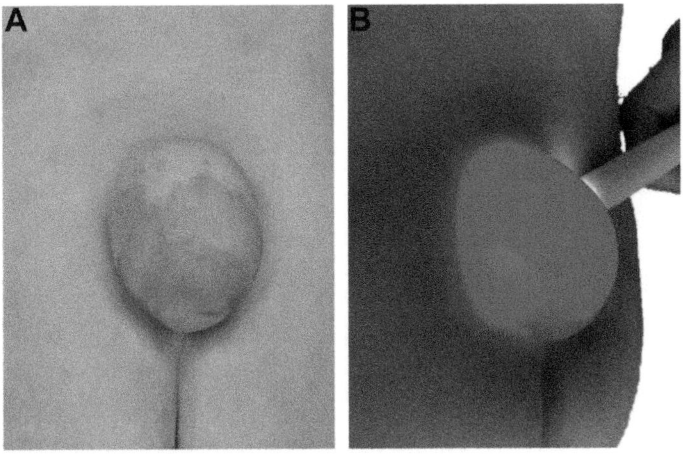

Fig. 5. Myelocystocele can comprise of cystic outpouching. (*A, B*) This patient has a myelocystocele, which can be further transilluminated to demonstrate the cystic component.

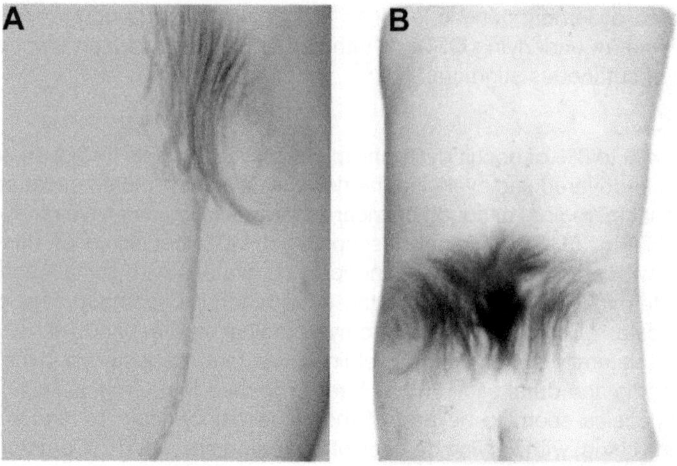

Fig. 6. Hypertrichosis has a wide presentation, and although patients with select spinal dysraphism often have a patch of hair, not all hair patches are associated with spinal dysraphism. Physiologic hair patches should be distinguished from that of pathologic presentation. (*A, B*) Prominent hypertrichosis of the lumbar spine, presenting as thick dark hair over the midline and extending to the lateral aspect symmetrically.

they can present with transient drainage, infection, and meningitis. These lesions not only tether the spinal cord (if the dermal sinus tract travels all the way to the spinal cord level) but may also allow entry of bacteria into the central nervous system (CNS). Given the risk of tethering and meningitis, all infants suspected of harboring a dermal sinus tract should undergo a spinal MRI.[39] Given the risk of meningitis, pediatric neurosurgeons recommend surgical excision of all dermal sinus tracts, as imaging may not detect the full extension intraspinal.

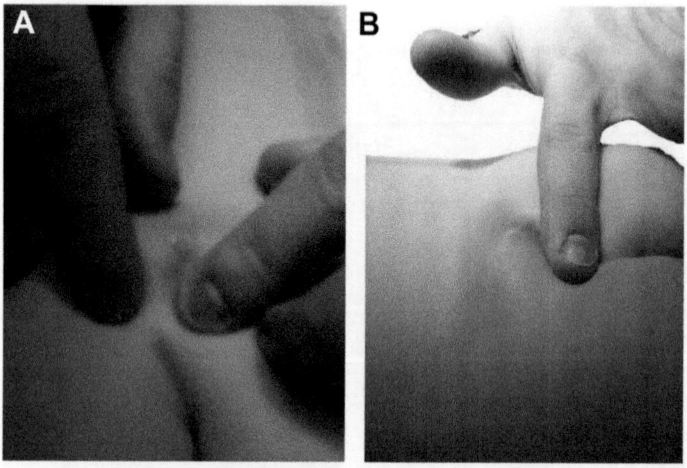

Fig. 7. Dermal sinus tract can present in a variable fashion; however, cutaneous findings are common. (*A, B*) Prominent infected dermal sinus tract with significant intradural involvement on radiographic imaging.

Meningocele manque, also referred to a as "cigarette burn" in the lumbar spinal midline, is a cutaneous finding of localized or widespread absence of skin and subcutaneous tissue (**Fig. 8**). Similar to a dermal sinus tract, this tract of aberrant tissue or tethering bands attaches the spinal cord to the overlying dura, soft tissue, or skin.[40] The clinical appearance ranges from a solitary erosion or ulcer to a glistening thin membrane at birth.[41] These lesions, commonly present in the lumbosacral region, are highly associated with underlying spinal dysraphism and spinal cord tethering.[25,26,42] This abnormal stalk of tissue attaching to the conus has been noted to consist of fibrous tissue, abnormal Pacinian corpuscles or peripheral nerves, adipose tissue, blood vessels, epidermal cells, cartilage/bone, smooth muscle, CNS tissue, and dermal/epidermal cysts when viewed microscopically.[12,23,43] Interestingly, the tethering bands do not commonly contain meningeal tissue.[40]

Midline cutaneous vascular lesions can also be considered a broad category for a range of physiologic and pathologic findings (**Fig. 9**). They make up a large portion of patients being referred for subspecialty evaluation of possible OSD. The difficulty in determining the risk of associated OSD stems from the ambiguity in classifying vascular skin lesions.[5] On occasion, they are referenced interchangeably with that of skin pigmentation as seen in port wine stain, salmon patch, strawberry nevus, vascular nevus, cutaneous angioma, and flat capillary lumbosacral hemangioma.[44] Given the broad number of patients who fall into this category, there have been contradictory results in the current literature as to the yield of screening these lesions for underlying SD. Although some investigators note a low correlation between cutaneous hemangiomas and OSD,[45] others deem hemangioma of infancy in the lumbosacral region highly indicates underlying spinal dysraphism.[10,27,46,47] A recent study by Guggisberg and colleagues found the most significant correlation with OSD was a spinal midline vascular abnormality in conjunction with another cutaneous stigmata.[23]

Lumbosacral dimples and coccygeal dimples (pit) of the midline spine are one of the most controversial areas in pediatric neurosurgery. Although frequently referred to as

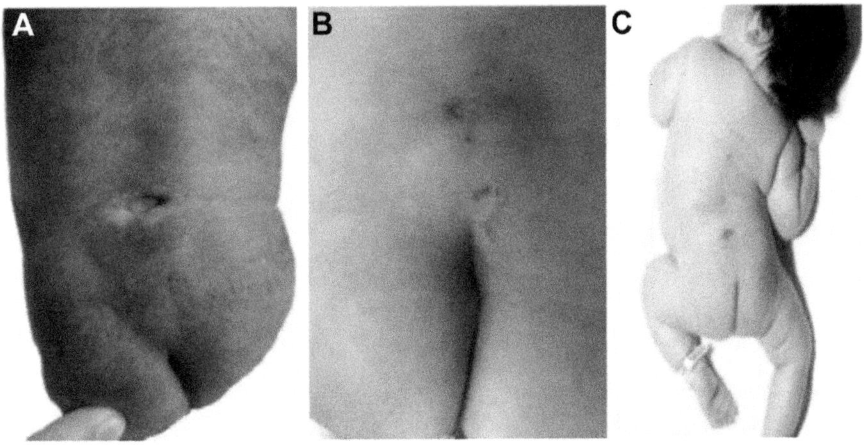

Fig. 8. Meningocele manque can be subtle or prominent skin findings that are not only limited to the superficial layers, rather extend to the subcutaneous region. (*A*) Cutaneous aplasia of the lumbar region with associated patch of hair inferior to the lesion. (*B*) A small region of cutaneous aplasia, hypertrichosis, vascular cutaneous lesion, and gluteal cleft deviation demonstrated in this patient. (*C*) Another demonstration of cutaneous aplasia without significant other skin stigmata.

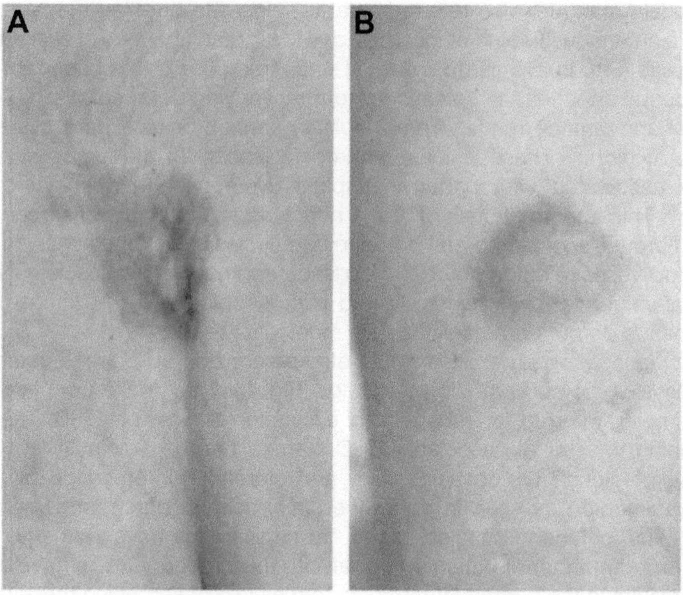

Fig. 9. (*A, B*) Variability in vascular lumbosacral cutaneous findings in isolation of any other abnormality.

"sacral dimples," the lesion is a whorl of skin that tracts to the coccyx (**Fig. 10**). At times, it may be noted higher in the gluteal crease overlying the sacrum, but with skin manipulation, it is apparent that the base is attached to the coccyx. These coccygeal dimples are the most common minor malformation in man, occurring in 4.6% of the population.[48] Controversy exists as to whether these lesions are associated with

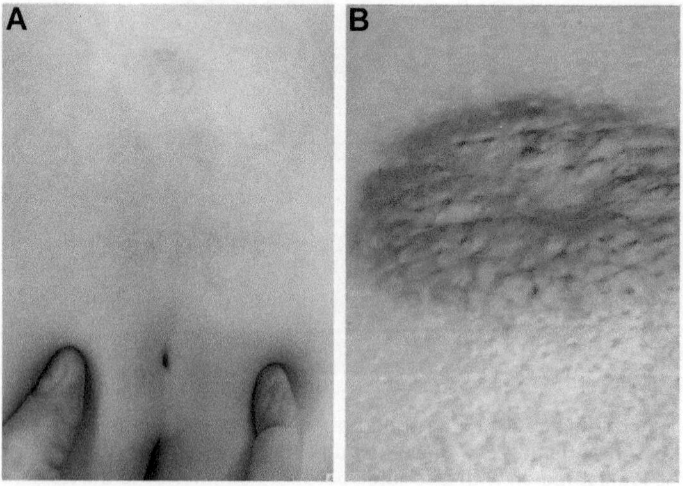

Fig. 10. Although pits seem to be benign in nature, they can be a sign of dangerous underlying lesions. (*A*) Prominent lumbosacral dimple is visualized within the gluteal crease, which indicates a more benign process. (*B*) A sacral pit with surrounding hemangioma.

an increased risk of OSD. Interestingly, lumbosacral dimples make up to 45% of the population undergoing imaging to evaluate for possible spinal dysraphism.[45] The size, location relative to the anus, and presence or absence of the dimples' terminus have been reported as contributing factors in determining risk of associated OSD. Large dimples with atypical appearance, ranging greater than 25 mm away from the anus are most likely to be associated with underlying pathology.[10,49–52] In one study, patients with dimples averaging 15 mm above the coccyx was correlated with presence of OSD, whereas patients with dimples positioned on average 12.2 mm above the coccyx did not correlate with having OSD.[45] Factors such as the location; depth of the pit; concurrent presentation with other cutaneous stigmata; and neurologic, urologic, or orthopedic abnormalities all increase the suspicion of an associated OSD.

Gluteal cleft deviation, although seemingly specific, contains a spectrum of definition ranging from minimal physiologic asymmetry to significant deviation with associated asymmetric glutes (**Fig. 11**). Of patients undergoing screening for OSD as part of cutaneous stigmata identification, up to 8% had asymmetric gluteal cleft deviation and 7% presented with Y-shaped gluteal cleft,[45] which makes up a significant portion (up to 25%) of referrals for OSD evaluation.[45,49] Some pediatric neurosurgeons are unsure as to the significance of an isolated deviated gluteal crease and would recommend evaluation for underlying pathology.[23]

Radiographic Imaging Workup

The ultimate goal for identifying and categorizing lumbosacral cutaneous stigmata is to further evaluate for underlying spinal dysraphism with spinal cord tethering (**Figs. 12** and **13**). Currently, there are no clear guidelines for radiographic assessment following identification of cutaneous stigmata; however, there is consensus in utilization of ultrasound and in some cases MRI for further radiographic evaluation (**Table 3**).

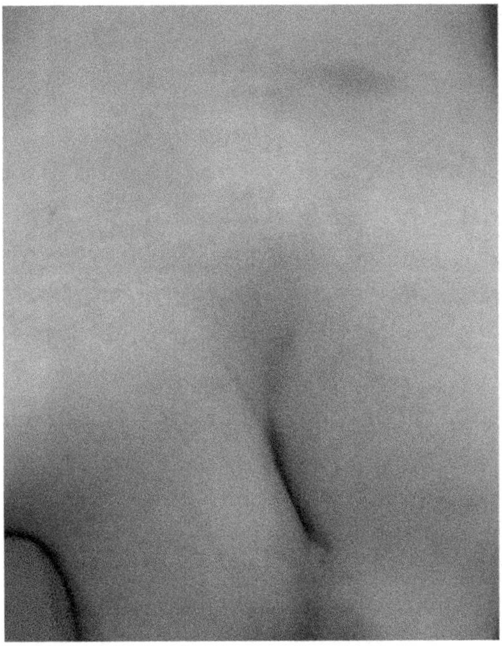

Fig. 11. Patient with clear gluteal cleft deviation.

The benefits and limitations of various imaging modalities in workup for spinal dysraphism in the setting of cutaneous stigmata are explored.

Current imaging modalities used for study of such pathology include plain radiographs, ultrasound, computed tomography, as well as MRI. Plain radiograph can be used for screening in the setting of prominent bony spinal abnormalities; however, it lacks the appropriate resolution to study subtle bony abnormalities. Furthermore, it offers no insight into the associated soft tissue abnormalities and exposes the newborn to unnecessary radiation. There is no evidence as to the utility of this imaging modality in screening for spinal dysraphism in the setting of identification of cutaneous stigmata. On the other hand, ultrasound allows for early visualization of soft tissue abnormalities and to some degree bony abnormalities, without exposing the newborn to unnecessary radiation. Ultrasound is used in the antenatal period, although its utilization is limited by a multitude of factors. Utility of ultrasound in study of spinal dysraphism depends on the age of the patient (younger than 6 months) and technician's skills. Computed tomography (CT) is yet another imaging modality that can provide information regarding the bony anatomy, with significant limitations in providing information regarding soft tissue or neuronal structures. Some of these limitations can be alleviated by intrathecal injection of contrast agents as seen in myelogram; however, the invasive nature of this procedure and high dose of radiation make it a poor initial study choice in newborns. Utility of myelogram and computed tomography imaging is particularly highlighted in the case of diastematomyelia, both in the diagnostic phase as well as surgical planning. Lastly, spinal MRI is a particularly sensitive and specific study in evaluation for spinal dysraphism, detailing the extent of soft tissue and neuronal structure involvement, while eliminating the risk of radiation exposure to the patient.[53] Limitations with utilization of MRI, aside from its lack of wide availability

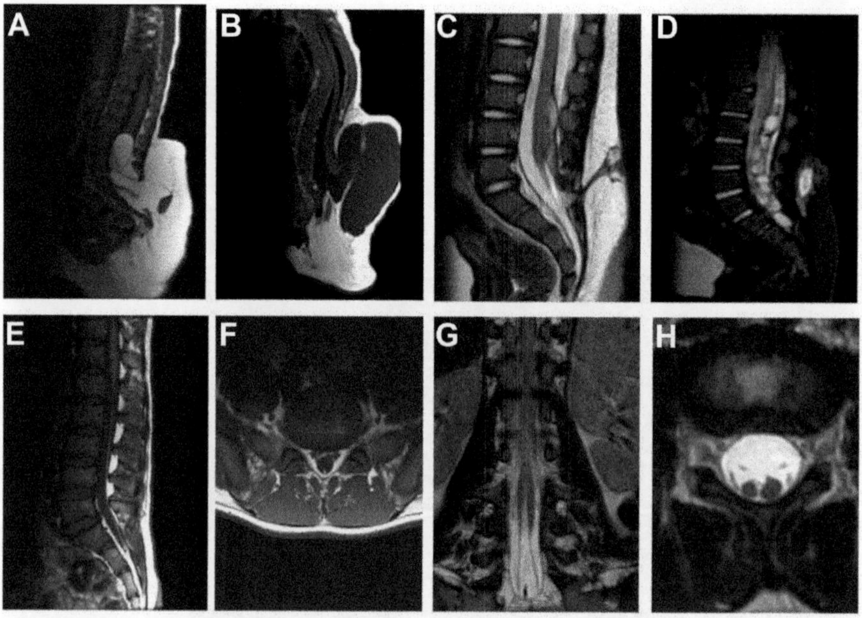

Fig. 12. MRI is the gold standard in assessment of spinal dysraphic findings. Patient with (*A*) lipomyelomeningocele, (*B*) myelocystocele, (*C, D*) dermal sinus tract, (*E, F*) fatty filum, and (*G, H*) diastematomyelia.

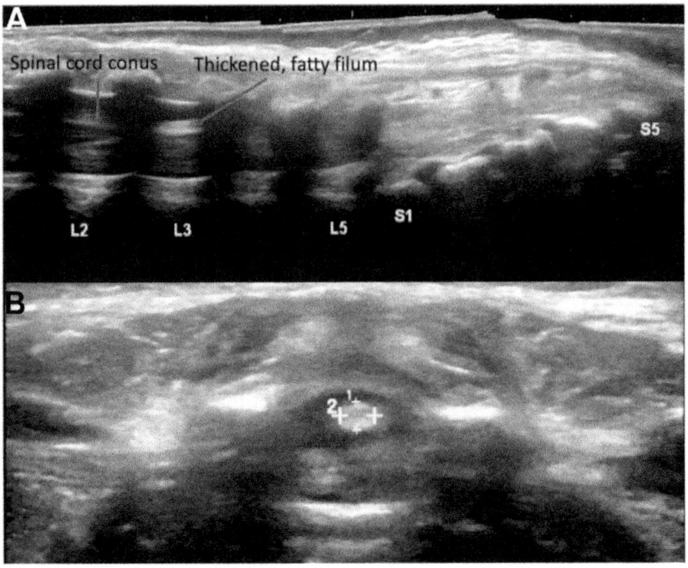

Fig. 13. Ultrasound imaging of a young patient with appropriate acoustic window, allowing visualization of (*A*) sagittal view of the vertebral body shadows, conus medullaris (*red straight arrow*), and thick/fatty filum terminale (*red slanted arrow*); (*B*) axial view of the thick/fatty filum.

in all institutions and high cost, is need for patient cooperation throughout the lengthy examination. Consequently, anesthesia or specified protocols for obtaining limited series in pediatric patients to avoid need for anesthesia is necessary. Common practice patterns consist of evaluation of suspicious lesions with ultrasonography in the newborn age group, where the acoustic window is conducive to study of neuronal and soft tissue structure. Should any abnormalities be noted or there is a high concern

Table 3
Imaging findings in ultrasound and MRI, respectively

Ultrasound Findings	MRI Findings
Highly dependent on presence of acoustic window and operator dependent	**Able to visualize anatomy at any age and not operator dependent*
Bifid spine	Bifid spine, neuronal anatomy, dural separation, and information regarding tissue within hemicords
Split cord	Position of cord
Low lying conus	• Ventral/dorsal dislocation
Fatty filum	• Location of conus termination
Cystic cavity	• Anatomy of the cord
Lipoma	• Anatomy of filum terminale (thickness, presence or absence of fat)
Syrinx	Nerve root anatomy
Minimal demonstration of vertebral body abnormalities	Anatomy of subarachnoid space
Genitourinary anatomy	Dermal sinus tract and subtle manque findings
	Vertebral body morphology
	Anatomy of sacrum in sacral agenesis
	Abdominal, genitourinary anatomy

for OSD not visualized on ultrasound, an MRI may be obtained.[54,55] MRI is particularly more sensitive than ultrasound in the setting of occult spinal dysraphism and subtle abnormalities.[56] MRI is the best modality to diagnosing spinal dysraphism and is relied on by pediatric neurosurgeons for presurgical planning for spinal dysraphism with tethered spinal cords.[39,53] Chapter 2 titled "Neuroimaging for primary care provider in your evaluation: radiographic imaging work-up paragraph," allows for thorough discussion of when and what modalities should be used in workup of OSD.

Therapeutic Options

The goal of surgical intervention is to safely release the spinal cord from tethering elements and resect aberrant bony structures and/or lipomatous masses/appendages. Once an underlying dysraphic abnormality with spinal cord tethering is identified, the child undergoes a workup to evaluate for neurologic, orthopedic, and/or urologic symptoms. This evaluation may, at the discretion of the care team, include additional providers. Lower extremity strength may be documented by manual muscle testing by physical therapist. An orthopedic surgeon may assess the child for musculoskeletal deformity or abnormal tone. A urologist may evaluate the child's bowel and bladder function in conjunction with cystometrogram and ultrasound. Lastly, a pediatric neurosurgeon may assess for pain and neurologic compromise of function. Presence of functional compromise in any of these areas warrants surgical intervention, aimed at untethering or relieving spinal cord tension. In some scenarios, surgical intervention is considered without presence of symptoms in order to prevent future decline in function. Although there is controversy in the literature regarding surgical intervention on asymptomatic patients, thorough baseline functional evaluation with a detailed discussion between the neurosurgeon and patient/parents is optimal. If nonsurgical, conservative management is deemed appropriate, long-term follow-up is recommended to detect any signs or symptoms of functional decline necessitating prompt, surgical intervention as the child grows and develops.

DISCUSSION

Presence of skin stigmata in the midline lumbosacral region has been associated with known underlying spinal dysraphism. These skin stigmata occur in early stages of embryogenesis. Understanding of these cutaneous findings can highlight the likelihood of their association with underlying pathology and allow for a management algorithm.[57] Once OSD is identified, the associated symptoms can be managed through either long-term monitoring or surgical intervention. Here the authors explore a range of cutaneous findings that prompt the referring physicians to seek subspecialty expertise to further workup these lesions. Not all cutaneous findings have the same likelihood of being associated with underlying OSD.[23] Guggisberg and colleagues showed a significantly increased risk of OSD in children with more than one cutaneous stigmata. Unfortunately, it is also impossible to clinically predict which patients with OSD have subtle evidence of tethering or who will develop it in the future. Hence, patients with evidence of OSD/tethered cord should be observed for evidence of neurologic decline as they grow and develop.

Factors contributing to the likelihood of underlying pathology depend on the type of stigmata itself, as well as the occurrence of multiple cutaneous stigmata in the same patient. In addition, presence of an associated mass or lipoma increases the likelihood of underlying pathology. In such patients, early imaging, early neurosurgical referral, and close monitoring are warranted. Lesion location is of importance when assessing for likelihood of a pathologic lesion. Lesions further away from the anus, particularly those above the gluteal crease, are much more likely to be pathologic in nature than ones closer to the anus and overlying the coccyx. All pits above the gluteal cleft should be evaluated immediately given concern for a dermal sinus tract, which may allow bacteria access to the CNS.

Once the decision to proceed with imaging is made, a realistic question facing the clinician is that of the specific modality of imaging to pursue. In a younger child, whose acoustic windows are amenable, a spinal ultrasound screening study may be obtained. In case of lower clinical suspicion with negative ultrasound studies, it is prudent to conduct follow-up with the patient's pediatrician on a routine basis. If there is a high

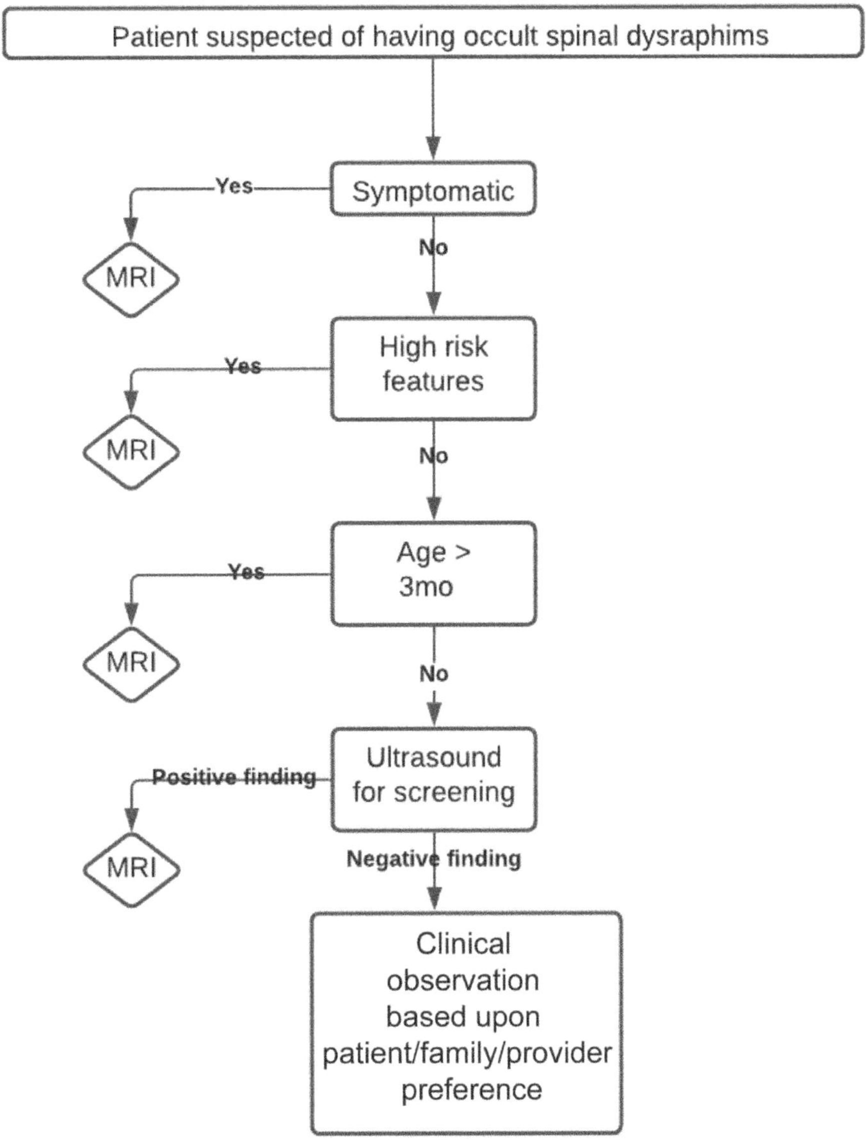

Fig. 14. Algorithm in choosing radiographic study for workup of spinal dysraphism.

clinical suspicion or there is positive screening ultrasound, the patient should undergo MRI and follow-up with a pediatric neurosurgeon. Inevitability, the timing, and modality of imaging highly depend on the patient's age (**Fig. 14**).

SUMMARY

Infants with evidence of spinal dysraphism on examination or radiologic testing, as well as children with symptoms that suggest OSD, benefit from neuroimaging and neurosurgical evaluation for clear diagnosis and subsequent treatment. Clear understanding of lesions with high likelihood of associated dysraphic pathology can help primary care physicians and referring physicians streamline their workup in a timely manner. Early diagnosis and treatment can allow for improved outcomes of neurologic, orthopedic, and urologic function.

Clinics Care Points

- Presence of soft tissue lesion or skin stigmata overlying the spinal midline increases the likelihood of underlying dysraphic pathology.
- MRI is the gold standard of imaging workup in evaluation for an underlying spinal cord or column abnormality in association with cutaneous stigmata.
- Controversy exists regarding the timing of surgical intervention for tethering spinal cord lesions; however, the goal remains preservation or improvement of orthopedic, neurologic, and urologic function.

DISCLOSURE

No disclosure.

REFERENCES

1. Yamada S, Zinke DE, Sanders D. Pathophysiology of "tethered cord syndrome". J Neurosurg 1981;54(4):494–503.
2. Gomi A, Oguma H, Furukawa R. Sacrococcygeal dimple: new classification and relationship with spinal lesions. Childs Nerv Syst 2013;29(9):1641–5.
3. Harada A, Nishiyama K, Yoshimura J, et al. Intraspinal lesions associated with sacrococcygeal dimples. J Neurosurg Pediatr 2014;14(1):81–6.
4. Tamura G, Morota N, Ihara S. Impact of magnetic resonance imaging and urodynamic studies on the management of sacrococcygeal dimples. J Neurosurg Pediatr 2017;20(3):289–97.
5. Guggisberg D, Hadj-Rabia S, Viney C, et al. Skin markers of occult spinal dysraphism in children. Arch Dermatol 2004;140(9):1109–15.
6. Gibson PJ, Britton J, Hall DM, et al. Lumbosacral skin markers and identification of occult spinal dysraphism in neonates. Acta Paediatr 1995;84(2):208–9.
7. Albert GW. Spine ultrasounds should not be routinely performed for patients with simple sacral dimples. Acta Paediatr 2016;105(8):890–4.
8. Rufener SL, Ibrahim M, Raybaud CA, et al. Congenital spine and spinal cord malformations— pictorial review. Am J Roentgenol 2010;194(3_supplement):S26–37.
9. Sadler TW. Embryology of neural tube development. Am J Med Genet C Semin Med Genet 2005;135C(1):2–8.
10. Acharya U, Pendharkar H, Varma D, et al. Spinal dysraphism illustrated; Embroyology revisited. Indian J Radiol Imaging 2017;27(4):417.
11. Ackerman LL, Menezes AH. Spinal congenital dermal sinuses: a 30-year experience. Pediatrics 2003;112(3):641–7.

12. Hettige S, Smart C, Bridges LR, et al. Paciniolipoma in congenital spinal dysraphism. J Neurosurg Pediatr 2012;9(3):280–2.
13. Al-Omari MH, Eloqayli HM, Qudseih HM, et al. Isolated lipoma of filum terminale in adults: MRI findings and clinical correlation. J Med Imaging Radiat Oncol 2011; 55(3):286–90.
14. Pang D, Hou YJ, Wong ST. Classification of spinal dysraphic malformations according to embryogenesis: gastrulation defects and split cord malformation. In: Textbook of pediatric Neurosurgery. Cham: Springer International Publishing; 2017. p. 1–53.
15. Choi SJ, Yoon HM, Hwang JS, et al. Incidence of occult spinal dysraphism among infants with cutaneous stigmata and proportion managed with neurosurgery. JAMA Netw Open 2020;3(7):e207221.
16. French BN. The embryology of spinal dysraphism. Neurosurgery 1983; 30(CN_suppl_1):295–340.
17. Joel Belzberg A, Terence Myles S, Lucy Trevenen C. The human tail and spinal dysraphism. J Pediatr Surg 1991;26(10):1243–5.
18. Wilkinson CC, Boylan AJ. Proposed caudal appendage classification system; spinal cord tethering associated with sacrococcygeal eversion. Child's Nerv Syst 2017;33(1):69–89.
19. Gupta DK, Mahapatra AK. Terminal myelocystoceles: a series of 17 cases. J Neurosurg Pediatr 2005;103(4):344–52.
20. Cohen AR. The mermaid malformation: cloacal exstrophy and occult spinal dysraphism. Neurosurgery 1991;28(6):834–43.
21. Radmanesh F, Nejat F, El Khashab M. Dermal sinus tract of the spine. Child's Nerv Syst 2010;26(3):349–57.
22. Tortori-Donati P, Rossi A, Cama A. Spinal dysraphism: a review of neuroradiological features with embryological correlations and proposal for a new classification. Neuroradiology 2000;42(7):471–91.
23. Kojc N, Korsic M, Popovic M. Pacinioma of the cauda equina. Dev Med Child Neurol 2006;48(12):994–6.
24. Caldarelli M, Castagnola D, Ceddia A, et al. [Spinal lipomas in childhood]. Minerva Pediatr 1992;44(9):437–44.
25. Schropp C, Sörensen N, Collmann H, et al. Cutaneous lesions in occult spinal dysraphism—correlation with intraspinal findings. Child's Nerv Syst 2006;22(2): 125–31.
26. Vanaclocha-Vanaclocha V, Saiz-Sapena N. [Neural tube dysfunction and cutaneous lesions]. Rev Neurol 1997;25(Suppl 3):S232–7.
27. Meling TR, Due-Tønnessen BJ, Lundar T, et al. [Occult spinal dysraphism]. Tidsskr Nor Laegeforen 2002;122(9):913–6.
28. McLone DG, Naidich TP. Terminal myelocystocele. Neurosurgery 1985;16(1): 36–43.
29. Kumar R, Chandra A. Terminal myelocystocele. Indian J Pediatr 2002;69(12): 1083–6.
30. Lemire RJ, Benjamin Graham C, Bruce Beckwith J. Skin-covered sacrococcygeal masses in infantsand children. J Pediatr 1971;79(6):948–54.
31. Chandra RVV, Kumar PM. Cervical myelocystocele: case report and review of literature. J Pediatr Neurosci 2011;6(1):55–7.
32. Muthukumar N. Thoracic myelocystoceles–two variants. Acta Neurochir (Wien) 2006;148(7):751–6 [discussion 756].

33. Weaver KB, Matthews H, Chegini S, et al. Vertebral column and spinal cord malformation in children with exstrophy of the cloaca, with emphasis on their functional correlates. Teratology 1997;55(4):241–8.
34. Keppler-Noreuil KM. OEIS complex (omphalocele-exstrophy-imperforate anus-spinal defects): a review of 14 cases. Am J Med Genet 2001;99(4):271–9.
35. Peacock WJ, Murovic JA. Magnetic resonance imaging in myelocystoceles. Report of two cases. J Neurosurg 1989;70(5):804–7.
36. Morioka T, Hashiguchi K, Yoshida F, et al. Neurosurgical management of occult spinal dysraphism associated with OEIS complex. Childs Nerv Syst 2008;24(6): 723–9.
37. Weprin BE, Oakes WJ. Coccygeal Pits. Pediatrics 2000;105(5):e69.
38. Drolet BA. Cutaneous signs of neural tube dysraphism. Pediatr Clin North Am 2000;47(4):813–23.
39. Tortori-Donati P, Rossi A, Biancheri R, et al. Magnetic resonance imaging of spinal dysraphism. Top Magn Reson Imaging 2001;12(6):375–409.
40. Schmidt C, Bryant E, Iwanaga J, et al. Meningocele manqué: a comprehensive review of this enigmatic finding in occult spinal dysraphism. Childs Nerv Syst 2017;33(7):1065–71.
41. Manning JR, Lee DH. Uncommon neonatal skin lesions. Pediatr Ann 2019;48(1): e30–5.
42. Higginbottom MC, Jones KL, James HE, et al. Aplasia cutis congenita: a cutaneous marker of occult spinal dysraphism. J Pediatr 1980;96(4):687–9.
43. Bale PM. Sacrococcygeal paciniomas. Pathology 1980;12(2):231–5.
44. Drolet BA, Boudreau C. When good is not good enough. Arch Dermatol 2004; 140(9):1153–5.
45. O'Neill BR, Gallegos D, Herron A, et al. Use of magnetic resonance imaging to detect occult spinal dysraphism in infants. J Neurosurg Pediatr 2017;19(2): 217–26.
46. Tubbs RS, Wellons JC, Iskandar BJ, et al. Isolated flat capillary midline lumbosacral hemangiomas as indicators of occult spinal dysraphism. J Neurosurg Pediatr 2004;100(2):86–9.
47. Goldberg NS, Hebert AA, Esterly NB. Sacral hemangiomas and multiple congenital abnormalities. Arch Dermatol 1986;122(6):684–7.
48. Sumanović-Glamuzina D, Bozić T, Brkić V, et al. Minor malformations: neonatal or anthropological story? Coll Antropol 2009;33(Suppl 2):31–5.
49. Aby J, Kim JL. A cross-sectional assessment of cutaneous lumbosacral and coccygeal physical examination findings in a healthy newborn population. Glob Pediatr Heal 2018;5. 2333794X1875613.
50. Kriss VM, Desai NS. Occult spinal dysraphism in neonates: assessment of high-risk cutaneous stigmata on sonography. Am J Roentgenol 1998;171(6):1687–92.
51. Ausili E, Maresca G, Massimi L, et al. Occult spinal dysraphisms in newborns with skin markers: role of ultrasonography and magnetic resonance imaging. Child's Nerv Syst 2018;34(2):285–91.
52. Sardana K, Gupta R, Garg VK, et al. A prospective study of cutaneous manifestations of spinal dysraphism from India. Pediatr Dermatol 2009;26(6):688–95.
53. Altman NR, Altman DH. MR imaging of spinal dysraphism. AJNR Am J Neuroradiol 1987;8(3):533–8.
54. Korsvik HE, Keller MS. Sonography of occult dysraphism in neonates and infants with MR imaging correlation. RadioGraphics 1992;12(2):297–306.

55. Pires CR, Medeiros JMM, Araujo Júnior E, et al. Occult spinal dysraphism in the presence of rare cutaneous stigma in a neonate: importance of ultrasound and magnetic resonance imaging. Case Rep Med 2013;2013:1–4.
56. Dhingani D, Boruah D, Dutta H, et al. Ultrasonography and magnetic resonance imaging evaluation of pediatric spinal anomalies. J Pediatr Neurosci 2016; 11(3):206.
57. Hand JL, Frieden IJ. Vascular birthmarks of infancy: resolving nosologic confusion. Am J Med Genet 2002;108(4):257–64.

Caring for the Child with Spina Bifida

Brandon G. Rocque, MD, MS[a,*], Betsy D. Hopson, MHSA[b], Jeffrey P. Blount, MD[a]

KEYWORDS

• Spina bifida • Myelomeningocele • Hydrocephalus • Chiari 2 malformation
• Transition of care

KEY POINTS

- Prenatal consultation with a specialty team, including maternal-fetal medicine specialists and neurosurgeons, can help parents understand what to expect and can reduce anxiety.
- Fetal myelomeningocele closure has been shown to reduce the rate of hydrocephalus in well-selected patients.
- Hydrocephalus occurs in approximately 80% of children with myelomeningocele. Signs and symptoms of hydrocephalus include headache, vomiting, lethargy, as well as other more subtle symptoms.
- Chiari 2 malformation is present in nearly all children with myelomeningocele. If brainstem symptoms develop, the first priority is to assure that hydrocephalus is adequately treated.
- Interdisciplinary clinics, including neurosurgery, orthopedics, rehabilitation medicine, urology, and other specialists, provide optimal care for children with spina bifida.

INTRODUCTION

Myelomeningocele (MMC) is one of the most complex congenital conditions that pediatricians will provide care for in their practice. It is also the most common, with an annual incidence of approximately 8 to 10 cases per 10,000 live births in North America. The incidence correlates directly with maternal red blood cell folate levels, so folic acid fortification remains an important public health opportunity in parts of the world where fortification still does not occur.

The characteristic lesion in MMC is the open blister–like defect over the spine, but the full spectrum of manifestations is broad and includes both cranial and spinal anomalies. More than 20 structural abnormalities of the nervous system characteristically accompany MMC. More importantly, the aberrant neurologic function arising from these anomalies imparts dysfunction of a variety of normal reflexes that

[a] Division of Pediatric Neurosurgery, Department of Neurosurgery, Children's of Alabama, University of Alabama at Birmingham, 1600 7th Avenue South, Lowder 400, Birmingham, AL 35233, USA; [b] Children's of Alabama, 1600 7th Avenue South, Lowder 400, Birmingham, AL 35233, USA
* Corresponding author.
E-mail address: Brandon.rocque@childrensal.org

Pediatr Clin N Am 68 (2021) 915–927
https://doi.org/10.1016/j.pcl.2021.04.013

predominantly but not exclusively affect the lower extremities and sphincters (bowel/bladder). As such there are a wide variety of clinical manifestations of MMC. Children often have multiple health concerns that require care from many medical disciplines, including Neurosurgery, Urology, Orthopedics, Physical Medicine and Rehabilitation, Developmental Pediatrics, and Sleep Medicine as well as Orthotists, Nurse Clinicians and Physical, and Occupational and Speech Therapists. Because of the complexity of care and the inherent interconnectedness of problems, care coordination is the central concept for the most highly effective clinics.

The pediatrician plays a crucial role in care of children with MMC. Although multidisciplinary clinics may be optimally designed to provide for the common needs that are specific to children with MMC, children with this condition also must have a primary care provider (PCP). Children with MMC and other forms of spina bifida require routine well-child care, as well as care for conditions that are outside the expertise of the specialists. Naturally, the PCP assures a holistic, patient-centered approach to care that can be at risk in highly subspecialized care models. The purpose of this chapter is to review the neurosurgical care of children with MMC, focusing on information that a PCP should be familiar with to serve as partner in the child's comprehensive care team.

DEFINITIONS

Spina bifida is a nonspecific term that refers to many distinct abnormalities of the spinal cord. Another collective term that is used for this family of conditions is spinal dysraphism. Fundamentally, all of these abnormalities are problems of the embryologic development of the spinal cord. The most severe type is MMC. This is caused by a failure of the primary closure of the neural tube, leading to an open neural placode on the infant's back, with no overlying skin coverage (**Fig. 1**). Neurologic function below the level of the lesion is lost—this is the most common type of spinal dysraphism. The term "spina bifida" is often used colloquially to describe MCC. However, for the purposes of this manuscript, the authors refer to open, non–skin covered spinal dysraphism as MMC.

Closed types of spinal dysraphism are caused by several different embryologic abnormalities. These abnormalities can be dramatic and obvious at birth, such as a large terminal myelocystocele (**Fig. 2**). Or they might show no outward signs of abnormality. **Table 1** shows many different types of congenital abnormalities that fall under the

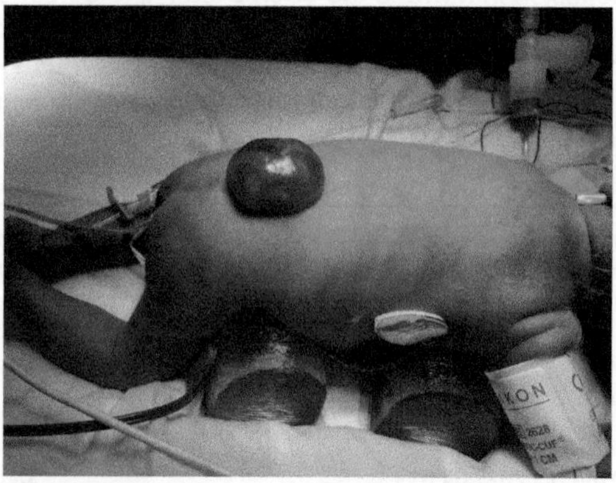

Fig. 1. A child with a cystic myelomeningocele.

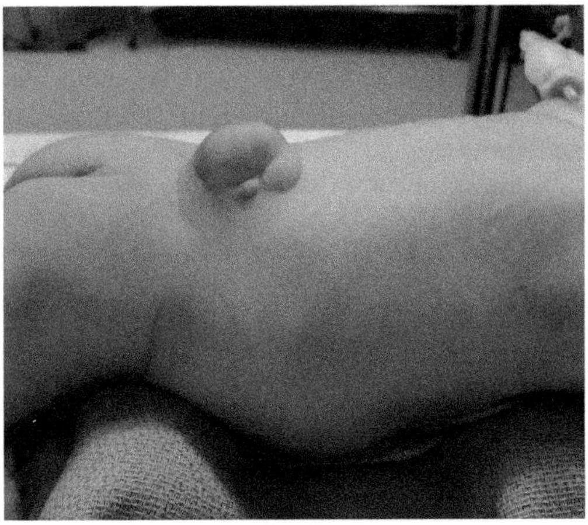

Fig. 2. A child with a skin-covered terminal myelocystocele.

broad term "spina bifida." Most of this chapter focuses on the care of children with MMC, with discussion of some specific issues surrounding other types of spina bifida. For a more detailed discussion of occult spinal dysraphism, the reader is referred to *Chapter 14: Cutaneous stigmata of the spine: a review of indications for imaging and referral*.

DIAGNOSIS

Prenatal Diagnosis

Initial diagnosis of MMC is usually triggered by elevated alpha-fetoprotein (AFP) level in maternal serum, performed for screening early in the second trimester. AFP is elevated in about 80% of cases. Diagnosis is confirmed on second trimester ultrasound, between the 18th and 24th week of gestation. High-resolution ultrasound is

Table 1
Types of spinal dysraphism

Diagnosis	Characteristics	Other Terms
Open Spinal Dysraphism		
Myelomeningocele	Open spinal cord, no skin covering	Spina bifida aperta
Closed Spinal Dysraphism		
Lipomyelomeningocele	Fatty mass, skin covered	Spinal lipoma
Split cord malformation	Duplicated spinal cord, focal hypertrichosis (hairy patch)	Diastematomyelia, diplomyelia
Terminal myelocystocele	Fluid-filled mass, skin covered	
Dermal sinus tract	Sacral dimple	Fibrovascular tract
Limited dorsal myeloschisis	Sacral dimple	Meningocele manqué
Neurenteric cyst	Ventral attachment to spinal cord, minimal cutaneous findings	
Spina bifida occulta	Incomplete closure of posterior bony arch of lower lumbar vertebrae. No clinical consequences	

often able to distinguish open MMC from other types of spina bifida, determine the anatomic level of the abnormality, and determine the presence of associated findings such as hydrocephalus. The Spina Bifida Association recommends that parents with a new diagnosis of MMC undergo prompt consultation with specialists who are dedicated to providing care to individuals with MMC and will be part of their long-term care team.[1] This consultation is often done with a collaborative, interdisciplinary approach to review the expectations for initial newborn management, including surgical closure of the defect as well as the long-term expectations for function.

Estimation of Lesion Level

Although it is impossible to predict a child's neurologic outcome before birth, there are generalizations that can be made based on the type of spina bifida and the anatomic level of the abnormality seen on ultrasound. Ultrasound-based estimation of the anatomic location of the lesion is typically accurate within 1 to 2 spinal levels. Therefore, estimations about future functions, such as ambulation and bowel and bladder function, can be provided during prenatal discussions. **Table 2** provides information about the likelihood of community ambulation for each functional lesion level for children with spina bifida.

This is a time of high anxiety for families. Learning accurate information can ameliorate some of the fear surrounding the diagnosis. The care team during the prenatal period can also aid the family in determining if they are a good candidate for prenatal MMC closure.

PRENATAL CLOSURE OF MYELOMENINGOCELE

Publication of the Management of Myelomeningocele Study (MOMS) in 2011 was a watershed moment for neurosurgical care of children with MMC. MOMS was a randomized controlled trial comparing standard open MMC closure with fetal repair.[2] The primary outcome was a composite of death or development of hydrocephalus requiring surgical treatment. Final results showed significantly fewer children reaching the composite endpoint in the fetal surgery group versus the standard care group. More impressively, although 82% of children in the postnatal surgery group underwent ventriculoperitoneal shunt placement for hydrocephalus, only 40% in the fetal surgery group were shunted. Other observed benefits to fetal surgery included improvement in motor function, given the anatomic level of the MMC defect, less severe hindbrain herniation (Chiari 2 malformation), and improved cognitive function. Fetal surgery was also associated with a higher rate of preterm delivery and uterine dehiscence than postnatal repair.

Based on these largely favorable results, many programs have developed fetal surgery centers, and the technique for fetal surgery has continued to evolve.[2–5] On the

Table 2
Myelomeningocele lesion level definition and likelihood of community ambulation

Lesion Level	Definition	Likelihood of Community Ambulation (%)
Thoracic	Flaccid lower extremities	<1
High-lumbar	Hip flexion present	7
Midlumbar	Knee extension present	44
Low-lumbar	Foot extension (dorsiflexion) present	79
Sacral	Foot plantar flexion present	95

other hand, the MOMS trial had very strict inclusion criteria. At many current centers, patients who would not have been candidates for enrollment may be offered fetal surgery. In addition, long-term follow-up shows that there may be unintended consequences for mothers after fetal surgery, such as problems with subsequent pregnancies. Detailed discussion of the nuances of fetal surgery is beyond the scope of this text. However, it is crucial for pediatricians to know that the option for fetal repair exists and that parents who are considering fetal surgery should be referred for specialist consultation.

PERINATAL CARE OF MYELOMENINGOCELE

Obstetric Care

For the infant who is not undergoing fetal surgery, routine obstetric care is delivered throughout the third trimester. Current recommendation is for scheduled cesarean delivery at 37 or 38 weeks.[6] However, this remains an area of controversy, and vaginal delivery remains a viable option. Although strong practice preferences exist in obstetrics, high-quality evidence demonstrating clear superiority of one route of delivery over another does not exist. Parents should be encouraged to discuss these issues with their obstetricians.

Neonatal Care and Myelomeningocele Surgery

After delivery, the child with MMC is admitted to the neonatal intensive care unit. Screening for other congenital abnormalities is typically performed, including echocardiogram and renal ultrasound. Surgical closure of the MMC defect is performed within 24 to 48 hours of birth. Before surgical closure, the child should be positioned prone, and the exposed placode kept covered and moist. Technical details of surgical closure are beyond the scope of this text, but briefly, the goals are to close the dura and skin over the neural elements. With large MMC defects, various techniques may be necessary to achieve adequate coverage of the defect with skin closure.[7]

Children born with a skin-covered lesion or closed form of spina bifida often will not have an initial surgery while in the neonatal intensive care unit; however, it is recommended that these children undergo similar monitoring and education to establish future treatment plans. Bowel and bladder management should be discussed even in the cases where surgical intervention is delayed.

NEUROSURGICAL CARE FOR THE CHILD WITH MYELOMENINGOCELE

The neurosurgical care of children with MMC centers around 3 distinct conditions with potential surgical treatment: hydrocephalus, Chiari 2 malformation, and tethered spinal cord.

Hydrocephalus

Incidence

Hydrocephalus is an abnormal accumulation of cerebrospinal fluid in the ventricles of the brain. It is the most common condition treated by pediatric neurosurgeons. Although there are many causes of hydrocephalus that differ in prevalence, MMC is one of the most common causes of hydrocephalus. Published data from small series note that hydrocephalus develops in 50% to 90% of children with MMC. In a national sample of more than 4000 children, enrolled in the National Spina Bifida Patient Registry (NSBPR), 80% of children had hydrocephalus requiring surgical treatment.[8] Furthermore, children with higher lesion level (thoracic or upper lumbar functional level) were found to have greater odds of having hydrocephalus compared with lower levels. It is very uncommon for closed spinal dysraphism (non-MMC forms of spina bifida) to be associated with hydrocephalus.

The primary outcome from the MOMS trial of fetal MMC closure was a complex composite outcome including death, cognitive test scores, and meeting criteria for the treatment of hydrocephalus. The trial was stopped early due to significantly better results in the fetal surgery group. A simple examination of the proportion of children who were treated for hydrocephalus in each group illustrates the important point: 40% of children with fetal surgery later underwent shunt placement for treatment of hydrocephalus compared with 82% in the postnatal surgery group.[2] Therefore, one of the primary potential benefits of fetal surgery is reduction in the need for treatment of hydrocephalus.

Signs and symptoms in infants

In infants, before closure of the cranial sutures, hydrocephalus produces characteristic signs, most importantly accelerated head growth and bulging of the anterior fontanelle (**Fig. 3**). Additional signs and symptoms may include impaired eye movements, especially paralysis of upward gaze, apnea or bradycardia, lethargy, and vomiting. The most severe symptom of hydrocephalus in newborns with MMC is stridor, which may exist in isolation or may accompany other signs of bulbar dysfunction, such as poor swallowing or secretion control. Inspiratory stridor in the newborn with MMC is a clinically urgent sign of brainstem distress. The acute threat is laryngeal dysfunction and respiratory obstruction from relaxation of the vocal cords. Hydrocephalus is a global stressor for the compromised nervous system, which is thought to tip a tenuous system out of balance and result in brainstem failure. This brainstem failure becomes manifest as stridor, a sirenlike wailing cry, and impairment of management of normal oral secretions. Therefore, stridor in an infant with MMC is considered an urgent indication for hydrocephalus treatment.

Signs and symptoms in older children

In older children, with fused cranial sutures, the primary symptoms of hydrocephalus are headache, nausea/vomiting, and lethargy. Importantly, children with MMC may have additional symptoms of hydrocephalus that are not common in children without MMC. These can include lower cranial nerve dysfunction, sleep apnea, swallowing dysfunction, or leakage of cerebrospinal fluid (CSF) from the MMC closure site. As stridor, lower cranial nerve dysfunction, swallowing problems, and sleep apnea are likely consequences of vulnerability of the brainstem, which is a result of the Chiari 2 malformation. When a child with MMC displays these symptoms, the first line of treatment is directed at hydrocephalus. Surgical decompression of the posterior fossa (Chiari 2

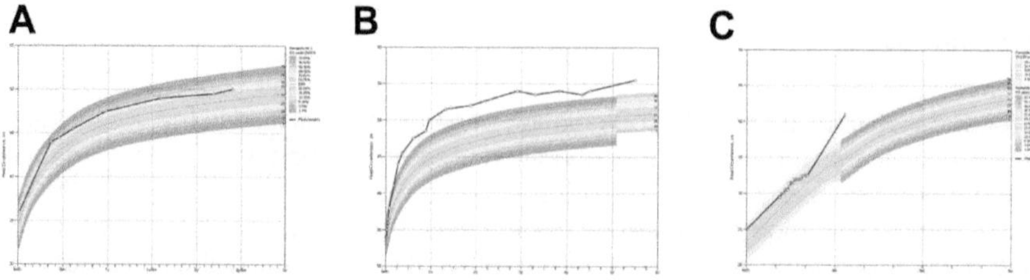

Fig. 3. (*A*) A normal head growth curve. (*B*) A macrocephalic but reassuring head growth curve. Note that although this represents a larger-than-average head, the growth trajectory is parallel to the normal curve. (*C*) A concerning head growth curve, with head growth trajectory crossing percentiles.

decompression) is only indicated once adequate treatment of hydrocephalus has been assured. In an older child or adolescent with MMC, inadequately treated hydrocephalus may also present as neck or back pain (**Table 3**).

Treatment

Ventriculoperitoneal shunting. The goal of hydrocephalus treatment is to maximize the growth and development potential of the child's brain. The mainstay of treatment is the ventriculoperitoneal (VP) shunt. A VP shunt consists of a ventricular catheter, a valve that regulates CSF flow and a distal catheter placed into the peritoneum. The VP shunt was invented and first used in the 1950s and has revolutionized the care of children with hydrocephalus. Before shunting, 90% of children born with hydrocephalus could be expected to die before age 10 years, and the other 10% were at high risk for severe developmental delay. Now, the goal for a newborn with hydrocephalus is their brain development and function to be as close to normal as possible (although possibly limited by other conditions). It should be noted that for many children with MMC, even when hydrocephalus is adequately treated, there are learning challenges. Nonverbal learning disorders, problems with fine motor skills, and behavioral difficulties are common.[9] Pediatricians should be aware of these commonly associated conditions, as children may benefit from focused academic assistance.

Although shunts are highly beneficial overall, they have shortcomings. Most importantly, shunts can become obstructed or disconnected, known as shunt failure. For reasons that are not entirely clear, shunt failure is more common in younger children.[10] However, shunt failure can occur at any age, throughout the lifetime. Shunt failure leads to symptoms of elevated intracranial pressure, as described earlier. Symptoms of shunt failure differ from one child to the next, even for multiple shunt failures in the same child. For some children, shunt failure may manifest with subtle symptoms, such as mild headache or decline in school performance. For others, shunt failure may be life threatening, with coma onset within minutes or hours. Most commonly, in a child who has multiple shunt failures, the failures will have similar symptoms. However, it is possible that a child will have different symptoms from one failure to the next. Therefore, providers caring for these children must be vigilant for all signs of shunt failure.

Table 3
Signs and symptoms of hydrocephalus

Infants	• Increasing head circumference • Vomiting/poor feeding tolerance • Irritability • Lethargy • Bulging fontanelle • Separated cranial sutures • Impaired eye movements (upgaze palsy) • Apnea or bradycardia
Older Children	• Headache • Nausea/vomiting • Lethargy • Bradycardia/hypertension • Eye movement abnormalities
Symptoms Unique to Myelomeningocele	• Stridor (infants) • Neck pain • Back pain

For most children, if the shunt fails, the cerebral ventricles will become larger. However, in some cases, there is no change in ventricle size. In these cases, the clinical presentation alone must guide decisions about surgical exploration of the shunt. A more detailed discussion of hydrocephalus can be found in Chapter 8: *Hydrocephalus and the Primary Care Provider.*

Endoscopic third ventriculostomy. Endoscopic third ventriculostomy (ETV) is an alternative procedure for treating hydrocephalus that does not require implanted hardware. ETV involves the use of a neuroendoscope to make a fenestration of the floor of the third ventricle, allowing passage of CSF from the ventricle into the prepontine cistern. Traditionally, ETV was used only as a treatment of obstructive hydrocephalus, such as that caused by posterior fossa tumors or stenosis of the cerebral aqueduct. The most important limitation of ETV is that it does not successfully treat hydrocephalus in all patients. Younger children and those whose hydrocephalus is caused by intraventricular hemorrhage or MMC are less likely to be adequately treated by ETV.[11] Recently, with the addition of choroid plexus cauterization (CPC), the combined procedure (ETC/CPC) has been shown to be successful in up to 70% of children with MMC.[12] Again, a more detailed discussion of ETV and ETV/CPC can be found in Chapter 8: *Hydrocephalus and the Primary Care Provider*. Children treated with ETV are not cured of their hydrocephalus, but rather they depend on the patent ETV channel. Therefore, they could become symptomatic if the ETV were to close. Although this is less common than shunt failure, it is still important to consider hydrocephalus as a possible problem, should these children develop symptoms that would be concerning for shunt failure.

Clinics Care Points

- Pediatricians should be aware of the signs and symptoms of hydrocephalus, in particular those that are unique to children with MMC, such as stridor.
- Pediatricians should recognize that these children are always at risk for recurrence of symptoms.
- Any signs or symptoms that are possibly related to hydrocephalus should be evaluated by a neurosurgeon.

Chiari 2 Malformation

The Chiari 2 malformation was originally described by Hans Chiari, along with his descriptions of other forms of hindbrain abnormalities that now bear his name.[13] The Chiari 2 malformation is fundamentally different from the Chiari 1 malformation, which is discussed elsewhere in this text (*Chapter 7: Chiari malformation*). According to the unified theory originally proposed by McLone, the open neural tube in MMC allows for venting of CSF during gestation. Therefore, the posterior fossa does not expand to its normal proportions, resulting in displacement of hindbrain tissue (brainstem and cerebellum) outside of the foramen magnum.[14] In addition to hindbrain herniation, there are numerous anatomic abnormalities that have been described as part of the Chiari 2 malformation, including beak shape of the midbrain tectum, interdigitation of the cerebral gyri, and disproportionate dilation of the posterior horns of the lateral ventricles (colpocephaly). It is typically thought that, although the degree of hindbrain herniation may vary, all children with MMC are born with some degree of Chiari 2 malformation present.

Signs and symptoms

The clinical manifestations of the Chiari 2 malformation can generally be attributed to abnormalities of the function of the brainstem. Symptoms include stridor, vocal cord paralysis, opisthotonos, sleep-disordered breathing (SDB), swallowing difficulties, absent gag reflex, or other lower cranial nerve palsies. In general, the severity of hindbrain herniation seen on imaging studies does not correlate with the severity of symptoms. Therefore, attention to the clinical situation is far more important than the imaging appearance of the posterior fossa.

In infants with MMC, one of the most important clinical signs to recognize is inspiratory stridor. Stridor in this setting is thought to occur because of impairment of vocal cord function, leading to adducted vocal cords on inspiration. There are many causes of stridor in infants.[15] Pediatricians and pediatric emergency medicine physicians may be accustomed to evaluating an infant with stridor. However, in the setting of MMC, stridor is typically considered a harbinger of potentially life-threatening brain stem dysfunction. Urgent neurosurgical evaluation and treatment is indicated.[16]

Treatment

First-line therapy for brainstem-related symptoms in children with MMC is always directed at assuring adequate treatment of hydrocephalus. The presence of elevated intracranial pressure from undertreated hydrocephalus is thought to place additional stress on the brainstem and lead to Chiari 2 symptoms. If symptoms persist, despite adequate hydrocephalus treatment, direct decompression of the Chiari 2 malformation can be performed, which involves surgical removal of the bone of the posterior foramen magnum, the posterior arch of the C1 vertebra, and sometimes additional removal of more caudal lamina. There is ongoing debate about whether expansile duraplasty in addition to bony decompression is beneficial. In a national sample of more than 4000 children with MMC, approximately 10% had undergone Chiari 2 decompression surgery.[17] More rostral lesion levels (thoracic level MMC, more than lumbar level, more than sacral level) were more likely to have undergone Chiari 2 decompression. This study, based on a large sample, also showed that children who underwent Chiari 2 decompression when younger than 2 years were more likely to also require tracheostomy. One interpretation of this finding is that some children with MMC have a congenitally dysfunctional brainstem, leading them to require tracheostomy for airway protection regardless of other interventions. Nevertheless, the treatment algorithm for Chiari 2 symptoms in modern use remains as follows: (1) treat hydrocephalus, (2) decompress Chari 2 malformation, and (3) consider additional support such as tracheostomy as needed.

It has recently been recognized that children with MMC may be at high risk for SDB[18,19]; this is another likely manifestation of the Chiari 2 malformation. Pediatricians should be alert for symptoms such as snoring, excessive daytime sleepiness, or irritability. However, even in the absence of these symptoms, because of the high prevalence of SDB among children with MMC, referral for screening polysomnography may be indicated.

Clinics Care Points

- Pediatricians should be aware of the manifestations of the Chiari 2 malformation, such as stridor, cranial nerve dysfunction, swallowing difficulties, or sleep apnea.
- There should be a low threshold for referral to neurosurgery if any of these symptoms are noted.

Tethered Cord

Definition

Tethered spinal cord, or tethered cord, refers to the concept that the spinal cord naturally exists within the thecal sac, bathed in CSF, and without any significant attachment to the surrounding tissue. Any type of spinal dysraphism can act as an attachment of the spinal cord to the surrounding structures, thus "tethering" the cord. The prevailing theory is that a differential between spinal growth or lengthening and somatic growth then results in traction on the tethered spinal cord, leading to a loss of function. When this manifests clinically, it is usually with back pain, leg pain, or loss of neurologic function in the legs and/or bladder.[20,21] In the case of MMC, the initial closure of the back is typically performed within 1 to 2 days of birth, but scar at the site of closure can result in spinal cord tethering later in life.

Diagnosis

For children with MMC, imaging studies are not useful in determining whether a spinal cord is tethered. Essentially all MRI scans of children who have a history of MMC closure will seem to be "tethered." Thus, the determination of whether a patient is experiencing a clinically relevant tethered cord must be made based on signs and symptoms alone. As noted earlier, typical symptoms are back pain, leg pain, and neurologic deficit referable to the caudal spinal cord, typically leg weakness or sensory loss or loss of bladder function (**Box 1**).

Treatment

Surgical treatment of tethered cord is referred to as tethered cord release (TCR). This procedure has wide variability in risk profile, depending on the complexity of the tethering lesion. Therefore, decisions about whether to undertake a TCR in any given patient must consider the severity and progressive nature of the symptoms as well as the anatomy of the tethering lesion. Furthermore, there must be clear understanding between surgeon and patient/family about the goals of surgical treatment. In general, surgical untethering is effective at relieving back and leg pain and for arresting progression of deficit but not effective at reversing neurologic deficit. Therefore, outside of surgeries performed because of pain, the TCR is a prophylactic operation, performed to reduce the risk of worsening function. Careful explanation of these factors is crucial for appropriate shared decision-making when considering a TCR in a patient.

Clinics Care Points

- Tethering of the spinal cord can occur after initial closure of MMC.
- Surgical release of the tethered cord can be performed to alleviate pain or prevent worsening neurologic function.

Interdisciplinary Spina Bifida Care

The Spina Bifida Guidelines produced by the Spina Bifida Association places a strong emphasis on interdisciplinary lifespan care for individuals with spina bifida.[22] Lifespan care can be characterized as a mechanism for delivering care where the provider embraces the idea that, although they might not be involved in the individual's care throughout their entire lifespan, the care that is delivered will affect the patient across the lifespan. Therefore, every effort should be made to promote independence and overall wellness and to empower the patient to reach their highest potential and quality of life. This care is optimal when delivered longitudinally across a continuum that begins during the prenatal consultation and continues through pediatric and then eventually to transition into adult years.[23]

A multidisciplinary approach is recognized as best practice among spina bifida clinics throughout North America. Most clinics include Neurosurgery, Urology, Orthopedics, Physical Medicine and Rehabilitation, and Development Pediatrics. A collaborative interdisciplinary approach to care has been linked to improved health

Box 1
Signs and symptoms of tethered spinal cord

- Back pain
- Leg pain
- Leg weakness
- Worsening of bladder function
- Decreased leg sensation
- Scoliosis

outcomes, decreased morbidity and mortality, and decreased cost of care for individuals with spina bifida.[24] A central component of multidisciplinary care includes the access to individualized care coordinator. Quality care coordination is an essential part of the multidisciplinary care team. The coordinator is often the link between the community pediatrician and the specialist medical team.

Transitional Care

In the United States there are 1500 new births of children with spina bifida every year, and 75% of those children will now survive well into adulthood.[25] Transition of care is not unique to individuals with spina bifida. There are many individuals with chronic conditions of childhood surviving into adulthood, which has resulted in the establishment of transition as a core outcome in the Healthy People Maternal Child Health Bureau (MCHB), as well as a focus of the American Academy of Pediatrics (AAP). The AAP has embraced the importance of good transitional care and has provided guidance and leadership under the "Got Transition?" initiative. Transition of care is a process that begins early in adolescence and involves more than transferring care and/or changing providers. Health care transition is defined as the organized process of supporting youth in acquiring independent health care skills, preparing for an adult model of care, and transferring to new providers without disruption of care. The goal of health care transition is to optimize health and assist youth in reaching their full potential.

This process of health care transition involves working with youth and their families/caretakers beginning by age 13 to 14 years. The care changes from a "pediatric" model of care where the parents make most of the decisions to an "adult" model of care where youth being taking responsibility for their decision-making and self-care. Transition of care has evolved and grown into a separate domain in Pediatric care for which the details exceed the scope of this chapter. However, a recognition that all efforts expended by the patient, family, and provider team results in an adult with successful strategies and capabilities to participate in the full range of adult spina bifida care gives rise to an awareness of the overarching importance of transition readiness throughout the scope of care.

DISCLOSURE

The authors have nothing to disclose.

REFERENCES

1. Adzick NS, Thom EA, Spong CY, et al. A randomized trial of prenatal versus postnatal repair of myelomeningocele. N Engl J Med 2011;364(11):993–1004.

2. Belfort MA, Whitehead WE, Shamshirsaz AA, et al. Fetoscopic Repair of Meningomyelocele. Obstet Gynecol 2015;126(4):881–4.
3. Tulipan N, Wellons JC, Thom EA, et al. Prenatal surgery for myelomeningocele and the need for cerebrospinal fluid shunt placement. J Neurosurg Pediatr 2015;16:613–20.
4. Bennett KA, Carroll MA, Shannon CN, et al. Reducing perinatal complications and preterm delivery for patients undergoing in utero closure of fetal myelomeningocele: further modifications to the multidisciplinary surgical technique. J Neurosurg Pediatr 2014;14(1):108–14.
5. Dewan MC, Wellons JC. Fetal surgery for spina bifida. J Neurosurg Pediatr 2019; 24(2):105–14.
6. Luthy DA, Wardinsky T, Shurtleff DB, et al. Cesarean section before the onset of labor and subsequent motor function in infants with meningomyelocele diagnosed antenatally. N Engl J Med 1991;324(10):662–6.
7. Lien SC, Maher CO, Garton HJL, et al. Local and regional flap closure in myelomeningocele repair: a 15-year review. Childs Nerv Syst 2010;26(8):1091–5.
8. Kim I, Hopson B, Aban I, et al. Treated hydrocephalus in individuals with myelomeningocele in the National Spina Bifida Patient Registry. J Neurosurg Pediatr 2018;34(1):1–6.
9. Dennis M, Barnes MA. The cognitive phenotype of spina bifida meningomyelocele. Dev Disabil Res Rev 2010;16(1):31–9.
10. Dupepe EB, Hopson B, Johnston JM, et al. Rate of shunt revision as a function of age in patients with shunted hydrocephalus due to myelomeningocele. Neurosurg Focus 2016;41(5):E6.
11. Kulkarni AV, Drake JM, Kestle JR, et al. Predicting who will benefit from endoscopic third ventriculostomy compared with shunt insertion in childhood hydrocephalus using the ETV Success Score. J Neurosurg Pediatr 2010;6(4):310–5.
12. Warf BC, Campbell JW. Combined endoscopic third ventriculostomy and choroid plexus cauterization as primary treatment of hydrocephalus for infants with myelomeningocele: long-term results of a prospective intent-to-treat study in 115 East African infants. J Neurosurg Pediatr 2008;2(5):310–6.
13. Abd-El-Barr MM, Strong CI, Groff MW. Chiari malformations: diagnosis, treatments and failures. J Neurosurg Sci 2014;58(4):215–21.
14. McLone DG, Knepper PA. The cause of Chiari II malformation: a unified theory. Pediatr Neurosci 1989;15(1):1–12.
15. Bhatt J, Prager JD. Neonatal Stridor: Diagnosis and Management. Clin Perinatol 2018;45(4):817–31.
16. Alford EN, Hopson BD, Safyanov F, et al. Care management and contemporary challenges in spina bifida: a practice preference survey of the American Society of Pediatric Neurosurgeons. J Neurosurg Pediatr 2019;1–10. https://doi.org/10.3171/2019.5.PEDS18738.
17. Kim I, Hopson B, Aban I, et al. Decompression for Chiari malformation type II in individuals with myelomeningocele in the National Spina Bifida Patient Registry. J Neurosurg Pediatr 2018;1–7. https://doi.org/10.3171/2018.5.PEDS18160.
18. Patel DM, Rocque BG, Hopson B, et al. Sleep-disordered breathing in patients with myelomeningocele. J Neurosurg Pediatr 2015;16(1):30–5.
19. Shellhaas RA, Kenia PV, Hassan F, et al. Sleep-Disordered Breathing among Newborns with Myelomeningocele. J Pediatr 2018;194:244–7.e1.
20. Hertzler DA II, DePowell JJ, Stevenson CB, et al. Tethered cord syndrome: a review of the literature from embryology to adult presentation. Neurosurg Focus 2010;29(1):E1.

21. Bowman RM, Mohan A, Ito J, et al. Tethered cord release: a long-term study in 114 patients. J Neurosurg Pediatr 2009;3(3):181–7.
22. Guidelines for the Care of People with Spina Bifida. spinabifidaassociation.org. Available at: https://www.spinabifidaassociation.org/wp-content/uploads/Guidelines-for-the-Care-of-People-with-Spina-Bifida-2018.pdf. Accessed September 30, 2020.
23. Hopson B, Rocque BG, Joseph DB, et al. The development of a lifetime care model in comprehensive spina bifida care. J Pediatr Rehabil Med 2018;11(4):323–34.
24. Kaufman BA, Terbrock A, Winters N, et al. Disbanding a multidisciplinary clinic: effects on the health care of myelomeningocele patients. Pediatr Neurosurg 1994;21(1):36–44.
25. Sawin KJ, Brei TJ, Buran CF, et al. Factors associated with quality of life in adolescents with spina bifida. J Holist Nurs 2002;20(3):279–304.

Review of Tone Management for the Primary Care Provider

Samuel G. McClugage III, MD[a,b], David F. Bauer, MD, MPH[a,b,*]

KEYWORDS

• Spasticity • Dystonia • Cerebral palsy • Intrathecal baclofen • Dorsal rhizotomy
• Pediatric movement disorders

KEY POINTS

- Movement disorders in the pediatric patient population represent a complex spectrum of problems, often overlapping and coexisting, that can lead to severe functional deficits in children, impeding quality of life.
- Cerebral palsy, related to premature birth or perinatal hypoxic injury, represents the most common cause of movement disorders in the pediatric patient population.
- Types of movement disorders in the pediatric patient include spasticity, dystonia, myoclonus, and choreoathetosis, all of which have unique causes and differences, requiring tailored therapy for each.
- The complex and often overlapping nature of the problems in these patients may require evaluation by a multidisciplinary team of practitioners, including physical and occupational therapists, physical medicine and rehabilitation physicians, neurosurgeons, and orthopedic surgeons to best evaluate and tailor individual treatment.

INTRODUCTION

Movement disorders of children encompass a multifocal spectrum of disease, often overlapping, related to underlying issues with development, neonatal, and perinatal insults, and both congenital and pathologic diagnoses. Spasticity and dystonia encompass most of the movement disorders encountered in children. Spasticity is defined as a "*resistance to externally imposed movement with increasing speed of stretch and varies with the direction of joint movement, and/or a resistance to externally imposed movement that rises rapidly above a threshold speed or joint angle*."[1] Dystonia, by comparison, is defined as "*involuntary sustained or intermittent muscle contractions causing twisting and repetitive movements, abnormal postures, or both*."[1] Cerebral

[a] Department of Neurosurgery, Baylor College of Medicine, Houston, TX, USA; [b] Department of Surgery, Division of Pediatric Neurosurgery, Texas Children's Hospital, 6701 Fannin Street, Suite 1230.01, Houston, TX 77030, USA
* Corresponding author.
E-mail address: dfbauer@texaschildrens.org

Pediatr Clin N Am 68 (2021) 929–944
https://doi.org/10.1016/j.pcl.2021.04.018 pediatric.theclinics.com

palsy (CP), a leading cause of spasticity and movement disorders in children, represents a collection of distinct disorders that can exhibit spasticity, dyskinesias, or both.[2] CP affects motor functionality, including postural changes and limitations on activities of daily living, but can also include issues with cognition, sensation, verbal speech, and behavior.[2] The prevalence of CP in United States is greater than half a million patients, with an incidence of 1 in 500 births having a diagnosis of CP.[3] CP is primarily associated with preterm birth and low birth weight in infants, but genetic factors have been implicated as a risk factor.[4,5] Motor dysfunction in CP can be further categorized based on the primary component seen in each patient (**Fig. 1**).[6]

The primary focus of treatment is improvement of motor symptoms with an emphasis on improving functionality, ability to ambulate, and ease of activities of daily living. Treatment interventions encompass a variety of medical, surgical, and rehabilitation services, tailored to the individual patient and symptoms, and frequently used in conjunction with one another for synergistic effect. This multifaceted approach demonstrates the importance of multispecialty teams being involved in the care of this patient population, including neurosurgeons, orthopedic surgeons, rehabilitation physicians, physical therapists, and primary care physicians, to ensure adequate evaluation and treatment of the many problems related directly and indirectly to the underlying cause of the movement disorder.

PATHOPHYSIOLOGY OF SPASTIC CEREBRAL PALSY

Spasticity is the most common movement disorder associated with CP, affecting more than 90% of patients.[7] A consistent association exists between the development of spastic CP and preterm birth/low birth weight, which has important implications in terms of the pathophysiology.[8] Spastic CP can, however, develop from any

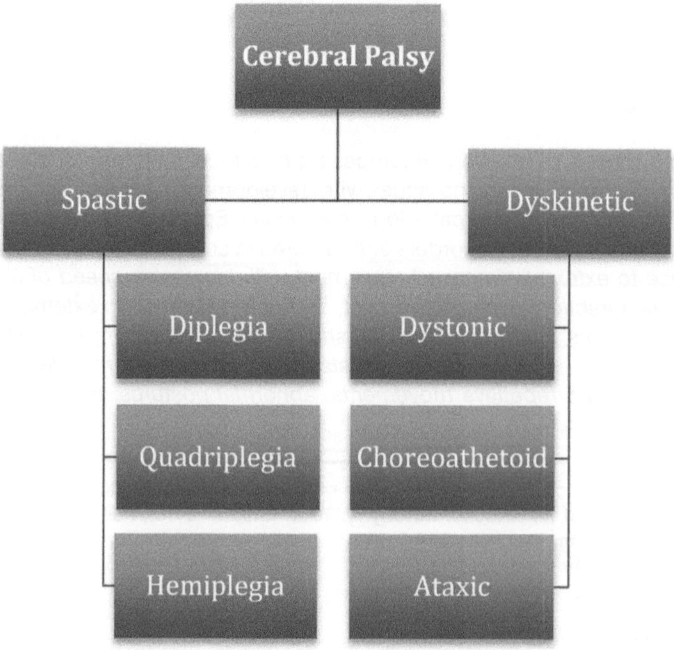

Fig. 1. Types of movement disorders in cerebral palsy.

permanent injury or disorder affecting primary motor pathways in children younger than 3 years.[9] The primary underlying cause of spastic CP results from injury to the upper motor neuron subcortical white matter tracts.[9,10] The most common MRI finding associated with spastic CP is periventricular leukomalacia (PVL) in the periventricular white matter tracts.[11] Spastic diplegia (legs affected more than arms) is the most common form of spastic CP, which makes anatomic sense, given the somatotopic organization of the white matter motor tracts in the periventricular region, with lower extremity motor pathways passing medially through the periventricular white matter (**Fig. 2**). More severe PVL, encompassing larger areas of white matter, can affect other extremity motor pathways, such as arms, resulting in more severe symptoms and spastic quadriplegia.

Symptoms of spasticity result from this primary central upper motor neuron dysfunction, which causes a loss of inhibition in the peripheral motor groups from the corticospinal and reticulospinal tracts, as well as a loss of primary motor function and control.[9] This loss of both primary motor control and secondary inhibitory control from the supratentorial centers results in the velocity-dependent resistance to muscle stretching associated with spasticity.[9] These pathophysiologic mechanisms involved in spasticity are targeted with current treatment options directed at decreasing uninhibited excitatory input (dorsal rhizotomy) or increasing inhibitory neurotransmitter

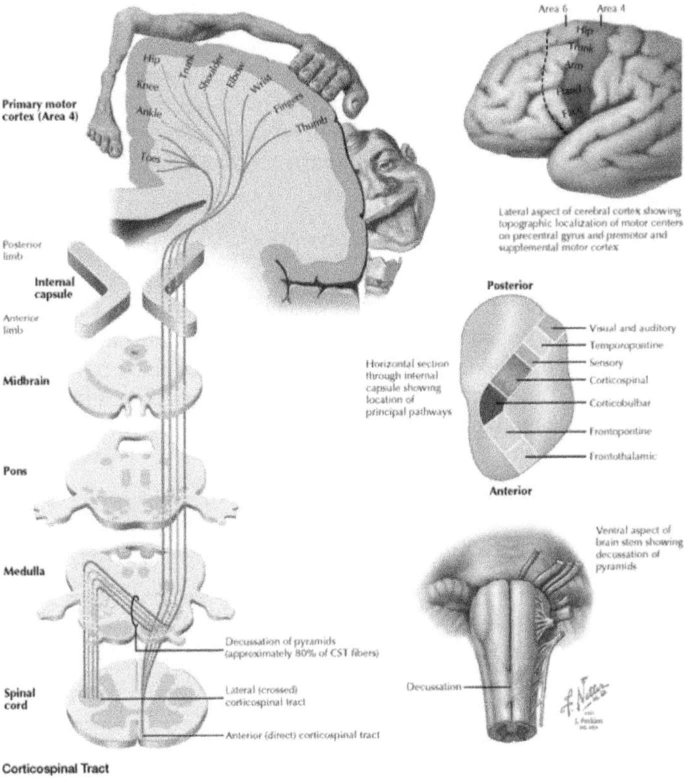

Fig. 2. Somatotopic organization of the corticospinal tract within the periventricular white matter. (*From* H. Royden Jones, Ted M. Burns, Michael J. Aminoff, Scott L. Pomerory. The Netter Collection of Medical Illustrations - Nervous System Part II. 2nd edition. © Saunders 2013; with permission.)

function (oral or intrathecal baclofen). Long-term untreated spasticity can cause fibrotic changes in the involved muscle groups, eventually leading to contractures and fixed deficits of the musculature.[12,13]

ASSOCIATED MEDICAL AND NEUROLOGIC DISORDERS IN SPASTICITY AND CEREBRAL PALSY

CP is associated with several secondary neurologic and general medical problems that are important to identify in the care of patients with spasticity as noted in **Table 1**. Visual disorders are frequently observed in children with CP, and children are often misdiagnosed with a cortical origin of visual impairment, which is untreatable.[14] More frequently, children with CP have very treatable disorders of vision, hence the importance of ophthalmologic evaluation for a thorough evaluation.[14] Aphasia and disorders of speech are common, occurring in 60% to 90% of patients, and correlate with the overall severity of the disease.[15] Epilepsy is a common secondary sequelae of CP, occurring in 15% with mild CP and up to 50% of patients with severe CP.[15,16] Cognitive and behavioral deficits are common and also correlate with severity of disease. Secondary effects of CP are also noted in **Table 1**. As a side effect of the constant muscle contractions seen in spasticity, patients are often malnourished because they require a higher caloric intake than a healthy child of similar age to maintain body weight[17]; this is compounded by other factors that can worsen caloric intake, such as swallowing dysfunction and disorders of cognition. Because of this, patients require evaluation by a nutritionist and frequently need gastrostomy tube placement. It is important to note that any systemic or local infection can temporarily worsen symptoms of spasticity and reduce the effectiveness of medications or intrathecal baclofen therapy. Patients presenting with symptoms of baclofen withdrawal or increased tone despite maintaining their normal medical therapy for tone control should be evaluated for other medical issues as a possible cause.

Clinical Evaluation of Patients with Spasticity

An important first step in the evaluation of a pediatric patient with a movement disorder includes classification of the tone abnormality as spastic, dystonic, choreoathetoid, ataxic, or mixed. Spasticity typically affects flexor muscles and muscles of internal rotation more than extensors, resulting in characteristic patterns of posture within the extremities. The most common classification for overall function is the Gross Motor Function Classification System (GMFCS) (**Fig. 3**), which evaluates a child's

Table 1
Sequelae of cerebral palsy

Primary	Secondary
Visual impairment	Pressure sores
Hearing impairment	Increased risk of bony fractures
Disorders of sensation/proprioception	Scoliosis
Epilepsy	Joint dislocations
Aphasia	Malnutrition
Developmental delay/cognitive deficits	Frequent infections (UTI, pneumonia)
Urinary dysfunction	Renal dysfunction
Dysphagia	Chronic pain

Abbreviation: UIT, urinary tract infection.

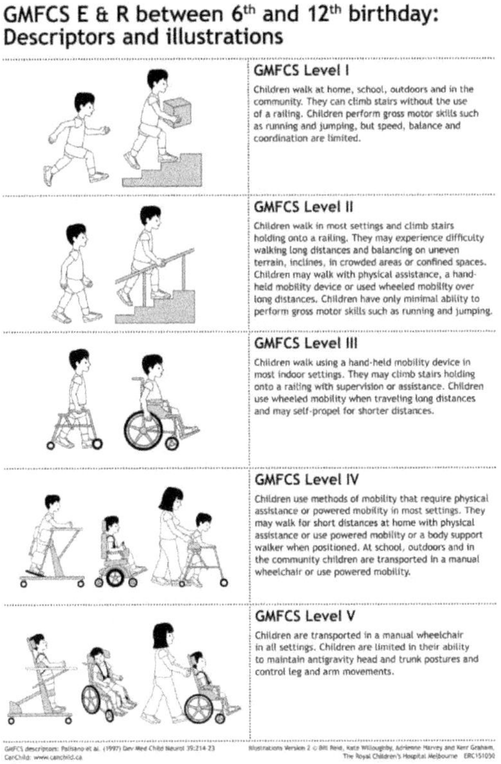
GMFCS E & R between 6th and 12th birthday: Descriptors and illustrations
GMFCS Level I
Children walk at home, school, outdoors and in the community. They can climb stairs without the use of a railing. Children perform gross motor skills such as running and jumping, but speed, balance and coordination are limited.
GMFCS Level II
Children walk in most settings and climb stairs holding onto a railing. They may experience difficulty walking long distances and balancing on uneven terrain, inclines, in crowded areas or confined spaces. Children may walk with physical assistance, a hand-held mobility device or used wheeled mobility over long distances. Children have only minimal ability to perform gross motor skills such as running and jumping.
GMFCS Level III
Children walk using a hand-held mobility device in most indoor settings. They may climb stairs holding onto a railing with supervision or assistance. Children use wheeled mobility when traveling long distances and may self-propel for shorter distances.
GMFCS Level IV
Children use methods of mobility that require physical assistance or powered mobility in most settings. They may walk for short distances at home with physical assistance or use powered mobility or a body support walker when positioned. At school, outdoors and in the community children are transported in a manual wheelchair or use powered mobility.
GMFCS Level V
Children are transported in a manual wheelchair in all settings. Children are limited in their ability to maintain antigravity head and trunk postures and control leg and arm movements.

Fig. 3. The gross motor function classification system. (Copyright Bill Reid, Kate Willoughby, Adrienne Harvey, and Kerr Graham, The Royal Children's Hospital Melbourne.)

ability to undertake normal daily tasks and the assistance required to do so.[18] The Modified Ashworth Scale is useful to assess tone specific to individual muscle groups and is used to assess the benefits of treatment over time (**Table 2**).[19] Imaging studies are not typically necessary in the evaluation of CP or spasticity; however, they can be

Table 2
Modified Ashworth scale

Score	Description
0	No increase in muscle tone
1	Slight increase in muscle tone, manifested by a catch and release or by minimal resistance at the end of the range of motion when the affected part is moved in flexion or extension
1+	Slight increase in muscle tone, manifested by a catch, followed by minimal resistance throughout the remainder (less than half) of the range of motion
2	More marked increase in muscle tone through most of the range of motion, but affected part is easily moved
3	Considerable increase in muscle tone, passive movement difficult
4	Affected part rigid in flexion or extension

Adapted from Bohannon RW and Smith MB. Interrater reliability of a modified Ashworth scale of muscle spasticity, *Phys. Ther.* Feb 1987 67(2) 206-7.

helpful when the diagnosis is unclear. Brain MRI findings typically show PVL in mild cases and cystic encephalomalacia in more severe cases.[11,15] Gait analysis can be useful in ambulatory children undergoing preoperative planning, and it can help determine the complex interplay between affected and unaffected muscles and joints.[20] Community ambulators with spasticity often use both affected and unaffected muscles to walk and stand upright, meaning that surgical treatment of spasticity may be detrimental to their ambulation if a careful evaluation and gait analysis has not been completed before surgery.

TONE MANAGEMENT IN SPASTICITY

Treatment of spasticity is optimized through the use of a multidisciplinary team of providers, working in conjunction, to determine an individualized plan for each patient. Treatment differs for each patient and is determined by the muscle groups involved, severity of the disease, goals of care, and the individualized needs of the patient and their family. Treatments are often combined to provide synergistic effect, such as Botulinum toxin (Botox) injections used in conjunction with bracing and physical therapy to improve tone.[9] Therapeutic options for spasticity include physical therapy, orthotic bracing, oral medications, intramuscular injections, and surgical interventions. Early surgical treatment of spasticity that is refractory to medical management is often advocated to address spasticity before permanent contractures and muscle fibrosis have developed,[9] which is typically when younger than 6 years and can often be considered as early as 2 or 3 years of age.

PHYSICAL THERAPY AND NONPHARMACOLOGIC INTERVENTIONS IN SPASTICITY

Physical therapy represents a mainstay of treatment of spasticity, and all patients should undergo evaluation with physical therapists, occupational therapists, speech therapists, and physical medicine and rehabilitation physicians at an early age. The goals of physical therapy include the following:

- Improve joint flexibility
- Increase muscle strength and conditioning
- Determine appropriate bracing and assist devices
- Improve the performance of activities of daily living
- Aid ambulation

Any pharmacologic or surgical treatments are reliant on physical therapy to help maximize their effects. Bracing and splinting is used primarily to prevent muscle shortening, reduce and prevent contractures, and improve functionality after surgery or percutaneous intervention. Bracing can also be used in the lower extremities to provide support for ambulation, such as ankle foot orthoses. Serial casting is used to increase muscle length in a spastic extremity, whereas temporary splinting serves to retain muscle length at a stable level.

PHARMACOLOGIC OPTIONS FOR SPASTICITY TREATMENT

Oral medications are typically first-line treatment of global tone management. These medications are typically used in patients with increased tone in multiple muscle groups as opposed to isolated tone issues. Appropriate patient selection is important, as initiating a medication to globally decrease tone may actually be detrimental to the performance of some activities of daily living (ADLs). The most common oral medications used in tone control include gamma aminobutyric acid (GABA) agonists and muscle relaxers, such as baclofen, diazepam, and tizanidine. Baclofen, a $GABA_B$ agonist, is the mainstay treatment of global tone disorders. It acts by increasing the centrally acting inhibitory reflex arcs within the spinal cord.[21] Dosage is titrated for effect, weighed against the side effects seen at increasing doses, such as somnolence, respiratory depression, hypotonia, and confusion.[21] Abrupt discontinuation of baclofen can cause severe withdrawal symptoms, such as hypertonia, fevers, seizures, and altered mental status, and baclofen must be tapered to avoid these complications.[22] Tizanidine is a centrally acting alpha-2 adrenergic agonist, which modulates excitatory neurotransmitter release. Diazepam is a benzodiazepine, which modulates $GABA_A$, has proven benefits in relieving spasms and decreasing tone in children.[23] Dantrolene is less commonly used currently, as studies have shown limited efficacy, but it has an increased effectiveness when used with diazepam.[24,25]

INTRAMUSCULAR INJECTIONS FOR NEUROMUSCULAR BLOCKADE IN SPASTICITY

Intramuscular injections providing neuromuscular blockade are used to treat focal spasticity and increased tone but can be used in patients with global spasticity to treat specific muscles. Botulinum toxin A (BTA), alcohol, and phenol have all been used with reasonable reductions in tone; however, alcohol and phenol have fallen out of favor, given a better side effect profile and improved efficacy with Botulinum toxin.[26] Neuromuscular blockade with Botulinum toxin weakens muscle contractions by blocking acetylcholine release at the neuromuscular junction, leading to improvement in tone. Frequently, BTA is used in conjunction with bracing, splinting, and physical therapy to help maintain muscle lengthening and relaxation after treatment. For example, BTA treatment of spastic muscles can be used to reduce tone, which allows for strengthening with physical therapy for the related antagonistic and unaffected muscle groups. Treatment is generally repeated in at least 3-month intervals, as needed, to avoid antibody formation and maintain efficacy.[27]

ORTHOPEDIC PROCEDURES FOR SPASTICITY

Many surgical procedures have been used for the management of secondary orthopedic deformities caused by chronic spasticity. Most commonly, orthopedic surgeons address focal fixed deformity in muscles and joints that have undergone fibrotic changes, preventing a benefit from less invasive measures such as oral medications, bracing, or injections. A list of common orthopedic sequelae seen in CP and the associated treatments are listed in **Table 3**. Previously, these orthopedic procedures were generally done on an individual or limited basis, as problems arose with particular muscle groups or joints at a single level. More recently, the concept of single-event multilevel surgery (SEMLS) has gained support, meaning that multiple orthopedic procedures are performed at multiple levels on both lower extremities under the same anesthesia.[28] SEMLS has the advantage of grouping multiple procedures under one hospital stay and one rehabilitation period, to minimize the need for multiple procedures with multiple instances of anesthesia over time, with the goal to maximize benefit from a rehabilitation standpoint.[28]

NEUROSURGICAL PROCEDURES FOR SPASTICITY

There are 2 main surgical treatments for spasticity: intrathecal baclofen (ITB) pump and dorsal rhizotomy. Treatments are typically reserved for patients with either spastic diplegia or spastic quadriplegia, and surgical decision-making must include the functional status of the patient and goals of the parent and child. In general, selective

Table 3
Common orthopedic sequelae of cerebral palsy and treatment options

Orthopedic Deformity	Treatment
Clubfoot deformity	Achilles tendon lengthening Gastrocnemius muscle lengthening Anterior tibialis tendon transfer Foot or limb osteotomies
Hamstring contractures	Hamstring lengthening
Hip dysplasia/subluxation	Adductor tenotomy Derotation osteotomy Pelvic osteotomy with open reduction
Scoliosis	Bracing Surgical deformity correction

dorsal rhizotomy (SDR) is used in patients with spastic diplegia who are ambulatory, to improve ambulation. Intrathecal baclofen therapy is typically used in patients with global or quadriplegic spasticity and more severe functional deficits, who are nonambulatory. Palliative combined dorsal and ventral rhizotomy is another option for more severely affected patients who are nonambulatory, with a goal of reducing leg scissoring and both strength and tone in the lower extremities to facilitate the care of nonambulatory patients. In clinical practice, there is variable use of both procedures because of parent wishes and provider biases. Many patients could benefit from both procedures, and procedural decision-making must reflect parental goals and biases. A major difference between these procedures is that dorsal rhizotomy is an ablative procedure that is permanent, whereas baclofen pump is a nonablative procedure that can be reversed in the future.

INTRATHECAL BACLOFEN THERAPY FOR SPASTICITY

Intrathecal baclofen treatment is widely used in patients with spastic diplegia or quadriplegia. It has the advantage over administration of a much higher concentration of oral baclofen in the cerebrospinal fluid (CSF) with minimal systemic effects.[29] The procedure consists of implantation of a programmable pump (**Fig. 4**) in the abdominal subcutaneous tissue with a tunneled intrathecal catheter inserted in the lower lumbar spine. Programmable pumps come with a multitude of options for different delivery schemes, allowing personalized treatment protocols and dosages for each patient's needs. Pumps have a battery life of 5 to 7 years, and the pump needs to be replaced before end of battery life. An intrathecal baclofen solution is replaced within the pump before running out of the medication or at least every 6 months; this is performed through an office-based sterile procedure accessing a subcutaneous port on the front of the device using a Huber needle and syringe. Before insertion of a baclofen pump, patients may undergo a baclofen trial, where ITB is injected via a simple lumbar puncture, with serial evaluation by a physical therapist to assess efficacy.[9] A successful baclofen trial with noticeable reduction in tone predicts a high likelihood of success with ITB pump placement.[9] Complications from ITB pump placement include erosion of the pump through the skin or peritoneum, CSF leak, surgical site infection, catheter misplacement, catheter fracture, catheter migration, or pump malfunction.[30] Malfunctions of the programmable pump or catheter can result in symptoms of baclofen withdrawal, which is a medical emergency. Despite the possible complications and the need for baclofen refills and pump replacement, ITB therapy has shown significant

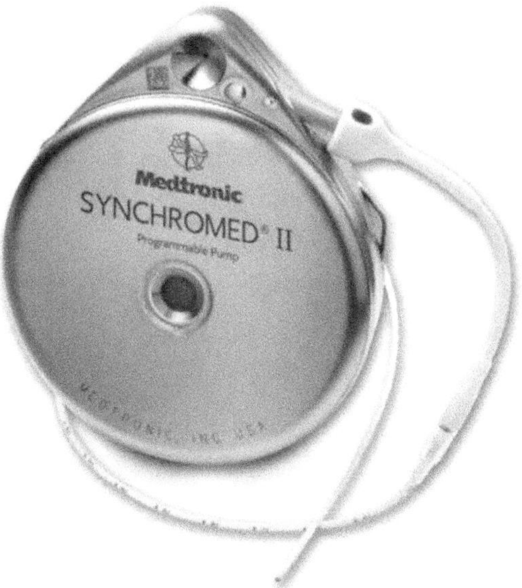

Fig. 4. Intrathecal Baclofen pump. (©2021 Medtronic. All rights reserved. Used with the permission of Medtronic.)

benefits in children with global CP and spasticity, improving transfers, lower extremity tone, ADLs, and even speech and feeding.[31,32]

INTRATHECAL BACLOFEN WITHDRAWAL: A MEDICAL EMERGENCY

Baclofen withdrawal can occur with any malfunction of the pump or fracture of the catheter and represents a medical emergency, as it can be life-threatening if not identified quickly.[31] Typical baclofen withdrawal symptoms include abrupt increase in tone, fever, somnolence, and irritability but can include a myriad of symptoms summarized in **Box 1**. Patients can progress to multiorgan system failure, disseminated intravascular coagulation, rhabdomyolysis, and even death if not treated quickly.[33] Other medical problems may mimic baclofen withdrawal, such as sepsis, urinary tract infection, or drug tolerance, and a high suspicion for baclofen withdrawal is indicated in any patient with an implanted baclofen pump and similar symptoms.[33] Initial workup for intrathecal baclofen withdrawal typically includes abdominal and/or chest radiographs to rule out a catheter fracture. Pump function is evaluated by the primary team managing the pump through telemetry to evaluate for battery failure or pump stall, through device reservoir aspiration and refill to assess adequate baclofen solution, and through side port aspiration or injection to ensure the catheter is functional and open to the intrathecal space. Other sources of increased tone should be ruled out, particularly sources of sepsis such as pneumonia or urinary tract infections. Initial management of baclofen withdrawal symptoms includes intravenous (IV) hydration and administration of oral baclofen or benzodiazepine such as diazepam. IV benzodiazepines may be necessary in severe cases or if oral supplementation proves inadequate. Typical withdrawal symptoms are self-limited over a few days. Replacement of a failed or clogged pump system is required in some cases to restore therapy.

Box 1
Symptoms of intrathecal baclofen withdrawal

- Increased muscle tone or return of baseline muscle tone
- Itching
- Altered mental status
- Seizures
- Fever higher than 38°C, often higher than 40°C
- Tachycardia
- Hypotension or hypertension
- Rhabdomyolysis
- Multiorgan system failure
- Disseminated intravascular coagulation (DIC)
- Cardiac arrhythmia

DORSAL RHIZOTOMY FOR SPASTICITY

Dorsal rhizotomy for spasticity control has been a therapeutic option since the 1970s and was popularized by the initial reports by Fasano and colleagues and Peacock and colleagues.[34,35] Selective dorsal rhizotomy (SDR) is used to treat ambulatory children to selectively decrease tone, which allows improvements in muscle strength and ambulatory function. Often, a child will improve one level on the GMFCS scale after SDR. More severely affected children may undergo palliative dorsal rhizotomy or palliative dorsal and ventral rhizotomy, which is an option for more globally affected patients who are nonambulatory, with the goal of reducing leg muscle tone, facilitating ease of care, and reducing leg scissoring.[36]

Selective dorsal rhizotomy is performed via a midline lumbar incision with intraoperative neuromonitoring that allows selective sectioning of affected sensory roots. A rehabilitation physician or physical therapist often provides real-time monitoring of leg function throughout the procedure. Dorsal sensory lumbar roots are sequentially stimulated. "Abnormal" roots are identified, which produce an abnormal motor response or clonus instead of a brief muscle contraction when stimulated. These abnormal dorsal roots are cut, which decreases the input signal into the spinal reflex and results in immediate reduction of tone in the lower extremity.[34] This surgery was first performed with a multilevel laminectomy, and more recently Park and colleagues[37] originated a less invasive approach using a 1- or 2-level laminectomy at the level of the conus medullaris.

Appropriate patient selection for SDR is very important, because this is an ablative surgery with permanent results. Candidates for surgery are typically between 4 and 12 years of age with spastic diplegia, adequate muscle strength in their legs, and few permanent contractures. Children younger than 4 years are still undergoing changes in brain development, which may reduce spasticity on their own. SDR is less effective in older children if the goal is improvement in function, because an older child's response to physical therapy and muscle strengthening may be limited by this time. Several randomized controlled trials have shown a significant improvement in lower extremity function and reductions in spasticity with SDR.[38,39] Although ITB pump placement was previously the preferred treatment of patients with global spasticity and GMFCS scores of 4 to 5, palliative dorsal or dorsal/ventral rhizotomy has gained support as a method of achieving permanent reductions in leg tone to facilitate ease of care. Leg scissoring is a common problem in severely affected patients with CP, which can make hygiene and urinary/bowel care difficult.[36] Palliative rhizotomy, where most of the lumbar dorsal nerve roots are sectioned, can produce permanent improvements in lower extremity tone to facilitate ADLs and care.[36]

PATHOPHYSIOLOGY OF DYSTONIA AND ASSOCIATED DISORDERS

Dystonia is defined as an abnormal muscle contraction, sustained or intermittent, resulting in abnormal posture and twisting of the extremities or body.[40] Dystonia can affect any of the extremities, head and neck muscles, and even muscles of the eyelid and eye movement.[41] Most commonly, dystonia results from lesions or disorders that disrupt the basal ganglia and cortical relay system, particularly lesions of the putamen.[42] This disruption of basal ganglia circuits and globus pallidus interna (GPi) results in abnormal activity from primary and supplemental motor cortex.[42] Dystonia can be categorized as either primary or secondary. Primary dystonia results from genetic abnormalities of the DYT gene, of which several dystonic disorders based on the different gene abnormalities have been identified.[43] Primary dystonia also includes disorders such as Segawa syndrome, a dopa-responsive form of dystonia that can be readily treated with oral levodopa, and should be ruled out in any child who presents with dystonia without an obvious cause.[44] Several degenerative disorders are also associated with the development of dystonia, including Huntington disease, Hallervorden-Spatz disease, Wilson disease, Leigh disease, and Rett syndrome.[45] Secondary dystonia, in contrast, is the most common form seen in children and typically results from structural lesions of the brain or basal ganglia, particularly the putamen.[42] Most commonly these result from premature birth or perinatal hypoxia, resulting in CP, traumatic brain injury, stroke, or mass lesions of the basal ganglia.[46] Secondary dystonia often worsens throughout childhood until adolescence, with more severe forms occurring at earlier ages.[45]

CLINICAL EVALUATION OF DYSTONIA

Aside from primary and secondary forms, dystonia can be further classified based on the body region affected. Focal dystonia involves only one isolated region of the body, such as one upper extremity or the sternocleidomastoid muscle, as is commonly seen with cervical torticollis. Hemidystonia affects the arm and leg on one side of the body and is usually caused by a structural brain lesion within the basal ganglia, such as a tumor, stroke, or vascular lesion, on the opposite side. Generalized dystonia, the most common pediatric form, affects the entire body and is most commonly seen after traumatic brain injury, premature birth, or perinatal hypoxic/ischemic injury. The most common grading scale used for pediatric secondary dystonia is the Barry-Albright Dystonia scale, which assesses levels of dystonia in each extremity, the head/neck, and eyes.[41] Typical assessment includes a detailed history and physical examination to elucidate possible causes for dystonia, with a focus on identifying primary versus secondary forms of dystonia. Brain MRI with and without contrast should be obtained to evaluate for basal ganglia lesions and typical findings of secondary or primary dystonia.[47] Genetic analysis and laboratory analysis of plasma and spinal fluid studies should be considered to rule out causes of primary dystonia, such as DYT gene abnormalities or the myriad of disorders associated with the development of dystonia, a comprehensive list of which has been published previously by Meijer and colleagues.[47] All patients with severe dystonia will likely benefit from evaluation by a focused multidisciplinary team, including a physical therapist, physiatrist, and neurologist.

MEDICAL THERAPY FOR DYSTONIA

Medical therapy is commonly initiated for pediatric patients with dystonia as a first-line therapy, but overall, medical therapy tends to be less effective compared with treatment of spasticity. First-line oral medication for pediatric dystonia includes baclofen, trihexyphenidyl, and carbidopa-levodopa. Muscle relaxers, such as benzodiazepines, are occasionally used, but these are less commonly used in pediatric dystonia compared with adult dystonia.[48] Baclofen is the most common medication used to treat secondary dystonia in children, and it has an added benefit of simultaneously treating spasticity, which is common in the patient population with CP who can exhibit both secondary dystonia and spasticity symptoms simultaneously.[48,49] Trihexyphenidyl is an acetylcholine receptor antagonist, which shows some efficacy in treating dystonia symptoms in children.[49] Carbidopa-levodopa is primarily used for dopa-responsive dystonia, a unique genetic form of primary dystonia, and this has significant clinical benefits with usage in this patient population.[50] Intramuscular injection of Botulinum toxin is well established as a treatment of focal dystonia, such as torticollis, single-limb dystonia, or blepharospasm, and is safe and effective in children.[48]

INTRATHECAL BACLOFEN THERAPY FOR DYSTONIA

ITB therapy for treatment of secondary generalized dystonia in children remains a mainstay treatment and produces response rates upward of 90% in patients, improving symptoms and dystonic movements by greater than 25% based on the dystonia scoring systems.[51] The surgical procedure for placement of a baclofen pump and catheter for ITB in patients with dystonia is the same as previously described for patients with spasticity. The exact mechanism of action providing benefit in patients with dystonia undergoing ITB treatment is not well understood, and both cortical and spinal sites of action have been implicated as a possible source.[51,52] ITB therapy for children with secondary generalized dystonia tends to require higher dosages of ITB than patients with spasticity to see a similar effect, and patients with dystonia often do not respond immediately to a single baclofen trial test dose. Symptoms abate with a longer infusion of baclofen, requiring a several day infusion through a lumbar drain to assess efficacy before pump placement.[45] ITB is an effective treatment of generalized secondary dystonia in children, seen most commonly in patients with CP, but tends to be less effective in patients with primary or genetic forms of dystonia.

CRANIAL NEUROSURGICAL PROCEDURES FOR DYSTONIA

Cranial surgical options in the treatment of dystonia have evolved rapidly with the more recent advent of functional stereotactic procedures to treat some forms of dystonia. Historically, pallidotomy, creating a destructive lesion within the globus pallidus, has been used to treat dystonia, and this has shown some benefit in children, but the creation of a permanent lesion in children coupled with the inability to tailor therapy once completed makes pallidotomy a rarely used option in children.[53] The advent of deep brain stimulation (DBS) and functional stereotactic procedures to treat dystonia has provided a better option for patients with refractory dystonia, which allows for tailored therapy and nonpermanent treatments. DBS involves the placement of a stimulating lead within the GPi, connected to a battery in the anterior chest wall via wires run under the skin. By placing a stimulating lead within the GPi, practitioners are able to make a functional nonpermanent deficit within the GPi, allowing for tailored therapy for each child. DBS for dystonia has been approved by the Food and Drug Administration for children as young as 7 years, but it is rarely placed in children before their teenage years, as dystonia symptoms are often variable and evolving before that point. Studies have shown a significant benefit and reduction in dystonic symptoms after DBS placement in patients with primary dystonia, but a similar benefit has not been noted in patients with secondary dystonia.[54] The reason for this difference is unclear but is likely related to underlying structural damage to the thalamic anatomy in patients with secondary dystonia, leading to a smaller beneficial response. For this reason, DBS remains a better treatment of patients with primary (genetic) dystonia that is refractory to medications, whereas ITB is probably a better treatment option in patients with refractory secondary dystonia. In patients with heterodegenerative forms of dystonia, such as Huntington disease or Hallervorden-Spatz disease, it is unclear whether DBS or ITB offers a better treatment option for refractory cases. In these cases, undergoing a baclofen trial and test dose to assess efficacy for ITB therapy is a reasonable option. Epidural motor cortical stimulation is a newer adjuvant treatment of refractory focal dystonia, used primarily to treat upper extremity dystonia refractory to medical therapy. This new treatment has shown benefit in patients with focal upper extremity deficits but is probably not an ideal option for generalized or secondary dystonia at this time.[55]

SUMMARY

The treatment of spasticity and dystonia in children is optimized through the collaborative effort of a multidisciplinary team of providers who specialize in the care of these children. Surgical treatment should be considered in children who have not had an optimal response to conservative therapy. A discussion of outcome goals with the family will facilitate the choice of treatment options. Use of the Modified Ashworth Scale, Barry-Albright Dystonia Scale, and GMFCS helps to follow the benefit of treatment over time, and it allows for a standardized way to perform serial assessment of these complex patients.

Clinics Care Points

- A multi-disciplinary care team specializing in movement disorders is of great benefit to children with tone abnormalities.
- Patients with global spasticity often have significant nutritional deficits due to tonic muscle contraction prior to surgical interventions to optimize wound healing. Consideration should be given for dietitian evaluation and gastrostomy placement.
- Baclofen withdrawal due to failure of a baclofen pump is a medical emergency and must be treated with referral to the emergency department, close monitoring, and treatment with muscle relaxants.
- Symptoms of spasticity may worsen temporarily in children with concomitant illnesses, such as pneumonia or urinary tract infection.
- Regarding the management of spasticity selective dorsal rhizotomy is preferred in patients with spastic diplegia who can ambulate and intrathecal baclofen is preferred in non-ambulatory patients with spastic quadriplegia.
- Regarding the management of dystonia ITB is preferred for secondary dystonia, whereas DBS is preferred for primary dystonia.

DISCLOSURE

No sources of funding or financial support were used in the production of this article. The authors have no conflicts of interest related to this article.

REFERENCES

1. Sanger TD, Delgado MR, Gaebler-Spira D, et al. Task Force on Childhood Motor Disorders. Classification and definition of disorders causing hypertonia in childhood. Pediatrics 2003;111(1):e89–97.
2. Rosenbaum P, Paneth N, Leviton A, et al. A report: the definition and classification of cerebral palsy April 2006. Dev Med Child Neurol Suppl 2007;109:8–14.
3. Clark SL, Hankins GDV. Temporal and demographic trends in cerebral palsy–fact and fiction. Am J Obstet Gynecol 2003;188(3):628–33.
4. O'Callaghan ME, MacLennan AH, Haan EA, et al, South Australian Cerebral Palsy Research Group. The genomic basis of cerebral palsy: a HuGE systematic literature review. Hum Genet 2009;126(1):149–72.
5. Kuban KC, Leviton A. Cerebral palsy. N Engl J Med 1994;330(3):188–95.
6. Surveillance of Cerebral Palsy in Europe. Surveillance of cerebral palsy in Europe: a collaboration of cerebral palsy surveys and registers. Surveillance of Cerebral Palsy in Europe (SCPE). Dev Med Child Neurol 2000;42(12):816–24.
7. Grether JK, Cummins SK, Nelson KB. The California Cerebral Palsy Project. Paediatr Perinat Epidemiol 1992;6(3):339–51.
8. Atkinson S, Stanley FJ. Spastic diplegia among children of low and normal birthweight. Dev Med Child Neurol 1983;25(6):693–708.
9. Koman LA, Smith BP, Shilt JS. Cerebral palsy. Lancet 2004;363(9421):1619–31.
10. Folkerth RD. Periventricular leukomalacia: overview and recent findings. Pediatr Dev Pathol 2006;9(1):3–13.
11. Okumura A, Kato T, Kuno K, et al. MRI findings in patients with spastic cerebral palsy. II: correlation with type of cerebral palsy. Dev Med Child Neurol 1997;39(6): 369–72.
12. Gracies J-M. Pathophysiology of spastic paresis. I: paresis and soft tissue changes. Muscle Nerve 2005;31(5):535–51.
13. Dietz V, Sinkjaer T. Spasticity. Handb Clin Neurol 2012;109:197–211.
14. Ghasia F, Brunstrom J, Gordon M, et al. Frequency and severity of visual sensory and motor deficits in children with cerebral palsy: gross motor function classification scale. Invest Ophthalmol Vis Sci 2008;49(2):572–80.
15. Bax M, Tydeman C, Flodmark O. Clinical and MRI correlates of cerebral palsy: the European Cerebral Palsy Study. JAMA 2006;296(13):1602–8.
16. Carlsson M, Hagberg G, Olsson I. Clinical and aetiological aspects of epilepsy in children with cerebral palsy. Dev Med Child Neurol 2003;45(6):371–6.
17. Caramico-Favero DCO, Guedes ZCF, Morais MB de. Food intake, nutritional status and gastrointestinal symptoms in children with cerebral palsy. Arq Gastroenterol 2018;55(4):352–7.
18. Palisano R, Rosenbaum P, Walter S, et al. Development and reliability of a system to classify gross motor function in children with cerebral palsy. Dev Med Child Neurol 1997;39(4):214–23.
19. Delgado MR, Albright AL. Movement disorders in children: definitions, classifications, and grading systems. J Child Neurol 2003;18(Suppl 1):S1–8.
20. Rasmussen HM, Pedersen NW, Overgaard S, et al. Gait analysis for individually tailored interdisciplinary interventions in children with cerebral palsy: a randomized controlled trial. Dev Med Child Neurol 2019;61(10):1189–95.

21. Tilton A, Vargus-Adams J, Delgado MR. Pharmacologic treatment of spasticity in children. Semin Pediatr Neurol 2010;17(4):261–7.
22. Verrotti A, Greco R, Spalice A, et al. Pharmacotherapy of spasticity in children with cerebral palsy. Pediatr Neurol 2006;34(1):1–6.
23. Mathew A, Mathew MC, Thomas M, et al. The efficacy of diazepam in enhancing motor function in children with spastic cerebral palsy. J Trop Pediatr 2005;51(2):109–13.
24. Joynt RL, Leonard JA. Dantrolene sodium suspension in treatment of spastic cerebral palsy. Dev Med Child Neurol 1980;22(6):755–67.
25. Nogen AG. Medical treatment for spasticity in children with cerebral palsy. Childs Brain 1976;2(5):304–8.
26. O'Brien CF. Treatment of spasticity with botulinum toxin. Clin J Pain 2002;18(6 Suppl):S182–90.
27. Russman BS, Tilton A, Gormley ME. Cerebral palsy: a rational approach to a treatment protocol, and the role of botulinum toxin in treatment. Muscle Nerve Suppl 1997;6:S181–93.
28. McGinley JL, Dobson F, Ganeshalingam R, et al. Single-event multilevel surgery for children with cerebral palsy: a systematic review. Dev Med Child Neurol 2012;54(2):117–28.
29. Heetla HW, Staal MJ, Proost JH, et al. Clinical relevance of pharmacological and physiological data in intrathecal baclofen therapy. Arch Phys Med Rehabil 2014;95(11):2199–206.
30. Albright AL. Intrathecal baclofen in cerebral palsy movement disorders. J Child Neurol 1996;11(Suppl 1):S29–35.
31. Winter G, Beni-Adani L, Ben-Pazi H. Intrathecal baclofen therapy-practical approach: clinical benefits and complication management. J Child Neurol 2018;33(11):734–41.
32. Albright AL, Barron WB, Fasick MP, et al. Continuous intrathecal baclofen infusion for spasticity of cerebral origin. JAMA 1993;270(20):2475–7.
33. Alden TD, Lytle RA, Park TS, et al. Intrathecal baclofen withdrawal: a case report and review of the literature. Childs Nerv Syst 2002;18(9–10):522–5.
34. Peacock WJ, Staudt LA. Spasticity in cerebral palsy and the selective posterior rhizotomy procedure. J Child Neurol 1990;5(3):179–85.
35. Fasano VA, Broggi G, Barolat-Romana G, et al. Surgical treatment of spasticity in cerebral palsy. Childs Brain 1978;4(5):289–305.
36. Davidson B, Schoen N, Sedighim S, et al. Intrathecal baclofen versus selective dorsal rhizotomy for children with cerebral palsy who are nonambulant: a systematic review. J Neurosurg Pediatr 2019;1–9.
37. Park TS, Johnston JM. Surgical techniques of selective dorsal rhizotomy for spastic cerebral palsy. Tech note. Neurosurg Focus 2006;21(2):e7.
38. McLaughlin J, Bjornson K, Temkin N, et al. Selective dorsal rhizotomy: meta-analysis of three randomized controlled trials. Dev Med Child Neurol 2002;44(1):17–25.
39. Tedroff K, Löwing K, Jacobson DNO, et al. Does loss of spasticity matter? A 10-year follow-up after selective dorsal rhizotomy in cerebral palsy. Dev Med Child Neurol 2011;53(8):724–9.
40. Fahn S. Concept and classification of dystonia. Adv Neurol 1988;50:1–8.
41. Barry MJ, VanSwearingen JM, Albright AL. Reliability and responsiveness of the Barry-Albright Dystonia Scale. Dev Med Child Neurol 1999;41(6):404–11.
42. Vitek JL. Pathophysiology of dystonia: a neuronal model. Mov Disord 2002;17(Suppl 3):S49–62.

43. Bressman SB. Dystonia: phenotypes and genotypes. Rev Neurol (Paris) 2003;159(10 Pt 1):849–56.
44. Gordon N. Segawa's disease: dopa-responsive dystonia. Int J Clin Pract 2008;62(6):943–6.
45. Albright AL, Adelson PD, Pollack IF. Spasticity and movement disorders. In: Principles and practice of pediatric neurosurgery. 3rd edition. Thieme; 2014.
46. Hartmann A, Pogarell O, Oertel WH. Secondary dystonias. J Neurol 1998;245(8):511–8.
47. Meijer IA, Pearson TS. The twists of pediatric dystonia: phenomenology, classification, and genetics. Semin Pediatr Neurol 2018;25:65–74.
48. Jinnah HA. Medical and surgical treatments for dystonia. Neurol Clin 2020;38(2):325–48.
49. Lumsden DE, Kaminska M, Tomlin S, et al. Medication use in childhood dystonia. Eur J Paediatr Neurol 2016;20(4):625–9.
50. Segawa M. Dopa-responsive dystonia. Handb Clin Neurol 2011;100:539–57.
51. Albright AL, Barry MJ, Shafton DH, et al. Intrathecal baclofen for generalized dystonia. Dev Med Child Neurol 2001;43(10):652–7.
52. Dachy B, Dan B. Electrophysiological assessment of the effect of intrathecal baclofen in dystonic children. Clin Neurophysiol 2004;115(4):774–8.
53. Speelman D, van Manen J. Cerebral palsy and stereotactic neurosurgery: long term results. J Neurol Neurosurg Psychiatry 1989;52(1):23–30.
54. Alterman RL, Tagliati M. Deep brain stimulation for torsion dystonia in children. Childs Nerv Syst 2007;23(9):1033–40.
55. Franzini A, Ferroli P, Servello D, et al. Reversal of thalamic hand syndrome by long-term motor cortex stimulation. J Neurosurg 2000;93(5):873–5.